Creative Interventions in Grief and Loss Therapy: When the Music Stops, a Dream Dies

Creative Interventions in Grief and Loss Therapy: When the Music Stops, a Dream Dies has been co-published simultaneously as *Journal of Creativity in Mental Health*, Volume 1, Numbers 3/4 2005.

Monographic Separates from the *Journal of Creativity in Mental Health*

For additional information on these and other Haworth Press titles, including descriptions, tables of contents, reviews, and prices, use the QuickSearch catalog at http://www.HaworthPress.com.

Creative Interventions in Grief and Loss Therapy: When the Music Stops, a Dream Dies, edited by Thelma Duffey, PhD (Vol. 1, No. 3/4, 2005). *Innovative therapies to help deal with loss.*

Creative Interventions in Grief and Loss Therapy: When the Music Stops, a Dream Dies

Thelma Duffey, PhD
Editor

Creative Interventions in Grief and Loss Therapy: When the Music Stops, a Dream Dies has been co-published simultaneously as *Journal of Creativity in Mental Health*, Volume 1, Numbers 3/4 2005.

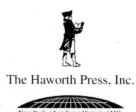

The Haworth Press, Inc.

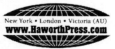

New York • London • Victoria (AU)
www.HaworthPress.com

Creative Interventions in Grief and Loss Therapy: When the Music Stops, a Dream Dies has been co-published simultaneously as *Journal of Creativity in Mental Health*, Volume 1, Numbers 3/4 2005.

The development, preparation, and publication of this work has been undertaken with great care. However, the publisher, employees, editors, and agents of The Haworth Press and all imprints of The Haworth Press, Inc., including The Haworth Medical Press® and Pharmaceutical Products Press®, are not responsible for any errors contained herein or for consequences that may ensue from use of materials or information contained in this work. With regard to case studies, identities and circumstances of individuals discussed herein have been changed to protect confidentiality. Any resemblance to actual persons, living or dead, is entirely coincidental.

The Haworth Press is committed to the dissemination of ideas and information according to the highest standards of intellectual freedom and the free exchange of ideas. Statements made and opinions expressed in this publication do not necessarily reflect the views of the Publisher, Directors, management, or staff of The Haworth Press, Inc., or an endorsement by them.

Library of Congress Cataloging-in-Publication Data

Creative interventions in grief and loss therapy: when the music stops, a dream dies / Thelma Duffey, editor.
      p. cm.
"Co-published simultaneously as Journal of creativity in mental health, Volume 1, numbers 3/4 2005."
      Includes bibliographical references and index.
      ISBN 13: 978-0-7890-3553-0 (hard cover : alk. paper)
      ISBN 10: 0-978-0-3553-7 (hard cover : alk. paper)
      ISBN 13: 978-0-7890-3554-7 (soft cover : alk. paper)
      ISBN 10: 0-7890-3554-5 (soft cover : alk. paper)
      1. Grief therapy 2. Loss (Psychology) 3. Arts–Therapeutic use. 4. Creative ability. I. Duffey, Thelma.
      [DNLM: 1. Creativeness. 2. Psychotherapy–methods. 3. Grief. 4. Life Change Events. W1 JO605 v.1 no. 3/4 2005 / WM 460.5.C7 C912 2007]
  RC455.4.L67C74 2007
  616.89'14–dc22
                                                               2006038349

The HAWORTH PRESS Inc.
Abstracting, Indexing & Outward Linking
PRINT *and* ELECTRONIC BOOKS & JOURNALS

This section provides you with a list of major indexing & abstracting services and other tools for bibliographic access. That is to say, each service began covering this periodical during the the year noted in the right column. Most Websites which are listed below have indicated that they will either post, disseminate, compile, archive, cite or alert their own Website users with research-based content from this work. (This list is as current as the copyright date of this publication.)

Abstracting, Website/Indexing Coverage . . . . Year When Coverage Began

- **CINAHL (Cumulative Index to Nursing & Allied Health Literature) (EBSCO)** <http://www.cinahl.com>. **2006**

- **MasterFILE Premier (EBSCO)** <http://www.epnet.com/government/mfpremier.asp> **2006**

- **Social Services Abstracts (Cambridge Scientific Abstracts)** <http://www.csa.com> **2006**

- **Social Work Abstracts (NASW)** <http://www.silverplatter.com/catalog/swab.htm>. **2006**

- **Sociological Abstracts (Cambridge Scientific Abstracts)** <http://www.csa.com> **2006**

- *(IBZ) International Bibliography of Periodical Literature on the Humanities and Social Sciences (Thomson)* <http://www.saur.de> **2006**

- *Alzheimer's Disease Education & Referral Center (ADEAR AD LIB Database)* <http://www.nia.nih.gov/alzheimers/Resources/ SearchHealthLiterature/> **2006**

- *Chartered Instituted of Library and Information Professionals (CILIP) Health Libraries Newsletter "Current Literature" (Published quarterly by Blackwell Science)* <http://www. blackwell-science.com/hlr/newsletter/> **2006**

- *Consumer Health Complete (EBSCO)* **2006**

(continued)

Bibliographic Access

- **Cabell's Directory of Publishing Opportunities in Psychology** *<http://www.cabells.com>*

- **MediaFinder** *<http://www.mediafinder.com>*

- **Ulrich's Periodicals Directory: International Periodicals Information Since 1932** *<http://www.Bowerlink.com>*

Special Bibliographic Notes related to special journal issues (separates) and indexing/abstracting:

- indexing/abstracting services in this list will also cover material in any "separate" that is co-published simultaneously with Haworth's special thematic journal issue or DocuSerial. Indexing/abstracting usually covers material at the article/chapter level.
- monographic co-editions are intended for either non-subscribers or libraries which intend to purchase a second copy for their circulating collections.
- monographic co-editions are reported to all jobbers/wholesalers/approval plans. The source journal is listed as the "series" to assist the prevention of duplicate purchasing in the same manner utilized for books-in-series.
- to facilitate user/access services all indexing/abstracting services are encouraged to utilize the co-indexing entry note indicated at the bottom of the first page of each article/chapter/contribution.
- this is intended to assist a library user of any reference tool (whether print, electronic, online, or CD-ROM) to locate the monographic version if the library has purchased this version but not a subscription to the source journal.
- individual articles/chapters in any Haworth publication are also available through the Haworth Document Delivery Service (HDDS).

As part of Haworth's continuing committment to better serve our library patrons, we are proud to be working with the following electronic services:

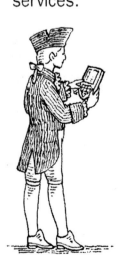

AGGREGATOR SERVICES

EBSCOhost

Ingenta

J-Gate

Minerva

OCLC FirstSearch

Oxmill

SwetsWise

FirstSearch

Oxmill Publishing

SwetsWise

LINK RESOLVER SERVICES

1Cate (Openly Informatics)

CrossRef

Gold Rush (Coalliance)

LinkOut (PubMed)

LINKplus (Atypon)

LinkSolver (Ovid)

LinkSource with A-to-Z (EBSCO)

Resource Linker (Ulrich)

SerialsSolutions (ProQuest)

SFX (Ex Libris)

Sirsi Resolver (SirsiDynix)

Tour (TDnet)

Vlink (Extensity, *formerly Geac*)

WebBridge (Innovative Interfaces)

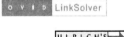

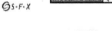

SerialsSolutions

Creative Interventions in Grief and Loss Therapy: When the Music Stops, a Dream Dies

CONTENTS

ABOUT THE EDITOR

Thelma Duffey, PhD, is Professor and Counseling Program Director at the University of Texas at San Antonio. Dr. Duffey spearheaded efforts to establish *The Association for Creativity in Counseling*, the newest division within The American Counseling Association, and serves as Founding President for the association. She also organized a series of conferences that focus on using creativity in mental health practices. She has served as Chair for *The Dr. Lesley Jones Creativity in Psychotherapy Conferences*, held in Texas, since 1999.

Dr. Duffey received two national awards during the 2006 American Counseling Association convention in Montreal. She was awarded the American Counseling Association Professional Development Award and the Counseling Vision and Innovation Award by the Association for Counselor Education and Supervision. The Professional Development Award recognizes an ACA member who has developed techniques and systems that have strengthened, expanded, enhanced, or improved the counseling profession and benefited counseling consumers. The ACES Counseling Vision and Innovation Award honors the individual who has shown exemplary commitment, vision, creativity, and future thinking; tolerated ambiguity and fear during innovations in preparation and practice; championed transformational leadership; defended visionary writing or publication; promoted trend-setting practice; and advocated for change in contemporary and futuristic service.

Dr. Duffey owns and operates a successful private clinical practice, working with individuals, couples, and families. Her areas of specialization include grief and loss counseling, relationship counseling, addictions, and gender issues. She has authored numerous publications in textbooks and refereed professional journals in the mental health field and is a frequent speaker and presenter at national conferences and workshops. She has developed graduate courses that address the use of the Enneagram Personality typology, Relational-Cultural Theory, and creative interventions in counseling. Dr. Duffey is a Licensed Professional Counselor, a Licensed Marriage and Family Therapist, and a Clinical Member of the American Association for Marriage and Family Therapists.

Preface

I am pleased to present to you this work which features creative ways of helping individuals, couples, and families transcend the loss of a dream. Each chapter includes relevant information on various forms of grief and loss experiences, including death, divorce, other relational losses, miscarriage, addictions, suicide, natural disaster, and diverse forms of trauma. This work also includes information on losses considered by some as disenfranchised, such as personal and professional betrayal, the dissolution of relationships not legally sanctioned, incarcerated parenting, and the death of a client. The authors provide unique insights into these experiences and illustrate creative ways to address them in counseling practice.

Distinctive to this work is the focus on the loss of dreams that accompany our grief experiences. No doubt, all of us have suffered losses of one form or another or counseled people through their losses and transitions. Many would say that, in addition to grieving our losses, a poignant and difficult aspect of our experiences involves making peace with our unrealized dreams and, in some cases, with our shattered illusions. It is through this process that we can honor our histories and experiences while creating space for a new dream's birth.

A song lyric introduces many of the chapters and sets the stage for the material. Chapters cite existing research on specific grief and loss issues and illustrate a clinical application for each situation, using music, ritual, bibliotherapy, writing, literature, psychodrama, and other creative mediums.

As we consider the grief and loss issues that people face, we must consider the contexts within which they are experienced. Culture,

[Haworth co-indexing entry note]: "Preface." Duffey, Thelma. Co-published simultaneously in *Journal of Creativity in Mental Health* (The Haworth Press, Inc.) Vol. 1, No. 3/4, 2005, pp. xxi-xxvi; and: *Creative Interventions in Grief and Loss Therapy: When the Music Stops, a Dream Dies* (ed: Thelma Duffey) The Haworth Press, Inc., 2005, pp. xv-xx. Single or multiple copies of this article are available for a fee from The Haworth Document Delivery Service [1-800-HAWORTH, 9:00 a.m. - 5:00 p.m. (EST). E-mail address: docdelivery@haworthpress.com].

Available online at http://jcmh.haworthpress.com

socio-economics, family structure, spirituality, education, and other considerations influence our experiences. It is important that as counselors and mental health professionals we develop our multicultural competencies and learn about diverse values, worldviews and customs. In that spirit of diversity, it also becomes critical that we avoid perpetuating stereotypes and develop our awareness of within-group diversity. In reading the chapters that follow, we caution our readers to consider a multi-dimensional perspective when hearing the stories that clients bring. Clients are the authors of their own stories and frame their experiences relative to their unique influences. The chapters in this publication carry representations of these voices through brief vignettes, disguised for purposes of anonymity. In listening to their stories against the backdrop of the literature, we become informed on the uniqueness and diversity characteristic of life and loss.

HIGHLIGHTS

The chapters in this book address various situations where people encounter the loss of a dream. Chapter 11 provides an overview of creativity as a function of healing and includes examples of how music, videography, visual arts, literature, drama, play, and altar-making can all be used to help clients work through difficult grief issues. The chapter addresses multicultural implications and describes how some cultures value the maintenance of a connection with the deceased. Uses of creativity to access and express complex emotions and to gain confidence in generating a new dream are discussed.

Creativity can be accessed to facilitate the grief process as it is expressed in various forms. For example, the death of some dreams comes to us through the relational ruptures and the disconnections we experience. In Chapter 1, we discuss some distinctive issues experienced by individuals who face the challenge of coming to terms with releasing a relationship of value. Although the process described in this manuscript may be experienced by people undergoing diverse losses, this work describes the loss involved in making peace with the release of an important relationship. An intervention using popular music is used to illustrate the means by which some people come to terms with these difficult decisions to cut their losses and move beyond painful situations.

In a similar context, Chapter 9 addresses the grief and loss experience that comes when we have made the decision to release important love relationships. It also addresses some important variables that must be in place for love to thrive and describes how addiction and commitment conflicts interfere with our capacity to enjoy loving relationships. Creative counseling interventions featuring writing, pictures, and other mediums are also included.

The costs to relationship loss are many. For example, feelings of anger and resentment commonly surface following the termination of a relationship. Chapter 7 describes some challenges for couples and families undergoing relationship dissolution and divorce. It includes a case study where a person attempts to reconcile her life choices with her religious beliefs and personal values. The chapter also presents the creative use of literary writing to help facilitate greater levels of empathy and forgiveness. Also included is a discussion on the disenfranchised grief experiences of couples whose relationships end without social or legal sanction. The feelings of isolation and marginalization that these losses can create are described.

Some of our losses come to us in our roles as professional counselors and mental health practitioners. Chapter 2 describes the loss experience of a counselor following the death of a client and illustrates how storytelling, journaling, and correspondence can be used to process this loss. This chapter is rich in personal accounts and provides voice for the counselor, the deceased client, and her loved ones. It also gives context to the excruciating pain and isolation that can come for some clients who struggle with eating disorders and to lesbian and gay couples whose relationships are not legally sanctioned.

Chapter 13 also addresses client death, but in this case, describes the experience of death through suicide and the impact that client death has on mental health practitioners. The chapter provides a succinct description of high risk suicide factors and a Pre-suicide Preparation Plan that mental health practitioners can use prior to a crisis.

Counselors and mental health practitioners suffer other forms of disenfranchised losses. Chapter 5 addresses the important role that we serve as gatekeepers to the profession and some of the emotional costs that counselor educators may inadvertently incur as a result of their efforts. This chapter addresses some experiences faced by counselor educators following their participation in a gatekeeping process and describes a creative methods used by some faculty to name their experiences and come to terms with them.

While some dreams are shattered because of disconnections and injustices that we encounter, other dreams are destroyed following the death of a loved one. The experience of adolescent death is discussed and described in Chapter 8. This chapter illustrates some of the experiences faced by parents who suffer this life-shattering loss and provides the reader with creative ways of addressing the utter helplessness and loss using books, songs, and tangible objects.

Children, too, suffer lost dreams through death, relocation, divorce, and other traumatic events. Chapter 17 describes the impact that traumatic loss can have on children and presents creative means for using bibliotherapy and storytelling in the therapeutic process. Examples, rich in expression, illustrate some sobering experiences that children face and describe the important value that forming relational connections and using available literary resources can bring.

While the losses of a child or a parent through death are universally recognized, some losses are ambiguous, disenfranchised, and not easily understood. Chapter 10 addresses the emotional and psychological impact that miscarriage can have on a woman and presents therapeutic and treatment implications for counselors working with women and their partners following the loss of a child through miscarriage. The use of ritual is addressed.

Another ambiguous and often disenfranchised loss involves the experiences of parents with special needs. Chapter 16 addresses common challenges faced by fathers with children who have special needs. It also presents "Redreaming" as an intervention to help fathers reappraise their dreams and visions for their children and validate their children in unique ways. A research study is presented.

Chapter 18 discusses the often disenfranchised experience of pet loss. Pets can be loyal, loving and entertaining members of a family. Their deaths are generally experienced as painful losses by the people who love them, even though this grief experience is often culturally disenfranchised. In this chapter, we discuss the role that pets can play in a person's life; the effects that pet loss can have on the people who love them; and some creative rituals for memorializing a beloved pet.

In addition to disenfranchised losses, we also experience a number of ambiguous losses. These losses come in many forms. For example, children who are adopted face distinctive gifts and losses that can be experienced as ambiguous. Chapter 15 describes common myths and misconceptions about the adoption experience and illustrates the search for identity that frequently ensues. It also describes a creative intervention, using super heroes and science fiction, to help children address and work through their experiences.

Identity issues also become salient for athletes, who have been groomed to succeed, become culturally celebrated, and acclaimed. Unfortunately, many are unprepared for life after sport. Chapter 6 gives context to some of the developmental challenges incurred by athletes and presents a unique approach, Emotional Freedom Therapy, to help athletes manage their experiences of loss when the game ends.

Other variations of the celebrated status bestowed on the rich and famous is brought to us daily through the media. Chapter 14 considers the parallels between the "celebutante" phenomenon and the superfluous man, an archetypal hero commonly described in Russian literature. The manuscript considers the impact of the infiltration of the often elusive celebutante experience on the dreams, values, and meaning-making experiences of young adults who belong to Generation Y. Written by a member of Generation Y, a literature-based exercise is included.

In another context, our meaning-making experiences and dreams are sometimes filtered through an addictive lens. In these cases, our dreams become distorted, disabled, and defunct. Chapter 3 discusses how people suffering from addictions experience a singular form of dream loss. It describes how addictions challenge perceptions, create smokescreens through denial, and impede connection, intimacy, and choice. This manuscript addresses the loss experience of addiction and provides creative intervention techniques for working through these losses. The use of psychodrama and other experiential exercises are illustrated.

Along the same vein, Chapter 12 addresses the challenges of incarcerated individuals with co-occurring mental health and substance use disorders. This manuscript illustrates how creativity can be used to help incarcerated clients negotiate grief and loss issues to re-create their dreams via a personal narrative, while increasing social integration, and augmenting psychological and physiological health.

Finally, there could not be a publication that addresses shattered dreams without including the grief issues involved in surviving a natural disaster. Chapter 4 includes the first hand experiences of counselors and counselor educators from the New Orleans area following the impact of Hurricane Katrina. This chapter provides an overview of the phases of disaster and discusses the ambiguous losses that people face during life-changing times. It also introduces ritual as a creative process and illustrates how ritual can be used in this context.

This material serves as a consolidated reference source on creative approaches to diverse issues encountered by clinicians in their practices. It is designed to provide practical clinical information for practicum, internship, and grief and loss courses offered in counseling and mental health training programs.

One goal of *When the Music Stops* is that our readers will deepen their insights into common problems faced by clients and develop a repertoire of innovative approaches for facilitating this work. Another goal of this book is that the material will help us assess and acknowledge our own rhythm and style for managing inevitable life tragedies and transitions. By deepening our understanding of our current patterns and vulnerabilities, we become more genuinely present in our connections with clients as they mourn their dream's death and find a new context for living.

Thelma Duffey
University of Texas at San Antonio

Acknowledgments

I want to thank you
Show my gratitude
My love and my respect for you . . .
For your selflessness . . . my admiration

(Merchant, 1995)

This book addresses the need for courage in the face of adversity
and the love and support that can help see us through it.
It is dedicated to my mother, Mary, my father, Richard,
and my children, Robby and Madelyn.

It was not long ago that my mother and I rushed across town in the middle of the night to be with my brother, Richard, and my little niece, Olivia. Two deputy sheriffs had come to the door to let them know that Laura, their beloved wife and mother, had been killed crossing the street while out of town on business. Laura was a beautiful person and a very beloved member of our family. The following year, my dear friend and mentor, Lesley, was killed driving home from work. Lesley left a legacy in our hearts and in our lives that I only hope she can see.

We all experience personal situations that cause us pain. Anyone who is in touch with their experience of loss knows of the sheer helplessness and isolation that can come with it. When we enter the profession of counseling, we assume the privilege of walking with people through their own pain, feelings of helplessness, and isolation. There could be no more fulfilling work.

Professionally, my clinical work began with children who were chronic and terminally ill and their families. What inspiring teachers they were and continue to be for me. Since then, my work has focused on being with people as they face life circumstances, such as relationship issues, addiction, career transitions, and divorce. Some face illness, family suicide, and other life-changing challenges. Daily, I am re-minded that difficult, even traumatic things, strike without a moment's notice. Life can turn on a dime, and with each tragedy, we encounter the loss of a dream.

What, then, do we learn from loss, given that our lessons are as unique as they are diverse? One lesson that I find personally important is recognizing the value of the relationships we share and making the most of our time with the people we love. We do this by appreciating them, nurturing their growth, and loving freely. With that said, I extend my appreciation to my greatest gifts in life: my mother, Mary; my father, Richard; and my children, Robby and Madelyn. They are the most amazing people anyone could ever hope to know. I have been truly blessed in this lifetime to have such a wonderful family. Their love, authenticity, humor, and good heartedness are fuel for my spirit.

I extend my appreciation to Mike, for whom I am always thankful; to my brothers, Richard and Jon; to Olguie; to Theresa, friend and colleague in every sense of the word; to Stella, for her care, loyalty, and unwavering friendship; to Marcheta; to Shane, Heather, Larry, Jerry, Chris, Albert, Michael, and Beth, for being the most genuinely collaborative faculty, colleagues, and friends, and for making work as much fun as it is meaningful. I extend my many thanks to Jen; to Kathy, for being such a delight and support; to Cindy, for all her hard work and organization; and to Lisa Marie, for coming into our lives at just the right time! The office looks wonderful. I give thanks to the contributors to this work, for sharing their experiences and insights with us; to my clients, who have been among my greatest teachers, and to my students, who stimulate my thinking and growth. I have much for which to be grateful.

Chapter 1

When the Music Stops:
Releasing the Dream

Thelma Duffey

SUMMARY. We each carry hopes, dreams, and visions of what our lives and relationships will look like. However, there are times when, in spite of our best efforts, these dreams remain unrealized. This manuscript addresses some unique issues faced by individuals experiencing a dream's death. Although the process described in this manuscript may be experienced by people undergoing diverse losses, this work details the loss experience as it relates to releasing relationships we value. An intervention using popular music is used to illustrate this process. doi:10.1300/J456v01n03_01 *[Article copies available for a fee from The Haworth Document Delivery Service: 1-800-HAWORTH. E-mail address: <docdelivery@haworthpress.com> Website: <http://www.HaworthPress.com> © 2005 by The Haworth Press, Inc. All rights reserved.]*

KEYWORDS. Dreams, grief and loss, creativity, counseling, relationships, music

Thelma Duffey is the Counseling Program Director at the University of Texas at San Antonio.

[Haworth co-indexing entry note]: "When the Music Stops: Releasing the Dream." Duffey, Thelma. Co-published simultaneously in *Journal of Creativity in Mental Health* (The Haworth Press, Inc.) Vol. 1, No. 3/4, 2005, pp. 1-23; and: *Creative Interventions in Grief and Loss Therapy: When the Music Stops, a Dream Dies* (ed: Thelma Duffey) The Haworth Press, Inc., 2005, pp. 1-23. Single or multiple copies of this article are available for a fee from The Haworth Document Delivery Service [1-800-HAWORTH, 9:00 a.m. - 5:00 p.m. (EST). E-mail address: docdelivery@haworthpress.com].

"I wonder if you know
I wonder if you think about it
Once upon a time
In your wildest dreams"

The Moody Blues
(Hayward, 1986)

We all carry music within us; a rhythm, melody, and beat that give us a unique presence in the world. The music can be seen in the sparkle in a person's eye, the warmth of their smile, their laughter, pain, and in their compassion. This music comes alive in our authentic expression, as we generate our hopes for the future, in our connections with others, and as we dream our dreams. Indeed, our capacity and inclination to dream evokes a chord and ignites within us a sense of life, energy, and direction.

Our hopes and dreams take on many forms. We dream of the life we want to live and of the people who will share this life with us. At times, we dream "big" and we are fortunate to see our wildest dreams become a reality. Certainly, there is no end to the excitement, energy, and sheer happiness that can come from having a dream come true. Dream-making evokes passion and creates a context for meaning. Our dreams reflect our values, and at their best, contribute to a life purpose. Although our dreams provide personal fulfillment, they are most satisfying when enjoyed and shared with others.

We begin to dream as children and experience anticipation. In time, we understand the action, investment, strength and courage it takes to make our dreams come true. Still, in spite of our best efforts, there are times when we inevitably fail to see our dreams realized. This, no doubt, evokes an experience of loss, as our dreams remain unrequited. Depending on our investment, the depth of care for the people involved, and our hopes for what the dream represents, coming to terms with a shattered dream can bring unspeakable pain.

Alternatively, there are times that we achieve our dreams and then receive the phone call, letter, or knock on the door that lets us know our dream is gone. Some dreams are shattered by death; others by abandonment, confusion, rejection, betrayal, or natural disaster. Shattered dreams are profoundly painful. They bring us face to face with the loss of potential and trigger immeasurable feelings of vulnerability, panic, and acute loneliness. We lose loved ones, homes, careers, and beloved pets. We lose our dignity, hopes for the future, livelihood, and reputations. With them, we lose our dreams. It is in these times that we hear–and feel–the music stop.

A DISCUSSION ON GRIEF

The death of a dream can be characterized as a powerful encounter with grief. Although Freud was the first to conceptualize the experience of bereavement (Marwit & Klass, 1995), variations of the grief and loss literature have evolved through the years (Kubler-Ross, 1969; Viorst, 1986; Worden, 1991). Theorists debate issues such as stage and task theories, cultural and gender influences, and other related points (Marwit & Klass, 1995). However, one point remains clear: none of us are exempt from the experience of loss and we will all face some variation of these notable challenges.

In this manuscript, we will discuss some challenges that come in accepting that the dreams we have hoped for and invested in will not be realized. Although our dreams are far-reaching and this article reflects a process for coming to terms with diverse dreams, the examples in this work will largely reflect the struggle to release important people and relationships from our lives. Further, the perspective of this manuscript is intentionally non-diagnostic. That is, its focus is not to address the experience or limitations of love, intimacy, or relational development. Rather, it discusses the challenges we experience when it becomes apparent that our dream will not be realized. With this as a focus, we will discuss counseling considerations and creative strategies using popular music as a resource for coming to terms with our losses and with our experiences of shattered illusions, fantasies, and unrequited hope.

TO LIVE IS TO DREAM

Each of our attachments carries with them a dream. For example, many of us dream of finding work that is satisfying and fulfilling. We dream of maintaining good health. We dream of having the time, energy, opportunity, and inclination to live into our dreams. We dream that if our lives are challenged by unexpected interruptions, we will have the resources to manage them and move forward.

Some of us dream of enjoying a "great love." We dream that we will encounter a person with whom we share passion, respect, friendship, and deep, mutual love. We dream of sharing with them time, comfort, pleasure, adventures, and the inevitable challenges life brings.

As parents, we dream that our children will be happy, healthy and wise. We wish them to be free of the health or physical limitations that can come with life. We hope they will feel connected in the world and experience the love, support, and friendship that give life meaning. We dream that we will see our children grow into adulthood with every benefit possible.

Still, some of us will lose our health, loved ones, security, and life as we've known it. Inevitably, some of our dreams will be shattered. How then, do we come to terms with that loss? How do we reconcile our lost dreams? How do we manage the feelings of grief, fear, anxiety, failure, rejection, and abandonment that can come with loss? When the challenge is great, how can we awaken from our nightmare to create a new dream? Moreover, if our experience involves rejection, betrayal, or other relational injuries, how will we risk including others in our dream again?

DENIAL, IDEALIZATION, AND OTHER COMMON COPING CHALLENGES

Although experiencing the loss of a dream is a universal experience, the way we respond to loss and cope with its effects varies and is influenced by a number of factors. For example, our personalities, worldviews, level of emotional and psychological functioning, past loss experiences, early childhood influences, family patterns (Covington & Beckett, 1988), and level of investment in the current dream all impact how we cope with life difficulties. In addition, culture (Parkes, Launagni & Young, 1997), gender (Greenspan, 2003), and the quality of our relationships with supportive others (Hartling, 2003; 2005) impact the ways we manage life. Each of these factors contributes to the manner in which we view our experiences. When our dreams are shattered, we lose some clarity of thought or emotion. However, as we proceed and work through our unrealized hopes, we become better able to negotiate them. What happens, however, if we deny our experience of loss and minimize its value in our lives? Or alternatively, what happens when we idealize our loss and confuse potential with reality? Ironically, these two coping styles, however diverse, create for us similar consequences: we remain stuck in our experiences.

Coming to terms with the loss of a dream requires that we access our well-developed coping capacities and strengthen those that are least developed in us. Although we vary in capacity and style with respect to how we manage our losses, there are patterns of coping that can be particularly problematic. For example, people who purportedly assume a practical position on loss and shut down on opportunities to genuinely grieve have a very different challenge from people who are aware of the loss they carry in their hearts and who feel "stuck" in the experience. Although both can be caught in their past losses, their lack of freedom to live life unencumbered by them is experienced and expressed in different ways.

In the first case, we rationalize or minimize the impact that the loss has had on us or avert our attention from the loss through entertainment, substances, and other distractions (Greenspan, 2003). We may use catch phrases such as "it wasn't meant to be" or "I live in the now" to circumvent pain and avoid genuine acknowledgment of the loss. Interestingly, although these statements and positions can be heartfelt expressions of strength and faith when expressed in an authentic context, they can also serve to superficially distance us from the value of the experience and the reality of the loss. In these cases, our optimistic perspective becomes a defense against pain or responsibility. Relational-Cultural Theory would say this position serves as a strategy for disconnection (Jordan, 2001), while Kubler-Ross (1969) would see this as an example of how we use denial to cope with life's losses and shattered dreams.

For example, when Frank is met with adversity, he tells himself that what he is losing is not what he wants or in his best interest. Although this perspective allows him to move quickly, it keeps him from truly valuing his experiences and the people he purports to care about. This is not Frank's only casualty. As he minimizes these losses, he becomes less clear on what is meaningful to him. Further, Frank becomes increasingly unhappy or dismissive when his relationships, at best, bring temporary relief. Although his unhappiness lifts as he directs his attention to new pleasures and opportunities, his sadness goes unnamed. In spite of Frank's cheerful demeanor, those close to Frank would see that his losses are palpably close to the surface.

Alternatively, some of us idealize our experiences or the people with whom we share them to such a degree that they hold a "bigger than life" imprint on our memories. This imprint keeps us from seeing them as they are and impedes our ability to grieve the reality of the loss. Sometimes we idealize our experiences after we no longer have them available. In a song popularized in the 1970s, Joni Mitchell sang, "Don't it always seem to go that you don't know what you've got till it's gone. They paved paradise and put up a parking lot" (Mitchell, 1970). In these cases and in others, it becomes difficult for us to release the idealized meaning we ascribe to the loss or the person who holds that projection (Covington & Beckett, 1988). Further, it becomes even more difficult for us to release our hope for the dream and our illusion or fantasy of what life could have been like had that dream come true.

MEANING

Part of the challenge in coming to terms with our shattered dreams and accepting life on life's terms involves how we make meaning of our experiences. According to Davis, Nolen-Hoeksema, and Larson (1998), we are better equipped to come to terms with our losses when we attribute to our experiences meaning and value. Thibault, Ellor, and Netting (1991) purport that an on-going task of mental health professionals is to help clients find and create meaning in life. Birren (1964), Butler (1963), and Erikson (1963) describe how the search for personal meaning and integrity is vital for successful adaptation to life and aging.

Fromm (1994) posits that we make life meaningful by living productively, and by using powers of love and reason to their fullest capacity. May (1994) describes how meaning is experienced when we live by our highest values, when we know our own intentionality, when we feel the power of our will to choose, and when we are able to love. Frankl writes, "A man who becomes conscious of the responsibility he bears toward a human being who affectionately waits for him . . . will never be able to throw away his life. He knows the 'why' for his existence, and will be able to bear almost any 'how' " (Frankl, 1963, p. 127).

We have an opportunity to make meaning of our experiences in ways that deepen our compassion for ourselves and others and that expand our possibilities for a new dream's birth. However, some people make meaning of their losses in ways that minimize the value of people and relationships they are releasing. People who assume this perspective also tend to rationalize their responsibilities for the losses they incur. On the flip side, other people make meaning of their losses by idealizing others and maximizing their own responsibility for the loss. In the first scenario, we "get ourselves off the hook" for the part we play in these losses and tell ourselves that our losses didn't matter much anyway. In the second scenario we "let others off the hook" and then "set ourselves up" to try harder to avoid the losses.

SPIRITUALITY AND A DREAM'S DEATH

The process of meaning-making, for many of us, is related to our spiritual belief system. Indeed, many of us who seek therapy during troubling times are also looking for clarification of our spiritual belief system and comfort within it. Interestingly, counselors and mental health professionals have not always been prepared for this process, and in some cases, have diverted their clients' attention from this need. For example, several years ago, Theresa, 32, was trying to come to terms with some important losses, and sought the help of her minister. Theresa's parents had recently divorced. Complicating matters, Theresa was experiencing conflict in her own marriage. She tried to make sense of her experiences through multiple lenses, including the spiritual, since this seemed to be where her core conflict was centered. Her pastor referred her to a well-respected counselor who could help her work through these issues. However, when Theresa attempted to approach the subject of spiritual confusion, her counselor became uncomfortable and said so. She told her that she could not help her discuss these issues, and suggested she talk to her minister. Since Theresa had already attempted to talk to her minister, she felt discouraged. She continued her work with the counselor and attempted to meet her needs for spiritual healing through other means.

Years later, she recalls that experience with bittersweet memories. "I felt so alone. I felt so guilty. I had wanted my parents to stay together more than anything, and did everything I knew on my part to make life better. Their divorce was such a hard pill for me to swallow." Theresa adds:

> I had tried so hard and was so angry at God. But I felt so guilty about being angry at God, and it scared me. I didn't want to have these feelings, but I didn't know how to work through them. In looking back, I can see how I became angry at myself. My parents were good parents and it was hard for me to see them suffer.

Theresa describes her experience:

My dream, since I was a child, had been that my family would remain a family. It was not until much later that I came to see the limitations of my dream. In time, I reconciled that perhaps God had a plan in mind, after all. I just couldn't know it and I couldn't accept it.

She smiles, and adds, "And, if it wasn't God's plan for them to part, I have accepted that it happened, and that even in the pain, He had His hand in making it better. We have lead lives I feel good about. I am grateful for the good." Considering the role that her spiritual beliefs have had on her healing, she concludes:

I couldn't have done it without coming to terms with God and my ideas about spirituality and what that means to me. I feel like I've taken the long road home–seeking spiritual clarification however I can. All I know is that I have had that yearning–to understand–to be at peace with an ending to a story that I would have so wanted to be different. I had to come to peace with God and with my hopes that He would save my family and my dream. I think I'm there and that is an amazing feeling.

Miller (1999) speaks to the spiritual competencies of counselors who work with clients on these issues. Spiritually competent counselors distinguish the relationship between religion and spirituality and consider these beliefs within a cultural context. They explore their own belief systems and consider these systems from a developmental perspective. As such, they are sensitive to diverse spiritual practices. Like Theresa's counselor, they identify the limits of their understanding; however, unlike Theresa's counselor, they refer appropriately when necessary and assess the relevancy of spiritual domain in the client's life. Finally, spiritually competent counselors have sensitivity and respect for spiritual themes and follow the client's lead in relating spiritual beliefs toward therapeutic goals (Miller, 1999).

More recently, The Council for Accreditation of Counseling and Related Programs (CACREP) has addressed this need in the 2001 Standards. In fact, religious and spiritual values are introduced within the social and cultural diversity section of the eight common core areas (CACREP, 2000). Coming to terms with our losses is no small feat. Reflecting on issues of spirituality during times of loss is a common need, challenge, and consideration. When counselors are comfortable and competent at facilitating this dialogue, clients, like Theresa, are able to more substantively address their losses and create a coherent context from which to move forward.

THE IMPACT OF THOUGHT ON REALITY

The spiritual realm is a significant factor that many of us must consider when creating context for and coming to terms with life experiences. In addition, some theorists purport that our perceptions, i.e., the way we perceive our losses, influence the way we experience and cope with them. This point is described in a documentary film entitled "What the Bleep Do We Know?" (Arntz, Chasse & Vicente, 2004). Posing a challenge to traditional thought and the concepts of certainty and perception, we see the protagonist enter a world of quantum uncertainty to find that her notion of reality is questionable. We witness her growing understanding of how her focus impacts her experience, which challenges her essential perspectives on life, relationships, and reality. It also prompts her to become a creative force in her own life.

Myss (1997) also speaks to how our thoughts create form and discusses how our deeper creative choices impact our attitudes, beliefs, resentments, and the manner and quality of our love. Although it is beyond the scope of this work to give more than mention to quantum uncertainty or thought forms (Arntz, Chasse & Vicente, 2004; Jahn, 2001; Myss, 1997), it is important to consider their role in relation to their impact on our experiences and the resolution of a dream's death. As we step back from our perspectives on how things are and take ownership in how our experiences evolve (Myss, 1997), we give broader context to the purpose our experiences have in our lives and to the creative ways we can grow in them.

As a cautionary note, when we are quick to rationalize our losses or behaviors, we may use the idea that "our perceptions create our realities" to deflect from our own pain or normalize coping styles of detachment or indifference. In addition, this perspective can provide us with an intellectual excuse when we create pain for others. The rationalization can come in the form of, "if our perceptions create our realities, it is the other person's perception, not our behaviors, that causes them pain." This worldview may circumvent immediate feelings of responsibility at the same time that it strengthens our egos and challenges our essential faith, purpose, and sense of life meaning. Further, it perpetuates the fantasy that our behaviors and choices do not impact others.

BARGAINING AND DESPAIR

Coming to terms with a dream's death can be heart-wrenching because it may require dealing with a fork in the road to leave behind people, places, ideas, and things that we love. It requires that we "give up" these dreams, and, at times, the people with whom we wanted to share them. For some of us, this experience of release can be among the most painful of our life experiences, bringing untold ambivalence and grief.

Given that, before we are ready to release a significant investment, some of us experience a desire to bargain. That is, we second guess ourselves and wonder if there is one more thing we can do to avoid this loss. We may wrestle with thoughts of "what if" or "if only" and undergo a process of negotiation with ourselves and with life. In short, we hope to negotiate an alternative ending to our loss.

If we are connected with our feelings, we may experience deep sorrow when our attempts at negotiation fail. This sorrow can trigger experiences of loneliness, hopelessness, and despair. Some people feel remorse or regret, and ruminate. Others experience guilt (Worden, 1991). Our energy may be drained and we might find ourselves tearful or irritable over inconsequential inconveniences. Other times, our despair can be experienced quietly. For example, we may say little about our experience, and at the same time, find ourselves unable to tolerate situations that create inconvenience, ambiguity, or risk of further loss. Our despair lives underneath the surface and impacts most areas of our lives (Worden, 1991; Greenspan, 2003).

Despair is also expressed as angry outbursts. The look in our eyes and the tone of our voices betray our attempts to dispel these experiences. We may use alcohol and other substances to ward off feelings of despair, masking our experience with a facade of palpable content (Nakken, 1996). Some of us show an act of bravado so no one will notice our perceived weaknesses or vulnerability. No doubt, unacknowledged despair has its costs.

RELEASING THE DREAM AND THE CREATIVE PROCESS

Some of us can release our dreams when we reach this place of despair. I heard from a client today who did all he knew to do to keep the job he had worked so hard to secure and maintain for over 30 years. In spite of growing evidence that problems out of his control existed at work, he tried harder to make himself indispensable. He invested in the dream of a successful career and comfortable retirement. Unfortunately, things did not work out as he hoped, and at 51, he found himself looking for a new job. In our time together, he worked through his feelings of shock, disbelief, depression, and despair. In time, he was able to release his need for "that" dream and found a new one. In fact, he now works as a well-compensated consultant and has more professional freedom and autonomy than he ever had with his former company. Release, for him, involved "giving up" the investment, understanding his gifts and opportunities, and taking the risk to start again.

Release, for many of us, involves genuinely working through our feelings of loss, cognitively revisiting our perceptions of what we are leaving behind, physically taking care of ourselves through the stress, and spiritually allowing ourselves to trust in a new dream (Myss, 2001). In addition, release involves looking at how our unrequited dream impacts our self-concept and working through the relational images (Miller & Stiver, 1993) we form about our own capacities and inherent potentials. Release involves adjusting to life without our dream and may involve seeing others seemingly live dreams that we had wished for ourselves. It involves stepping back from our fantasies and idealizations and adjusting to life with realism and centered hope. Release involves making new choices and befriending the discomfort of missing the people, places, and situations of which our dreams were made. Finally, release entails exploring whatever fears are evoked in the face of new opportunities as we embark on our road to a new dream.

COUNSELING CONSIDERATIONS

Adjustments come, but first, the challenge for counselors is to help clients alter their emotional positions to the loss and to the illusions that came with it. As we are able to alter these emotional positions, we are better able to manage our fears. Unfortunately, there are no simplistic remedies for achieving this release. And, for most of us, change must come on myriad levels to be substantive.

For example, we must first understand the claims that our unrequited dreams have on our hearts and the ways they prevent us from living fully and freely. Regardless of how autonomous and independent we may appear, our freedom to thrive may remain elusive if we are controlled by ghosts, shadows, and illusion from our pasts. These experiences may come in the form of previous marriages, childhood losses, or other life disappointments. Although some of us become numb or distant from these situations, their impact on our lives remain. As a result, we must have access to our heart and to the aches that it feels if we are to achieve release. Otherwise, why would we invest in this effort? Or, alternatively, how do we release something we do not know controls us? Ironically, our heart must first hurt for us to identify our loss and to then engage the process of release.

Next, we must acknowledge how our thought forms, beliefs and perspectives impact our experiences. According to Myss (2001), our thoughts affect our attitudes, beliefs, resentments, and the manner and quality of our love. Myss also addresses the impact of our ambivalent natures on our choices. She wonders, "How many parts of us are creating simultaneously? How much of us are in conflict, unaware of what we are doing?" How difficult is it to release a dream if there are parts of us that want to keep the dream alive? (Myss, 2001).

One way to accomplish this is for us to become aware of the narrative or story we carry about our dream. Many of us invest in trying to understand what went wrong and why our dream is not available to us, but this exercise is fruitless. Rather, as we see the story we carry and how that story impacts the meaning we ascribe to our dream, we can begin to distinguish between what we have had from what we hoped for. We have an opportunity here to remove ourselves from the illusion and to look at the facts. Reconciling these distinctions assists us in reconciling our ambivalence.

A part of the reconciliation process involves shifting our focus from the past to the present moment. If we do not make this shift, we will spend our energy and creativity holding the past in place rather than in investing in a new present. Shifting our focus to the present does not mean that we will not miss our dream or the people with whom we hoped to enjoy it. Nor does it mean that we forget the dream or discount its importance in our lives. No doubt, some of us may live with a bittersweet memory of the loss that reminds us of our humanness and of how our tenacious passion can become ignited. Rather, this challenge suggests that we genuinely come to terms with life as it presents itself so we can live in gratitude and a spirit of receptivity as new opportunities arise.

USING POPULAR MUSIC IN THERAPY

Popular music is one tool that counselors can use to help people distinguish fantasy from reality and reconsider challenging relational situations. Music can be used in a variety of ways toward this end, including a process I refer to as *A Musical Chronology and the Emerging Life Song* (Duffey, Lumadue, & Woods, 2001; Duffey, 2006). Below is a case that describes how music is used to help us move through the confusion and ambivalence that releasing a relationship we desire can bring. Following the case is a description of this model and a brief summary of the chronology steps.

The Case of Leah

Leah has been in a long term relationship that is very important to her. Although the relationship has brought her experiences of great happiness, joy, comfort and fun, it has also caused her deep pain, confusion, feelings of rejection and bewilderment. She is committed to the relationship and genuinely loves Tom, so thoughts of leaving the relationship are painful. Leah's words and some selections of her music are included in this section to show the complex, intense, and ambivalent nature that the notion of release can carry. The following is her interpretation of her experience. It may provide counselors with an inside view of the challenge that some clients can experience as they struggle with failed efforts and unrequited dreams.

Leah's chronology begins with Roy Orbison's (1989) rendition of "You Got It," which is followed by Johnny Cash's (1955) "Walk the Line." Both speak of love and passion and hope. She adds Bob Dylan's (1966) "I Want You," Bruce Springsteen's (1984) "Cover Me," Tom Petty's (1989) "You're So Bad," and Foreigner's (1984) "I Want to Know What Love Is." These songs set the tone for her work as Leah describes the passion, friendship, and fun she experienced with Tom. She describes how connected she has felt to him and how fortunate she perceives them to be to have found one another.

In the next breath, Leah sadly describes some limitations of the relationship and acknowledges that perhaps she has not been willing to look at these. She selected the following popular country western song lyrics to illustrate this point:

> And he's just an ordinary guy
> Like you and I
> And she's looking at him with her heart
> And not her eyes.

(Conley, 1996)

Sometimes, when we care about and love someone, or when there are qualities in a relationship that we especially appreciate or desire, we can overlook the limitations. We may convince ourselves that the limitations are not important. Because Leah genuinely loves Tom and because she perceives them to share many happy, loving, and endearing times together, she has tried to manage and minimize difficult aspects of the relationship. There are times, however, when she is reminded of her pain and of restrictions that feel unbearable. She finds words for her pain in another popular song:

> I wonder how it's going to be
> When you don't know me
> How's it going to be
> When you know I'm not here

> (Third Eye Blind, 1997)

Coming to terms with this relationship has been difficult for Leah. In fact, she becomes uncharacteristically speechless as she tries to describe it and the impact it has had on her life. In her attempt to put words to her experience she says:

> I respect and admire Tom. Right now he is showing his crusty, defensive side, but I know him and I know his heart, and it is a sweet one. And–I believe he loves me. But he has these relational rules that aren't very loving, and I don't know that I can live with them anymore. He seems to need things in a relationship that I've never heard of before . . . things I can't imagine anyone being O.K. with. And then, he turns around and is amazingly wonderful. It's been confusing and I am tired.

Later, Leah considers another position:

> I don't know. What if I have made myself believe that Tom had good intentions and that the relationship was a good one because I didn't want to bear thinking otherwise? Why would he encourage me to remain in the relationship on such one sided terms? I can't imagine he wouldn't know better. I don't like this.

Then she remembers the mixed messages she received when his words would say one thing and his actions another:

I love you but don't ask me to remember your birthday or celebrate it with you. You're wonderful, but let's not acknowledge Valentine's Day. You are important to me but I'll travel with others and not you. Don't crowd my space but please come over and keep me company. I want my freedom but don't leave.

Seeing his needs in a new light, she feels overwhelmed by what she couldn't deliver and wouldn't want to:

> No, no, no, it ain't me, babe
> It ain't me you're looking for, babe

> (Dylan, 1964)

Leah remembered the connection they shared in their passion for music and how they would sing together on the drives they would take. Then, as memories of KC and the Sunshine Band came to mind, she was reminded of basic pleasures that she hoped to enjoy with Tom but didn't –memories of seeing Tom dance with others, an experience he did not share with her. With others, he "sings the songs that remind him of the good times; he sings the songs that remind him of the better times" (Chumbawamba, 1997), times he shared with her only through the stories he would tell. With all that said, she recalls the uncomfortable and absurd way she would be left feeling that *she* needed too much.

These recollections brought with them a torrent of grief. Still, she did not want to remain confused or trapped in her grief and asked herself, "What was this? What am I grieving? What have I lost?" Further, given that Leah has invested in believing that Tom, too, loved and cared for her, she began to feel foolish as she took in the very real facts of the relationship. Now she wonders whether her fear of naming it for less than what she perceived it to be has kept her attached to a perspective clouded by fantasy.

And, still, there were tender moments:

> Want to get myself back in again
> The soft dive of oblivion
> Wanna taste the soul of your skin

> (Third Eye Blind, 1997)

Leah explains, "I miss him at the same time that I am angry and amazed at both of us. I am angry at myself for not wanting to look at anything but what I wanted to see. I didn't have context for the mixed messages I got. Perhaps I didn't want to. I guess if I had, this would have ended a long time ago, and for a number of reasons, I didn't want that." Leah is working on her own relational challenges. She is also coming to understand how she enjoyed and valued aspects of the relationship and loves and cares for Tom at the same time that the rigid structure and unusual limitations he required cause her pain. She adds U2's (1998) "Still Haven't Found What I'm Looking For" and then Kenny Roger's (1978) "Gambler" to her chronology:

> You've got to know when to hold 'em
> Know when to fold 'em
> Know when to walk away
> Know when to run

(Rogers, 1978)

At the same time, she laments, "He is a part of me . . . a part of my history. I don't know how to let go of the relationship and keep the good memories in tact. And, I don't like thinking that, after all we've shared, we will end up apart and perhaps, even strangers." Running from something or someone she loves is not Leah's strong suit. Still, there are cases where we treasure people, places, and things at the same time that irreconcilable restrictions impede our capacity to sustain them (Carter & Sokol, 2004). And, when our investments are substantial, it becomes more difficult to come to terms with the prospect of release. Further, the longer we invest in the experience, the more disappointing coming to terms with the release can become.

Thinking of Tom and of her investment in their relationship, song lyrics that describe her feelings toward him run through Leah's mind:

> I gave her my heart but she wanted my soul
> Don't think twice, it's alright

(Dylan, 1963)

Leah feels anger, shame, and disappointment. She muses:

> I ain't saying you treated me unkind
> You could have done better but I don't mind
> You just kinda wasted my precious time

> (Dylan, 1963)

Her perspective softens:

> Still, I think about the years since I first met you
> And the way it might have been without you here

> (Black, 1996)

Finally, Leah finds compassion for herself, for her tenacity, and gains some context for her dream:

> Just like some old nursery rhyme your mama told you
> You still believe in some old meant-to-be

> (Black, 1996)

Leah selected songs that resonate with her challenges in the relationship. Because she invested with her heart, Leah is grieving her investment. This exercise is but one opportunity for her to move forward, grieve the very real and important losses she faces, and leave her feelings of failure and rejection behind.

There are times when, like Leah, we are forced to release the people, places, and things that our dreams are made of; people, places, and things we love. For some, this form of release takes a great act of courage. Using favorite music as a metaphor, Leah reports:

> Sure, I want the "ring of fire" (Cash, 1963) and to walk in the "fields of gold" (Sting, 1993). It's what I thought I had with Tom. It's what I wanted. Neither of us are perfect people, and this hasn't been easy. I don't think I've ever been more upset with anyone in my life but that probably speaks to the good I thought we had together. He brought joy and laughter and happiness to my life, no doubt.

Thinking further about the relationship and her experience, she adds:

But the relationship had to be on his terms, and he didn't seem to consider how his behaviors would impact me. I wanted a relationship that took the needs of both people into account, but in our relationship, his needs and desires mattered most. I am trying not to take it personally. I believe he meant what he said when he professed his love, even in the end. It was excruciatingly painful.

She adds:

And now, reality is hitting me in the face and I'm thinking of the future. How hard will it be if I look back ten years from now and see that this is the life I chose? I think I could more easily look back at the two of us with some hope for warm feelings and compassion if I accept the reality of what he offered and heal my heart while I still have it in me to do that.

A MUSICAL CHRONOLOGY

Like Leah, many of us carry within us a repertoire of music that influences our love stories, relational worldviews and self-perceptions. Our music becomes, in one sense, archetypally bound, and can drive our actions in relationship to others (Duffey, Lumadue, & Woods, 2001; Duffey, 2006). The music we carry within us also influences the dreams we create for ourselves. If our thoughts create our reality, becoming aware of the relational storyline we carry through song provides us with a context for the roles we play in our relationships and for the choices we make relative to them.

The Chronology Process

One avenue for exploring our relational storyline is found in music. A Musical Chronology provides one context for this work. Given the relational nature of this process, A Musical Chronology is best employed within the context of a comfortable, growth-fostering relationship (see Jordan, 2001) between counselor and client. Indeed, part of the power of this work comes as we connect with our authentic experience and share this experience with someone who will respect and appreciate our struggles (see Greenspan, 2003); someone who can be moved by our experience (see Hartling, 2003; 2005). It is through this process that we grow in compassion for ourselves and our life challenges.

Clients begin the chronology process by identifying musical selections that have been important to them or that trigger for them associations to important life events, beginning with their earliest recollections. They compile the list of musical selections and arrange the song titles chronologically. After finding the lyrics to the songs they choose to include in their chronology, they compile a CD or audiotape and bring the tape to therapy session. This compilation is akin to a musical scrapbook. Clients play the compilation of music, and with the counselor, comment on thoughts, memories and associations that the music evokes. The counselor listens, engages with clients and enjoys the music with them. When moved, the therapist relates this experience to the client (see Hartling, 2003; 2005). Indeed, the therapist's experience is used to help the client move deeper into clarity and connection (see Jordan, 2001). Both therapist and clients engage in a client-led "revisiting" of historical events while listening to the music. Clients report what they feel in their hearts and notice their pain and how it relates to where they are now. They listen for relational themes and restrictive narratives or limiting perceptions they hold about themselves and their lives. Together, client and counselor work to create the possibility of alternate perspectives (Duffey, Lumadue, & Woods, 2001; Duffey, 2006).

At this point, clients identify a song that reflects their current situation which helps frame their current responses to historical events. Finally, through the chronology, clients find and play a song that represents their hopes, dreams, and goals for the future. This step is an intentional attempt to consciously re-author personal relational narratives and expand their relational images through song. Music, in this context, serves as a catalyst to our work in identifying thoughts, feelings, perceptions, and unproductive narratives about life. It also provides a context by which we can consciously create a new dream (Duffey, Lumadue, & Woods, 2001; Duffey, 2006).

BLESSINGS AND VISUALIZATION

As we work through feelings of anger, frustration, and disappointment that unrequited dreams can engender, some people choose to give the situation their blessing. Indeed, affirming its value in our lives is an important component of release and can be done through ritual. According to Gersten, "It is the goal of most therapies to help us learn to live in the moment, to learn to love others, to learn to love ourselves and to learn to forgive" (Gersten, 2005). Libby Gordon-Dartez, complementary therapist and founder of the Heartwell Healing Centre in Melbourne, Australia speaks to this process. She suggests that we visualize the person or situation that represents our loss, and holding that image, repeat to ourselves, "Heart to heart; unconditional love; no agenda; no control; heart to heart." This exercise is an acknowledgment of our Soul's journey and the Divine Light we share. Although there is no agenda for release in this ritual, the process recognizes our state of being and gives honor to it (L. Gordon-Dartez, personal communication, February 25, 2006).

CONCLUSION

In this manuscript, we examine some thoughts, feelings, and experiences of people whose lives are impacted by shattered dreams. We also look at the process some people undergo to reconcile them. Releasing a dream often involves releasing our grip on hope, reconciling feelings of faith, and ceasing our attempts at bargaining with ourselves and with life. To release our dream, we must have the courage to give up our struggle with aspects of the dream that are based in fantasy and choose to live in real life. With that said, part of this work not only involves letting go of our hope for the dream but also of the disappointment that can come with our illusions.

There are a myriad of creative resources that facilitate this work, including music, the media, scrapbooking, journaling, rituals, and visualizations, among others. In addition, there are a number of alternative and complementary therapies that can be utilized, including Emotional Freedom Therapy (Craig, 2006; Look, 2005), Cutting the Ties that Bind (Krystal, 1998), and The Circle 8 (Krystal, 2001). These and other therapies can be useful to clients who feel stuck in their experiences of loss. As with any therapy, the relationship with the therapist facilitates this process and it is through their mutual encounter that these therapies can best be effective.

Some people question what propels us to strive for a dream that hurts. Although there are a many possible ways to address this issue (Covington, 1994; Covington & Beckett, 1988; Carter & Sokol, 2004; Peabody, 2005), it is beyond the scope of this work to address these. Rather, this work has focused on the painful process involved in releasing our shattered dreams and unrequited experiences and creative ways for addressing them.

The old adage that time heals our wounds is, in some cases, a myth. Time may help us put some issues away for moments in time, but many of us need more than time to move past our hurts. Depending on the circumstances, some of us need to release our hope that our dreams will be realized. Further, while some dreams are lost by death or other concrete losses, other unrequited dreams remain seemingly available. Releasing these dreams requires courage and strength. Fortunately, we can find these qualities of courage and strength within ourselves and through the support of other important relationships where we are included, wanted, and valued.

This process requires us to be honest about our anger or hurt and to authentically work through these feelings. In so doing, we can give our dream a meaningful place in our lives without bitterness or willful determination to avoid having a comparable dream again. As we experience relief from our suffering, we accept our vulnerabilities and free ourselves to again risk trusting that a new dream is possible. Freedom to risk, from this perspective, saves us from meandering through a lost dream and creates the potential for us to experience a new, more fulfilling one.

I guess I just woke up from my American dream

(Taylor, 1997)

REFERENCES

Arntz, W., & Chasse, B. (Producers/Writers), & Vicente, M. (Director). (2004). What the bleep do we know? [Motion picture]. United States: Lord of Wind Films.
Birren, J. E. (1964). *The psychology of aging.* Englewood Cliffs, NJ: Prentice-Hall.
Black, C. (1996). Better man. On *Clint Black–The greatest hits* [CD]. New York, NY: RCA.
Butler, R. N. (1963). *Life review: An interpretation of reminiscence in the aged. Psychiatry*, 4, 1-18.
CACREP. (2000). *http://www.counseling.org/capcrep/main.htm*
Carter, S., & Sokol, J. (2004). *Men who can't love: How to recognize a commitment-phobic man before he breaks your heart.* New York, NY: M. Evans.
Cash, J. (1963). Ring of fire. On *Ring of Fire–The Best of Johnny Cash* [CD] New York, NY: Sony.
Cash, J. (1955). Walk the line. On *The Essential Johnny Cash* [CD] New York, NY: Sony.
Chumbawamba (1997). Better times. On *Tubthumper* [CD]. Seattle: Universal.

Comstock, D., & Duffey, T. (2003). Confronting adversity. In J. A. Kottler & W. P. Jones (Eds.), *Doing better: Improving clinical skills and professional competence* (pp. 67-83). Philadelphia: Brunner/Rutledge.

Conley, E. T. (1996). What she is (Is a woman in love). On *The essential Earl Thomas Conley*: [CD]. AMG: RCA.

Covington, S. (1994). *A woman's way through the twelve steps*. Center City, MN: Hazleden.

Covington, S., & Beckett, L. (1988). *Leaving the enchanted forest: The path from relationship addiction to intimacy*. Boston, MA: Harper Collins Publishers.

Craig, G. (2006). Thriving now: Transforming pain into optimal health. Retrieved from *http://www.thrivingnow.com/for/Health/gary-craig/* on February 7, 2006.

Davis, C. G., Nolen-Hoeksema, S., & Larson, J. (1998). Making sense of loss and benefiting from the experience. *Journal of Personality and Social Psychology*, 75, 561-574.

Duffey, T. (2005). Grief, loss and death. In D. Comstock (Ed.), *Diversity and development–Critical contexts that shape our lives and relationships* (pp. 216-245). Toronto: Wadsworth Publishing.

Duffey, T. (2006). A musical chronology and the emerging life song. *Journal of Creativity in Mental Health*, 1(1), 107-114.

Duffey, T., Lumadue, C., & Woods, S. (2001). Reframing the refrain: A musical chronology and the emerging life song. *The Family Journal, 9*, 398-406.

Dylan, B. (1963) Don't think twice, it's alright. On *Freewheelin' Bob Dylan* [CD]. New York: Sony.

Dylan, B. (1966). I want you. On *Blonde on Blonde* [CD]. New York: Sony.

Erikson, E. H. (1963). *Childhood and society*. New York: W. W. Norton.

Frankl, V. E. (1963). *Man's Search for Meaning*. New York: Washington Square Press.

Foreigner. (1984). I want to know what love is. On *Agent Provcateur* [CD]. New York, NY: Atlantic.

Fromm, E. (1994). *The art of being*. Boston: Continuum International Publishing Group.

Gersten, D. (2005). Alternative medicine: The source of personal power. Retrieved from *http://www.lightconnectiononline.com;Archive/jan05_colums.htm_on* February 7, 2006.

Greenspan, M. (2003). *Healing through the dark emotions: The wisdom of grief, fear, and despair*. Boston & London: Shambala.

Hartling, L. (2003). Prevention through connection. *Work in Progress*, # 103. Wellesley, MA. Stone Center Working Paper Series.

Hartling, L. (2005). CITE - In D. Comstock (Ed.), *Diversity and development–Critical contexts that shape our lives and relationships* (pp. 337-354). Toronto: Wadsworth Publishing.

Hayward, J. (1986). Your wildest dreams. On *The other side of life* [record]. New York: Polygram Records, Inc.

Jahn, R. G. (2001). The challenge of consciousness. *Journal of Scientific Exploration, 15*(4), 443-457.

Jordan, J. (2001). A relational-cultural model: Healing through mutual empathy. *Bulletin of the Menninger Clinic*, 65(1), 92-103.

Krystal, P. (1993). *Cutting the ties that bind*. KY: Thorsons/Element.
Krystal, P. (2001). *The cirle 8*. KY: Thorsons/Element.
Kubler-Ross, E. (1969). *On death and dying*. New York: Springer.
Look, C. (2005). Abundance with EFT: Emotional Freedom Techniques. California: Authorhouse.
Marwit, S., & Klass, D. (1995). Grief and the role of the inner representation of the deceased. *Omega: Journal of Death and Dying, 30*(4), 283-298.
May, R. (1994). *The discovery of being*. Scranton, PA: W. W. Norton & Company.
Mitchell, J. (1970). Big yellow taxi. On *Ladies of the canyon* [record]. New York, NY: Columbia Recording Studios.
Miller, G. (1999). The Development of the Spiritual Focus in Counseling and Counselor Education. *Journal of Counseling and Development, 77*(4), p. 500.
Miller, J. B., & Stiver, I. P. (1993). Relational images and their meanings in psychotherapy. *Work in Progress*, No. 74. Wellesley, MA: Stone Center Working Paper Series.
Myss, C. (1997). *Anatomy of the spirit: The seven stages of power and healing*. New York, NY: Three Rivers Press.
Myss, C. (2001). On *Anatomy of the spirit: The seven stages of power and healing*. [CD]. New York, NY: Sounds True, Inc.
Nakken, C. (1996). *The addictive personality: Understanding the addictive process and compulsive behavior*. Boston: Hazelden Publishing.
Orbison, R. (1989). You got it. On *Mystery Girl* [CD]. KY: Virgin Records.
Parkes, C., Launagni, P., & Young, B. (1997). *Death and bereavement across cultures*. London: Routledge.
Peabody, S. (2005). *Addiction to love: Overcoming obsession and dependency*. PA: Ten Speed Press.
Petty, T. (1989). You're so bad. On *Full Moon Fever* [CD]. New York, NY: MCA.
Rogers, K. (1978). The gambler. On *The Gambler* [CD]. Nashville, TN: Capitol Records.
Springsteen, B. (1984). Cover me. On *Born in the USA* [CD]. New York, NY: Sony.
Sting. (1993). Fields of gold. On *Ten Summoner's Tales* [CD]. Hollywood, CA: A&M Records.
Taylor, L. (1997). American Dream. On *First Row, Third Coast* [CD]. Stephenville, TX: Boatfolk Records.
Thibault, J. M., Ellor, J. W., & Netting F. E. (1991). A conceptual framework for assessing the spiritual functioning and fulfillment of older adults in long term care settings. *Journal of Religious Gerontology, 7*(4), 29-45.
Third Eye Blind. (1997). How's it going to be. On *Third Eye Blind* [CD] Redwood City: CA.
Tolle, E. (2005). *A new earth: Awakening to your life's purpose*. New York, NY: Dutton Adult.
U2. (1987). Still haven't found what I'm looking for. On *The Joshua Tree* [CD] New York: Island.
Viorst, J. (1986). *Necessary losses: The loves, illusions, dependencies, and impossible expectations that all of us have to give up in order to grow*. NY: Simon and Schuster.
Worden, W. J. (1991). *Grief counseling and grief therapy*. NY: Springer.

doi:10.1300/J456v01n03_01

Chapter 2

When Clients Die:
Using Storytelling, Journaling
and Correspondence in Times of Loss

Thomas R. Scofield

SUMMARY. The contexts of loss are as numerous as they are varied. This article reflects upon loss within the context of the helping relationship and illustrates how storytelling, journaling, and correspondence can be used to process the experience of a counselor's loss. The richness of personal accounts, interwoven and connected, provides voice and place to the experience of the deceased and their loved ones. Through such a process, the counselor is assisted toward an integrative healing intervention that can be used to work through their shattered dreams following the death of their clients. doi:10.1300/J456v01n03_02 *[Article copies available for a fee from The Haworth Document Delivery Service: 1-800-HAWORTH. E-mail address: <docdelivery@haworthpress.com> Website: <http://www.Haworth Press.com> © 2005 by The Haworth Press, Inc. All rights reserved.]*

KEYWORDS. Creativity, counseling, storytelling, journaling, client correspondence, loss

---

Thomas R. Scofield is affiliated with the University of Wisconsin-Oshkosh.

Address correspondence to: Thomas R. Scofield, Department of Counselor Education, College of Education and Human Services, University of Wisconsin-Oshkosh, 800 Algoma Boulevard, Oshkosh, WI 54901-8663.

[Haworth co-indexing entry note]: "When Clients Die: Using Storytelling, Journaling and Correspondence in Times of Loss." Scofield, Thomas R. Co-published simultaneously in *Journal of Creativity in Mental Health* (The Haworth Press, Inc.) Vol. 1, No. 3/4, 2005, pp. 25-39; and: *Creative Interventions in Grief and Loss Therapy: When the Music Stops, a Dream Dies* (ed: Thelma Duffey) The Haworth Press, Inc., 2005, pp. 25-39. Single or multiple copies of this article are available for a fee from The Haworth Document Delivery Service [1-800-HAWORTH, 9:00 a.m. - 5:00 p.m. (EST). E-mail address: docdelivery@haworthpress.com].

Available online at http://jcmh.haworthpress.com
© 2005 by The Haworth Press, Inc. All rights reserved.
doi:10.1300/J456v01n03_02

Be my friend
Hold me, wrap me up
Unfold me . . .
Warm me up and breathe me

(Sia, 2004)

When therapists accompany clients through the darkness of their pain, at best, a mutual understanding develops and relationship is formed. Therapists are trained to conceptualize client issues, while being with them in their pain (Cummings, Hallberg, Martin, Slemon, & Hiebert, 1990; Kagan, 1998; Worden, 1991). They are also trained to assist clients in all phases of their recovery (Humphrey & Zimpfer, 1996). Moreover, therapists who have the privilege of walking this path with their clients grow to "know" the person of the client and become moved by their mutual and deepened connection (Jordan, 2001; Miller & Stiver, 1993). Therapists' training, however, does not typically include the experience of coming to terms with their clients' deaths. What happens, then, when in spite of our best efforts we lose the battle of a qualitative and reasoned balance of mental health for those to whom we provide therapeutic service? How do we negotiate the loss of our dream when we cannot, for reasons and dynamics outside our control, free our clients from the insidious characteristics of their difficulties?

Counselors are vulnerable and humbled to know that even with our most empathic, well-intentioned interventions and empirically validated methods, we arrive at a place where our therapeutic power is simply preempted. We are left to depart from a place where no more can be done. How then are the lost struggles and broken relationships transformed into an experience of deep appreciation and personal and professional humility?

According to Grad, Zavasnik, and Groleger (1997) professionals will respond to the suicide of a patient in different ways, depending on factors such as personality, gender, vocation, acquired experiences, and legal litigation. While sharing some of the more common experiences associated with physical loss, the process of healing and subsequent reorganization of the professional follows a unique blueprint. Therapists are likely to feel guilt, shame, and denial that is compounded because of who they are and because of what they do (James, 2005).

Anderson (2005) recounts her confrontation of denial within the grieving process by employing poetry and utilizing writing as a coping mechanism. Like many therapists, she did not seriously consider the possibility that her clients would engage in self-harming behavior. Indeed, most therapists are ill prepared professionally for such a traumatic experience and emotional aftermath. Weiner (2005) offers that:

> No one had ever taught me what to do when (or if) this ghastly event was to occur. . . . When I learned of the large number of therapists who had experienced a client's suicide, I was astounded that I had never knowingly spoken with a person who had had a client kill her- or himself. (Weiner, 2005, p. 1)

Even with documented examples of professional survivorship, many would most likely agree that their training did not prepare them for the death of a client. And yet, we know such a tragedy will most assuredly affect us both professionally and personally. Rubel (2004) poignantly writes:

> Each of these people had been seeing me for many years and I had been highly invested in each of them . . . Their relationships with me were, in some respects, more open and intimate than their connections with their families. I knew their secrets, their struggles, their aspirations. When they died, I was left with an enormous residue of personal grief, but without any formalized way to express it or a satisfactory connection to the usual mourning process. . . . My sadness, though private, was profound. (Rubel, 2004, p. 2)

Still, what if this loss comes, not because of suicide, but in the form of some threatening protracted struggle as with cancer, AIDS or eating disorder? Duffey (2005) tells of her experience in working with children who were chronic and terminally ill. She writes about Jeffrey, who fought a valiant fight against cancer, and of his family's difficult challenge:

> Jeffrey is a part of my experience, a part of me. So are his parents and sisters. During our time together, they shared such courage, vulnerability, authenticity, and humanness. They faced not only an adjustment to life without him, but also faced reconciliation with a spiritual belief system and a faith they no longer understood. (Duffey, 2005, p. 266)

I too, experienced the death of a client, Jodi, and the present article addresses her internal struggle and the impact of that struggle on me, as her counselor. Through the perspectives of her parents, her life partner, Amy, and Jodi's own writings, an attempt is made to convey the depth and breadth of her battle and to help others dignify the experience of lost working relationships with creative repose. In this article, I will illustrate how storytelling, journaling, and correspondence, in various forms and contexts, can be used to process the experience of a counselor's loss, while giving voice and place to the experience of the deceased and their loved ones.

First, I will introduce Jodi's experience through her own voice, and then my own, in the form of a metaphorical story I wrote prior to Jodi's death. Throughout the article, I will document Jodi's struggle using her own words, and to give further context to the experience of loss, blessings, and grace, I will use the writings and correspondence of Jodi's parents and life partner. This "first hand" accounting is not only an intervention that counselors can use to work through their shattered dreams following the death of their clients. Additionally, it becomes a more accurate means for counselors to create a space of honor and understanding for the clients who trusted them with their stories; clients who are no longer here to tell them.

The death of a client is probably one of the most painful experiences that we will encounter as professionals. And, as tragic and disquieting as that thought is, many of us will encounter this experience. During our work together, Jodi brought to me her life. It was understandable, then, that as a practicing professional, I would feel a sense of isolation in my loss following her death. At the same time, I have also developed a sense of hope that I touched and have been touched by the richness of another person's life struggle. In this case, Jodi's struggle is evidenced by a personal story replete with shame, guilt, loss and grief. In her own words:

JODI'S SEARCH AND STRUGGLE

Since childhood, I have been searching, as I'm fairly sure we all do, for myself. It has been a search fraught with numerous obstacles. High expectations, failures, and lack of trust pulled at my life. Rather than being an active participant, I merely retreated to the inner-sanctum of my illness, the friend who has "built me up" when nothing else seemed to. The friend that defined me when I did not know who I was, the friend of 16 years, changing and yet constant: my eating disorder. I've clung to this disorder as if it were life itself. All these years, using it as an identity, an alias to hide behind and protect the fragile, vulnerable, scared, but knowing little girl. I am tired of living in a cage. I'm exhausted from wearing my heavy mask. I'm afraid of dying before I actually know what it means to live authentically and unashamed. I want to be the person I am without excuses or regrets.

Although Jodi could not overcome its suffocating embrace, she found no difficulty articulating the internal struggle of self-loathing she fought daily.

. . . Coat of armor, steeled and hardened, whispering perpetual promises of protection against pain, humiliation, shame, sadness, and all the ugly feelings I wanted to be free of. Conniving and deceiving, once the armor was on, it was mine. . . . I chose apathy in "a pathetic" attempt to rid myself of the horrors of my feelings, to escape being responsible for this existence I lead, as well as its affects on others I love. If I am not to blame, as evidenced by choosing not to decide, then I would not have to suffer being scrutinized or being wrong. I could just fade into the background and live like the victim I have grown comfortable with. . . . my silence was merely perpetuating violence against myself.

She continues:

But I was frightened, paralyzed and persisted in believing that I had no power and could not change my existence. I felt that any action I took was merely setting myself up for failure and its accompanying feelings, which I feared the most. In the meantime, my life happened around me, and I became comfortably acquainted with accepting whatever happened. . . . The pathetic irony is the pain I attempted to avoid became heightened and magnified. Rather than avoiding feeling, I was now feeling within the shell of the armor I had placed around me, unable to move or breathe. . . . fraudulent indifference, which others perceived as calmness and passivity.

Jodi grieves:

The fight raged inside, but I could not stand up to it. . . . Apathy, the tool I once sought for protection, now keeps me locked in its prison. . . . numerous hospitalizations for my eating disorder, my ongoing addiction with food, living a fraudulent life (to include marrying and having children), poor relationship choices, poor relationships with family, acting out to belong, working at a "thankless" job, loss of custody of my children, loss of creativity, ambition, spontaneity, and passion, as well as failure to build a strong identity complete with beliefs, values and opinions. . . . I want out.

HOW CAN I HELP?: A COUNSELOR'S CHALLENGE

Jodi's presence, her struggle for life, and our relationship in that struggle brought forth from me a short story; a fable of sorts, that metaphorically addressed the complexities she faced. I wrote the story because of my earnest regret and sustained sense of helplessness. The story, the "gift" I hoped would summon Jodi's spirit to pause and consider developing a revitalized sense of inner strength and personal advocacy. I wished for her a compassionate internal voice and an intolerant declaration against the erroneous self-image she clung to. The story provided us with a means to explore the turbulence beneath the surface of her difficulties and to also communicate the profound ways in which she impacted me.

METAPHOR AND STORYTELLING: THERE'S A WOLF AMONG US

Once upon a time, a small, yet fragile looking girl was asked to tend a flock of sheep. Although having no experience in how to do such a thing, she agreed because it made her feel important and powerful to be asked. During her watch, however, the flock was attacked by a wolf and one of the youngest and most helpless of lambs was devoured. The young girl was heartbroken and devastated. She was scorned and shamed by the elders who said, "You should have known better!" "You should have done something!" This came even in the face of her pleading and forthright justification, "But I did not know there was any danger!" "No one told me what to watch for!" No matter, they found fault and blamed her just the same. She, perhaps wiser, yet not knowing quite for sure why, found no fault with the wolf for devouring the innocent lamb. Nor did she find fault with herself for not knowing. She trusted her personal truth. No one had told her of the dangers, nor how to keep the lamb out of harms way.

All living creatures must feed themselves in order to survive. "Well," she thought, "like other living creatures, when I am hungry, I, too, know exactly what to do, and I do it. And, there are times when people have found fault with that. Either I have eaten too much, or too little; not enough of one thing–too much of another." It is so confusing sometimes to see how people take the natural order of things and make them questionable. And then suddenly, a simple but profound thought occurred to her. It came upon her, "How natural a thing to do!" "I will feed and nurture the wolf." "I will make him not hungry by filling him up!"

So at every watch hence, the young lady would leave a plate of food at the edge of the meadow where she had often caught a glimpse of the wolf. Her curiosity teemed! "Will he actually be drawn to what I have left him?" "Can I teach him to eat only what is on his plate?" So strong her interest, that she studied the wolf's every movement. She watched how cautiously he approached the edge of the meadow. He looked so frightened, vulnerable, so apprehensive approaching the very thing that would help him survive. "He must be looking for danger, taking his time not to be caught in a trap or physically attacked," she thought. "There must be truth in this." "Surely he had never encountered this sort of thing before." "It had to be completely unknown to him." But above all her ponderings she remained patient.

Well as you already understand, the wolf began to eat readily from the dish. And the young shepherd came not to fear the wolf and began placing the dish closer and closer to her person. In return, the wolf became less and less frightened of the shepherd. In time they became close and loving of one another. One cannot fully understand or say why, and yet they were very protective of the other; so much so, that one day a vicious wolf, separated from its pack, roamed too close to the flock. He was immediately and summarily driven off by the young shepherd's companion.

For a long time after, there had been no further encounters such as that. But even so, one day her elders visited the shepherd quite unexpectedly. They had come to make certain that she had not failed in her assigned task. When they approached the shepherd, however, her companion immediately moved to protect and defend his master by snarling at the approaching danger. Frightened, they cried out, "Kill it!" "Destroy it, before it can attack and devour us!" The young woman rose to her feet, more like a wisdom figure than shepherd, turned toward the huddled elders. Speaking from a voice of knowing and personal truth she said, "Hold fast!" "You have nothing to fear, save your misguided perceptions. The animal you see before you is clearly not attacking you but defending me, as any guard dog is so trained. One need only look to make note of it. Look carefully and you will know that my words are true." So the elders did her bidding, and as they considered her words more carefully, a consensus was reached. Indeed, what they saw before them was something quite different, something strange but remarkably familiar and their hearts were quieted.

A PARTNER'S CHALLENGE

My time with Jodi was brief but meaningful. I am left with a profound sense of humility for the impact she and those who loved her have had upon me. Her partner, Amy, graciously shared her thoughts and an approximate chronology leading to her loss. It is this chronology, documented through Jodi's writings, my story, and correspondence with her family and partner that have facilitated my own healing (Comstock & Duffey, 2003; Davis, Nolen-Hoeksema, & Larsen, 1998). In her personal communication Amy writes:

> That spring she was . . . complaining about her clothes looking bad and I noticed that she was really little. . . . then it just got worse. . . . I asked her if she wanted me to cut her hair before I took her to the hospital, so she had a choice, about the haircut but not about going to the hospital. I had to carry her down the stairs because she was too weak. She didn't think the hospital would even admit her. She was in for a couple days to pump up electrolytes then out again. This was about the time when we were trying to get her into treatment. She said she wanted to go but was very certain she wouldn't get accepted because she was too fat.

Amy adds:

> The first possibility of treatment for Jodi was not really feasible because she would have had to provide a very large sum of money up front and sign a contract to pay an additional sum after treatment for aftercare. With the help of a social worker, Jodi was able to be placed on Medicaid and eventually accepted. . . . By then she weighed 52 lbs. She looked so horrible, like a walking skeleton. When we stopped, people would stare . . . the looks in their eyes were pretty scary. The next day she was admitted and taken to the intensive care unit . . .

She continues:

> I didn't get privileges . . . because our partnered relationship was not recognized. As she began to gain weight and increased health, Jodi requested I . . . attend some family counseling sessions. During her treatment she seemed to learn a lot. It was really great in some ways but also painful in others. For example, she began remembering things that she blocked out. She also had some good conversations with her mom over the phone with her social worker. Jodi felt good about her work with her mom.

Jodi's condition worsens:

> During partial inpatient (treatment) Jodi reached over 100 lbs . . . She was asking for . . . medications because she was having so much trouble with all the stuff going through her mind. The treatment team decided that Jodi would be kicked out of treatment if she didn't gain 2 lbs. every week. She had already doubled her weight in a little over 3 and half months.

As time passed:

> Jodi was given a pass to come home and celebrate Thanksgiving. When she got back she had only gained 1.8 lbs, so she was kicked out. She was very upset and felt like there was nothing she could do. . . . Still she seemed to be doing all right at first, looking for a job getting settled in our new apartment. As it got closer to Christmas she began to struggle again. By January she became noticeably thinner again. She finally agreed to go to the free med clinic. Her decision brought her some hope. She was given medication in the dose she felt worked. She was happy. The attending physician wanted her to go to the hospital to get her electrolytes pumped up but she refused.

Amy describes the final moments:

> At the hospital I gave them Jodi's information. They took me into a room and the doctor came in and said she was gone and did I want to see her. I said I did, so we waited. Then my neighbor went to find out what was going on. They took her away so I didn't get to see her. The doctor never came back. Kind of wonder if that was

because I wasn't really family, even though Jodi said I was her partner . . . I never saw her again.

THROUGH JODI'S EYES

In addition to Amy's solemn recollections, she shares access to more of Jodi's own thoughts. They have become threads of a broader tapestry of suffering and provide brief glimpses, through unobstructed portals, into the weakening atrophy of Jodi's body and her life force. These entries came only weeks before her life ended. Again, through Jodi's voice:

> At one time in my life I believed that my diagnosis of Anorexia Nervosa meant that I merely had an eating disorder, but it was not until recently that I realized the implications and the complexities that hid underneath it all. My life has not merely been plagued by this malady, but conversely my mental illness manifested itself under this title, as well as those of Borderline, Depression and the countless others that have skillfully (and sometimes not so skillfully) been added to my repertoire of diagnoses. Mental Illness in and of itself is something I would not willfully place upon any life, but one that I would happily wish every individual could experience without the exasperation of owning it. Unfortunately I own it, and would graciously rid myself of it if a way existed; and then celebrate the triumph and the freedom of mental stability that I have never known.

Jodi ponders:

> My daughter's 7th birthday–oh how I love her and yearn to be with her daily, but this illness of my psyche has prevented that from happening. If I ponder the many things I have lost and am missing in my life the depression will grow worse and become unbearable as it sometimes gets. At this moment I can see the pendulum swinging back and forth, which really equates to up and down. . . . a few days of good and then plummeting into the depths of my personal hell. Each day is a transitional piece on this journey to where? I am uncertain of the destination that at one point was crystal clear like a sparkling jewel in my mind's eye. What happened? Where did it go?

The darkness:

> It's really dark today. No matter how I try to push away the clouds, they remain. Confusion and desolation overtake me, and I feel failure and disappointment all around me. I am screwing up and disappointing everyone again, and again and again. I am meaningless–I am nothing, worth nothing, a sad disappointment of a person. Lazy and ignorant, I must bring it on myself that is all I can figure out that must make me different from the masses. What happened to me? What happened to my visions, the future, the dreams that were at one time making a reality? Where did I lose it all? Why did I screw it all away?

The despair:

> I used to have answers, keys, insight, but it is futile and worthless it seems, as it gets me no further along the journey. I could easily tell each of these soul mates the way home, but it seems I have none, home that is. I belong nowhere right now, not a mother, not a daughter, a sorrowfully lacking girlfriend. . . . where did it all go and why? So many questions–so little wisdom. . . . Hurting myself, others, the world in general. My existence brings nothing. No hands or mind that write eloquently any longer, no mind that challenges, just a weary body and aching mind that longs for what I do not know.

JODI FALLS: HER MOTHER SPEAKS

Jodi died February 23, 2001. She was 29 years old. After her death and following the dedication of a piece of artwork presented by her parents, I had an opportunity to share the story, "There's a Wolf Among Us" with them. Later, Jodi's mother sent me a handwritten card and a copy of Jodi's obituary. She began her letter:

> The experience of the dedication of the "Fall" in the memory of Jodi really touched our hearts. We were overwhelmed once again by the goodness and kindness of others, and by our own emotions. Even though it's been two years since she died, we miss her still so much. For so long, we lived in fear of the disease that gripped her– always feeling that somehow we had failed her–despite how hard

we tried. Of course, we've come to understand that it wasn't up to us anyway. Jodi was a beautiful, precious soul that came through us; but she was on her own journey. We stand in awe, the more we realize the strength and courage she showed in dealing with life.

I sent a letter to Jodi's parents last month asking their permission to use this letter and Jodi's email for this manuscript, one I hoped would offer consolation and support to other practicing professionals. To a greater degree, I also hoped to bring further dignity to my friend, to those she loved and to those who love her. I closed my request to Jodi's parents with an invitation to contribute anything they wished. In her response Jodi's mother wrote:

> Dear Tom,
> Thank you for your letter, and especially for sending a copy of Jodi's e-mail. It made me cry to read her words–her voice, really. How special for us that it arrive just two days before the fifth anniversary of her death–today. She continues to make her presence known. We were thrilled to hear of your plan to write about her. You're welcome to use my letter, in conjunction with your story, and Jodi's e-mail. As you said–it may help someone else.
> We celebrate Jodi's life often and remember how beautiful, how funny, how intense, how sensitive she was–and how much she suffered. As hard as it is to be without her, we mostly just remember her greatness–and the right she had to her own journey. It's hard not understanding why everything happened the way it did–but it is not essential that we understand. We know that the love we shared transcends even death–and that's what matters. Again, thank you for your care and concern for Jodi–in life and in death–for the story you wrote, and for the piece you will write. We look forward to reading it.

CONNECTIONS AND INTERCONNECTIONS

Can there be any doubt that our lives are inextricably bound to others any time there is a struggle and we choose to become involved? It is confounding that we should have so little written in the area of client death and even less to draw upon professionally as we face these challenges. When faced with the loss of a client through death many questions remain regarding what we might have done differently. We have no way of knowing what could have been. I am left with the knowledge of a horrible struggle for life that ended.

Certainly, we are not simply involved in the everyday world of our clients. And although we want to be helpful, our desire does not guarantee that our intent will be realized. How do we, then, as practicing professionals, process this strange disparity between our well-intended efforts and the emotional aftermath of their limitations? No doubt, feelings emerge. Although the intensity of my loss has lessened over time, my feelings have ranged from anger to deeper levels of hurt, shame, and guilt. These were followed by feelings of resentment, lingering self-doubt and second-guessing. And, while these feelings are related to the common response of most who suffer loss and grief (Kagan, 1998; Worden, 1991; Viorst, 1986), no common template exists to traverse the meaningless landscape of the tragedy.

How do you help another to rejoin the spirit at the point where it has been displaced? Perhaps now, it involves a willingness to take what newfound knowledge lies before me, without denying, diluting, rationalizing or regretting the experience I have encountered. I have come to believe that my continued healing involves staying empathically connected to family and significant others, along with acknowledging, in all humility, that I tried to help.

A former client sent a copy of a short story, another "writing" that supports this challenge of integrating loss and a dream's death into our experience. The metaphor, again involving wolves, illustrates the choices we have when faced with loss.

FINDING PEACE:
A STORY OF TWO WOLVES

According to this story, a Grandfather from the Cherokee Nation was talking with his grandson. "A fight is going on inside me," he said to the boy. "It is a terrible fight and it is between two wolves. One wolf is evil and ugly: He is anger, envy, war, greed, self-pity, sorrow, regret, guilt, resentment, inferiority, lies, false pride, superiority, selfishness and arrogance. The other wolf is beautiful and good: He is friendly, joyful, peace, love, hope, serenity, humility, kindness, benevolence, justice, fairness, empathy, generosity, true, compassion, gratitude, and deep vision. This same fight is going on inside you, and inside every other human as well." The grandson paused in deep reflection because of what his grandfather had just said. Then he finally cried out, "Grandfather, which wolf will win?" The elder Cherokee replied, "The wolf that you feed" (Anonymous, 2006).

Counselors feel a gamut of emotions when faced with the death of a client. Although it is important to respect and work through these emotions as they come, we have a choice regarding which emotions we will feed. By giving place to a client's life through word and by being authentic about what the experience of life and loss mean to us, we have an opportunity to nurture, among others, the emotions of empathy, compassion, and grace. In doing so, we give value to the loss and come closer to placing our own dream's death to rest.

REFERENCES

Anderson, G. O. (2005). Who, what, when, where, how, and mostly why? A therapist's grief over the suicide of a client. In K. M. Weiner (Ed.), *Therapeutic and legal issues for therapists who have survived a client suicide: Breaking the silence* (pp. 25-34). New York: The Haworth Press, Inc.

Anonymous. The Story of Two Wolves. Retrieved February16, 2006 from http://www.rainbowbody.net/Ongwhehonwhe/cherokee.htm

Comstock, D., & Duffey, T. (2003). Confronting adversity. In J. A. Kottler & W. P. Jones (Eds.), *Doing better: Improving clinical skills and professional competence* (pp. 67-83). Philadelphia: Brunner/Rutledge.

Cummings, A. L., Hallberg, E. T., Martin, J., Slemon, A., & Hiebert, B. (1990). Implications of counselor conceptualizations for counselor education. *Counselor Education and Supervision, 30,* 120-134.

Davis, C. G., Nolen-Hoeksema, S., & Larson, J. (1998). Making sense of loss and benefiting from the experience. *Journal of Personality and Social Psychology, 75,* 561-574.

Duffey, T. (2005). Grief, loss, and death. In D. Comstock (Ed.), *Diversity and Development: Critical contexts that shape our lives and relationships* (pp. 253-268). Belmont, CA: Thompson Brooks/Cole.

Grad, O. T., Zavasnik, A., & Groleger, U. (1997). Suicide of a patient: Gender differences in bereavement reactions of therapists. *Suicide and Life-Threatening Behavior, 27*(4), 379-386.

Humphrey, G., & Zimpfer, D. (1996). *Counseling for grief and bereavement: Counseling in Practice Series.* London: Sage.

James, D. (2005). Surpassing the quota: Multiple suicides in a psychotherapy practice. In K. M. Weiner (Ed.), *Therapeutic and legal issues for therapists who have survived a client suicide: Breaking the silence* (pp. 9-23). New York: The Haworth Press, Inc.

Jordan, J. (2001). A relational-cultural model: Healing through mutual empathy. *Bulletin of the Menninger Clinic, 65*(1), 92-103.

Kagan, H. (1998). *Gili's book: A journey into bereavement for parents and counselors.* New York: Teachers College Press.

Miller, J., & Stiver, I. (1993). A relational approach to understanding women's lives and problems. *Psychiatric Annuals, 23*(8), 424-431.

Rubel, R. (2004). When a client dies. *Psychoanalytic Social Work, 11*(1), 1-14.

Sia. (2004). Breathe Me. On *Colour the small one*. [CD]. New York: Polygram Music.

Viorst, J. (1986). *Necessary losses: The loves, illusions, dependencies, and impossible expectations that all of us have to give up in order to grow*. New York: Simon and Schuster.

Weiner, K. M. (2005). *Therapeutic and legal issues for therapists who have survived a client suicide: Breaking the silence*. New York: The Haworth Press, Inc.

Worden, W. J. (1991). *Grief counseling and grief therapy: A handbook for the mental health practitioner*. New York: Springer.

doi:10.1300/J456v01n03_02

Chapter 3

Facing the Music:
Creative and Experiential Group Strategies
for Working with Addiction Related
Grief and Loss

Shane Haberstroh

SUMMARY. This article outlines how group practitioners can harness creative strategies to assist addicted clients in verbalizing and addressing the losses associated with addictive disorders. This article overviews the implementation of an experiential process that includes a warm up activity, a psychodrama, and utilization of empty chair techniques to address addiction related grief and loss. In addition, these models assist clients to discuss change and healing from the interpersonal devastation of addiction. Finally, the appropriate use and timing of these models are discussed and a case study is included to illustrate these principles in action. doi:10.1300/J456v01n03_03 *[Article copies available for a fee from The Haworth Document Delivery Service: 1-800-HAWORTH. E-mail address:*

Shane Haberstroh is Assistant Professor in the Department of Counseling and Educational Psychology at the University of Texas at San Antonio.

Address correspondence to: Shane Haberstroh, Department of Counseling, Educational Psychology, Adult & Higher Education, University of Texas at San Antonio, 501 Durango Boulevard, San Antonio, TX 78207 (E-mail: shane.haberstroh@utsa.edu).

[Haworth co-indexing entry note]: "Facing the Music: Creative and Experiential Group Strategies for Working with Addiction Related Grief and Loss." Haberstroh, Shane. Co-published simultaneously in *Journal of Creativity in Mental Health* (The Haworth Press, Inc.) Vol. 1, No. 3/4, 2005, pp. 41-55; and: *Creative Interventions in Grief and Loss Therapy: When the Music Stops, a Dream Dies* (ed: Thelma Duffey) The Haworth Press, Inc., 2005, pp. 41-55. Single or multiple copies of this article are available for a fee from The Haworth Document Delivery Service [1-800-HAWORTH, 9:00 a.m. - 5:00 p.m. (EST). E-mail address: docdelivery@haworthpress.com].

Available online at http://jcmh.haworthpress.com
doi:10.1300/J456v01n03_03

<docdelivery@haworthpress.com> Website: <http://www.HaworthPress.com>
© 2005 by The Haworth Press, Inc. All rights reserved.]

KEYWORDS. Creativity, addiction, group counseling, psychodrama, experiential

Larger than life is your fiction
In a universe made up of one
You have been drifting for so long
I know you don't want to come down
Somewhere below you, there's people who love you
And they're ready for you to come home
Please come home

(McLachlan, 2003)

At age 17, on a cold February morning, covered in grease from changing oil, I found myself at a crossroads. While many of my friends were spending this last year of high school preparing for college and seemingly bright futures, I was driven to a state of despair that left me considering the worth of my life. On that February morning, as I stood with my back to a dingy mechanic's bathroom, the loneliness and isolation I felt were palpable. I remember glancing at Mark, the resident crack addict employee, who furtively kept an eye on me. His stash was buried in a hole in the bathroom wall. Mine was close by. As we made eye contact, I foresaw myself ten years in the future, alone, high, and struggling to merely survive. In that moment, a quiet inner voice, one that I had numbed out, reminded me that this could all stop. For some reason I was ready to listen; that day I called an old friend and asked for help.

Nearly twenty years later, as I reflect on my journey, I am reminded that authentic relationships have been the key to finding meaning, purpose and fulfillment in my life. I am also reminded that addictive behaviors can only provide a sense of pseudo intimacy, ultimately leading to isolation and disconnection from others. It is from this context that I write this article.

Loss is the hallmark of the addictive process. The course of addiction often results in marked impairments in physical, relational and psychological functioning (De Alba, Samet, & Saitz, 2004; Harwood, 2000; Watkins et al., 2004). Oftentimes, addicted individuals are ostracized from nurturing social support systems (Nakken, 1996) and experience self-rejection as they compromise personal values and beliefs (Wilson, 2000). As this profound alienation from self and others grows, addicts seek amelioration from the very cause of their isolation, exacerbating the cycle of destruction. True empathic connections with others become negligible as the addict's life becomes increasingly shrouded in secrecy, shame, and self-centeredness.

Because addicts tend to anesthetize their emotions, the cognitive awareness and emotional experience of their loss and grief are minimized (Dayton, 2005). Thus, when addicted individuals seek treatment and begin to abstain from addictive behaviors, personal losses come into sharp focus and the urge to deaden the resulting emotional pain may rise. As a result, clients may turn to familiar defense mechanisms and rationalize their return to previous self-destructive behaviors. Many times, frustrated loved ones may confront an addict about the imminent consequences of relapsing. Arguing, cajoling or rationalizing with an addict about their addiction rarely works (Miller & Rollnick, 2002). Consequently, creative interventions aimed at building relationships, while supportively addressing losses are needed when working with these clients. In this article, I outline group-based strategies to invite addicted clients with various forms of addictions to verbalize, experience, and work through the many facets of their grief and loss (Dayton, 2005).

ADDICTION AND LOSS OF INTIMACY

Addiction is relational. In many ways, addictive disorders can be characterized as uninspired and uncreative ways of relating with the world. A core feature of addiction is loss of control over desires and impulses to engage in compulsive behavior. This loss of control is multifaceted, involving biochemical, environmental, genetic and psychological etiologies and processes (Orford, 2001; Spanagel & Heilig, 2005). Accordingly, as this disorder progresses, an addicted person's attention is driven away from nurturing and reciprocal social interactions and focuses more and more on the addictive behavior (Nakken, 1996). Given that human beings have only a finite amount of time and energy to spend on intimate relationships, these limited resources quickly become sapped during the course of the addictive process. As a consequence, true intimacy with others becomes an impracticable proposition (Keane, 2004).

Families and loved ones often suffer considerably from the destruction of addictive disorders. For example, Schneider (2000) noted that the relational consequences of cybersex addiction on spouses included feelings of betrayal, inadequacy, stagnated intimacy, and sexual rejection. Similarly, Collins, Grella, and Hser (2003) summarized the extant literature demonstrating strong links between parental substance use, parental-child bonding issues, and family dysfunction. Likewise, significant associations exist between parents' drug use and neglect of their children (Barnard & McGeganey, 2004). Thus, as social service and criminal justice systems intervene in the lives of substance addicted individuals, families are driven apart, institutionalized and subjected to further isolation and alienation (Barnard & McGeganey, 2004; Hanlan, O'Grady, Bennett-Sears, & Callaman, 2005). As families are shattered by addiction, the ensuing relational vacuum becomes a significant risk factor for youth's entry into addictive and maladaptive behaviors (Brook, et al., 2002; Phillips, Burns, Wagner, Kramer, & Robbins, 2002). This cyclical and self perpetuating process necessitates systemic interventions, and underscores the importance of relational prevention and intervention strategies.

GRIEF AND ADDICTION

People suffering from problems of addiction cope with numerous losses (Dayton, 2005). On the surface, they have lost tangible facets of their lives. For some, these losses include jobs, homes, finances, marriages, friends, and personal freedoms (Dayton, 2005; Rohrbach, Sussman, Dent, & Sun, 2005). Furthermore, researchers have conceptualized an addiction-grief model that assesses losses from a developmental perspective (Beecham & Prewitt, 1996). Understanding a person's grief and loss as a continuum that includes pre-addictive losses, losses resulting from active addiction, and losses as a result of treatment illustrates the compounded grief that these individuals may face. Pre-addictive losses may include unresolved grief related to histories of trauma, loss, or abuse (Dayton, 2005), loss of childhood innocence and opportunities for success and self actualization. In fact, Skolnick (1979) conceptualized addiction as pathological mourning for losses experienced early in life.

Likewise, active addiction takes its toll on both tangible and intangible aspects of a person's life. Readily observable losses are apparent for some addicted individuals. However, other losses may be less apparent. For example, Duffey (2005) explores the concept of functioning addicts. These individuals are able to maintain a semblance of personal responsibility attending to family and work tasks. However, functioning addicts may experience ambiguous losses related to finding meaning in life and maintaining authentic relationships with themselves and others. Finally, losses in treatment include disassociating with using peers, loss of comfort and familiar ways of coping, and admitting loss of control over addictive impulses and urges (Orford, 2001; Spanagel & Heilig, 2005).

RELATIONAL COUNSELING APPROACHES FOR ADDICTIVE DISORDERS

Recognizing the systemic and multilayered nature of addictive disorders, research strongly supports the use of relationally based modalities for treatment (Liddle, 2004; Markoff et al., 2005). Building upon principles of the Relational-Cultural Theory developed at the Stone Center of Wellesley College (Miller & Stiver, 1993), Markoff et al. propose a model of relational systems change for women suffering from co-occurring substance use disorders and trauma histories. In this approach, nurturing relationships serve as the catalyst for enacting systemic changes at all levels. Given that systems are comprised of people, these authors propose that healing addictive disorders can be facilitated through authentic, empowering and mutually collaborative relationships among clients, service providers and social systems.

Family Therapy Approaches

Further illustrating the power of relational interventions, Liddle (2004) overviewed the literature supporting family based therapies for treatment of addictive disorders. Specifically, this research shows that family treatment models encourage flexibility, increased treatment adherence, robust treatment engagement, and more efficacious outcomes than traditional therapies. Given the pervasive and systemic nature of addiction, family models allow clinicians to assess and influence family structures, communication patterns, and roles that members may play in dysfunctional families. In discussing change for adolescent clients, Liddle summarized how various contextual and ecological factors contribute to both dysfunction and recovery.

Group Models

Group based models have been the mainstay of addiction treatment for the past several decades (Weiss, Jaffee, de Menil, & Cogley, 2004).

Generally, therapeutic benefits of group therapy include a sense of belonging and cohesion, interpersonal learning, instillation of hope, cathartic expression, and finding meaning and purpose in life (Nerenberg, 2000; Yalom, 1995). These concepts and activities differ greatly from interactions familiar to addicts. The social ecology of addiction often centers on multiple individuals manipulating others to meet self-centered needs. In contrast, group therapy offers addicted clients an avenue to explore relational tasks in a supportive and collaborative context.

Twelve Step Programs

Twelve Step programs can be also conceptualized as helping diverse addicted individuals forge new, collaborative, and meaningful relationships (Hillhouse & Florentine, 2001). In these programs, addicts are invited to (a) attend and share in support groups, (b) identify an individual (i.e., a sponsor) to support and guide them through the program, (c) define and establish personal spiritual development, (d) give back to others through service, and (e) practice behaviors based upon principles such as honesty, willingness, forgiveness and acceptance (Alcoholics Anonymous World Services, Inc. [AAWSO], 1976; Narcotics Anonymous World Service Office [NAWSO], 1988). Although widely used in addiction treatment, twelve step models have limitations and do not meet the therapeutic needs for every client, especially those for whom personal spirituality holds little value. Nevertheless, it is apparent that 12 step models, group approaches and family therapy share a similar focus on developing and encouraging new and authentic ways for clients to relate with self and others (Covington, 1994).

EXPERIENTIAL WORK IN GROUPS
WITH ADDICTED CLIENTS

A major aim of counseling is to encourage and assist clients find and establish creative solutions to longstanding problems (Jacobs, 1994). Prior to working as a counselor educator, I worked for many years as an addiction counselor in several treatment centers. In my work with groups, I found that experiential techniques allowed clients to express genuine emotions underlying their unresolved addiction-related grief. Specifically, these strategies helped clients verbalize the losses resulting from their addictive behaviors. These experiences follow findings in the literature that support action oriented approaches in addiction groups (Blume, 1989; Dayton,

2005; Dushman & Bressler, 1991). In the following section, I will over-view the structuring of experiential activities for addicted clients that spans three group sessions.

Group Stages and Therapeutic Factors

When working with clients in groups, counselors should be cogni-zant of group developmental stages (Corey & Corey, 2006), and be able to identify the expression of therapeutic factors among members and the leader (Yalom, 1995). Therefore, I recommend that these strategies are only implemented after a group has reached the working stage (Corey & Corey, 2006), and members have expressed that the group is a cohesive and safe environment (Yalom, 1995). In addition, it is essential that group leaders receive ongoing supervision and consultation when im-plementing new and innovative techniques in group settings. Finally, counselors should always strive to promote the welfare of their group clients (American Counseling Association, 2005), respecting their au-tonomy and right to participate in experiential activities at their own comfort level.

THE CASE OF BILL

For illustrative purposes, I will share about Bill (pseudonym). Bill was a Caucasian male in his late forties, who owned a small, but failing business. Recently, he had been arrested for drunk driving, lost his driver's license, and was in the process of being divorced by his wife. He entered into treatment and was generally well liked among his peers; however, he received feedback from peers on numerous occasions that he minimized the consequences and losses of his alcoholism. Given this information, he wanted to explore his emotional detachment from his addictive process. He shared quite frequently in group about his intel-lectual awareness of the losses related to his alcohol use, but he had dif-ficulty "really seeing" the seriousness of his situation. The following section will follow Bill through three group sessions as he begins to come to terms with losses related to his addiction.

Activities to Demonstrate Relapse Risk and Commitment to Change

After the group has demonstrated cohesive behaviors (Yalom, 1995), the leader can begin to implement activities that encourage interpersonal risk taking and self-disclosure. The following activities follow the work of Jacobs (1994) and encourage clients to carefully consider their relationship to addiction and recovery principles. As with all experiential activities, the initial instructions invite clients to participate at their own comfort level, yet encourage them to take interpersonal risks.

Identifying the problem. The leader asks the group members to gather at one end of the room. Across from them, the leader places an object on the floor, and shares with the group that this item represents the idea of relapse. Next, the leader asks the group to consider how close they each are to relapsing. Once the members evaluate their connection with this behavior, they are invited to stand in a spot that represents their personal relapse risk (Figure 1). For this particular activity, Bill stood within inches of relapsing. The group members created a constellation of self assessed relapse risk, with some standing shoulder to shoulder with Bill, and others moving across the room.

Concretizing change. Next, the leader asks the members to visualize moving one step away from relapse. Once visualized, the members are asked to take a step backward. During this activity, clients may be asked to assess what factors are inhibiting change and facilitating relapse. All members are asked to rejoin the group and process their experience with this activity. During this processing, Bill identified his ambivalence and

FIGURE 1. Activity to Illustrate Addiction and Recovery Principles

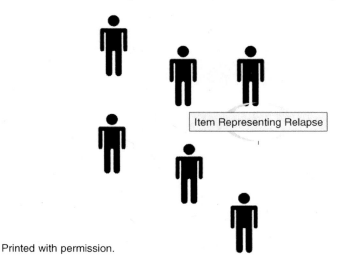

Item Representing Relapse

received supportive feedback from other members of the group. When asked how the group could help him, Bill stated " . . . to help me get to the bottom of this. To help me stay sober." At this point, the concept and structure of a psychodrama was introduced to the group, and Bill believed that this approach could help him come to terms with his losses. The psychodrama was scheduled for the next group session.

Implementing a Recovery-Focused Psychodrama

Blatner (2005) provides a cogent synopsis of psychodrama principles outlining the history, philosophy, and specific techniques for implementing this approach in counseling practice. Blatner reminds us that psychodrama blends the creative aspects of theatre, spontaneous self-expression, and movement to facilitate therapeutic change. Specific elements of psychodrama include (a) the director, (b) the protagonist, (c) the auxiliary ego(s), (d) the stage, and (e) the audience (Blatner, 2005). In addition, psychodramas follow a process that includes the warm up, the psychodrama, and the follow-up debriefing (American Society of Group Psychotherapy & Psychodrama [ASGPP], 2004; Dushman & Bressler, 1991). In working with addicted clients via psychodramatic approaches, Dayton (2005) overviews detailed instructions for implementing these strategies in groups. The following psychodrama builds upon strategies discussed by Dayton and illustrates the creation of an intervention for Bill, who reported struggling with rationalizing his return to using alcohol.

Setting the stage and warm up. In this stage, the counselor orients the group about the forthcoming psychodrama activity. This involves providing members with an overview of the general process of the exercise and answering any questions that members may have about the exercise. Like Bill, members who volunteer to serve as the protagonist in the psychodrama usually indicate a desire to expand their awareness and growth related to relapse, struggle with addictive thoughts, or desire more insight into the dynamics of their particular addiction.

The protagonist is asked to select two members of the group who will provide support and encouragement during the process. Once selected, these auxiliary egos are asked to help the protagonist share honestly about their emotions and experiences. From a 12 step perspective, these auxiliary egos take on the role of sponsors (Narcotics Anonymous World Service Office [NAWSO], 1988), and encourage the protagonist to deeply explore their relationship with addiction.

Finally, once this cast is chosen, a member from the group is asked to volunteer as the addictive voice. In my experience, it is imperative that this person volunteers for this persona rather than be chosen by the protagonist. Taking on this role carries psychological significance, and members may feel vulnerable playing this particular personification. Accordingly, all members are given permission to discontinue the activity at their discretion.

Snapshot of a psychodrama in an addiction group. Once the actors are identified, the physical format of the group changes (Figure 2) so that the protagonist faces the addictive voice, the auxiliary egos move close behind the protagonist, and the audience gathers around the pending psychodrama. Reminding the auxiliary "sponsors" to encourage authentic and honest communication, the director, or group leader, invites the protagonist and addictive voice to begin a conversation. Following is an example of Bill's conversation with his addictive voice:

"I don't know where to begin . . . we've had some fun I guess." Bill states plaintively with a demure smile on his face; his ruddy façade remains intractable. His smirk seems frozen, a disarming defense to keep people from truly seeing his pain.

FIGURE 2. Physical Arrangement of a Psychodrama in Addiction Groups

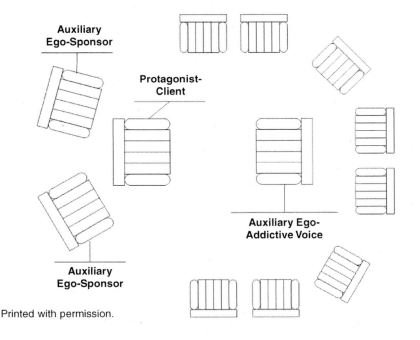

Auxiliary Ego-Sponsor

Protagonist-Client

Auxiliary Ego-Addictive Voice

Auxiliary Ego-Sponsor

Printed with permission.

"Oh yes, I don't know why the hell we're wasting our time in here. You know where I want to go." The addictive voice is almost soothing, yet seems to seethe with resentment. The member speaking from this role appears a little disturbed at the ease of these words flowing from his mouth.

"Uhm . . . " Bill stutters. He is entranced by memories of his favorite bar. Almost immediately, the familiar smells, faces of old friends and the lure of emotional relief flood his awareness. He begins to think this *treatment stuff* is too hard.

Quietly to his left, a voice urges "Tell him you are tired."

"I am tired." Bill seems unconvinced, but his voice begins to quiver. Behind his right shoulder another whisper, this one feminine, gently insists, "Tell him you are tired of being alone. That he took the only things you truly loved."

"You took my wife and daughter from me." Bill begins to panic as authentic feelings of loss wash over him in waves. He feels like his face is cracking from the inside out. He tries his hardest to force a smile, which seems oddly out of place. The audience looks on empathetically. This is a turning point.

"Bill . . . " he looks up at the sound of the director's voice. They lock eyes. He sees acceptance and genuine concern.

"You can let go." At that moment, he feels a hand gently touch his left shoulder, sees the other group members identifying and nodding. He stops fighting his feelings, and cries for the first time in over a decade. His tears roll in hitching sobs as his cheerful demeanor cracks revealing his true emotions of loss and pain.

Group process and debriefing. From the example given, it is obvious that all members have the opportunity to process the psychodrama (American Society of Group Psychotherapy [ASGPP], 2004; Blatner, 2005; Dushman & Bressler, 1991), with significant time allowed for the protagonist and auxiliary egos to share their experiences. Furthermore, allowing the member playing the addictive voice ample time to debrief is crucial, as these individuals may report feelings of guilt and increased sensitivity to their own relapse focused thinking. What becomes clear during this process is that the agenda of the addictive voice is to avoid authentic expression of emotions. In my experience, as the protagonist begins to share genuine feelings and experiences, the addictive voice's rationalizations appear transparent, insipid and the addictive agenda becomes obvious. Thus, it is important to allow the member who played this role reconnect with the group in an authentic way. Finally, after all actors have shared, the leader reconvenes the group into a circle and process the experience with a group round (Corey & Corey, 2006), allowing ample time for discussion.

Using the Empty Chair Technique to Solidify New Perspectives

As clients are given time to process the awareness that emerged from the psychodrama, follow-up focusing activities using empty chair techniques (Yontef & Jacobs, 2005) may help clients explore and verbalize new perspectives. In this activity, the leader invites the protagonist to dialogue with their ambivalent self from the new position of self honesty and genuineness. The leader structures the activity so that the client faces an empty chair that represents their relapse bound persona. For example, Bill volunteered to engage in an empty chair conversation with his relapse prone self. From his new perspective of self awareness and emotional connection to his loss, he spoke authentically to his struggling polar self.

"I know now in your heart that losing your family is almost too painful to feel." His voice is clear and calm. He continues, "It's easier to disappear in a bottle, to forget about all you lost. Now that I have felt the losses in my gut, I have a sense of relief that is true. The pain is still there, but we both know that our addiction lies to us. There will never be peace in a drink."

Clearly, experiential group work offers potent strategies for encouraging the expression of emotions and unresolved grief in the treatment of addiction. In the above example, Bill continued to process his grief, anger and sadness with the group. This particular group had experienced a high degree of cohesiveness before the psychodrama, and Bill's emotional risks and growth in group fused the group together in such a manner that they continued to meet for years after treatment ended.

DISCUSSION

Given that substances of abuse profoundly affect individuals at many levels, working with these issues requires sensitivity and knowledge of the neurobiological, social and psychological correlates of addictive behaviors. Furthermore, because addiction treatment may occur in correctional or coerced contexts (Hanlon, O'Grady, Bennett-Sears, & Callaman, 2005), it is essential that experiential activities are fully voluntary and the client's level of participation in no way affects treatment status. In addition, because there is limited empirical evidence on the use of psychodrama in addiction groups, more research is warranted to explore the implications of this practice with diverse clients and settings. Therefore, this article only overviews my professional experience, and other clinicians and group formats may yield different outcomes.

There are several other possible creative iterations for implementing group psychodramas in addiction treatment. For example, follow-up psychodramas with Bill could focus on rebuilding relationships with his estranged family, having a conversation with his authentic self, or reversing roles and engaging as an auxiliary ego. The point of these examples is to show there are many creative ways to help clients uncover and verbalize inner experiences in a supportive format. Furthermore, countless possibilities exist for using and modifying experiential techniques in groups with addicted clients. These kinesthetic activities make principles, decisions, emotions, and ambivalence tangible concepts, opening the group for meaningful and constructive dialogue (Jacobs, 1994).

These kinds of strategies allow group members to participate in new ways of communicating about themselves and with each other. Because addiction usually devastates interpersonal relationships, encouraging empathic dialogue and honest self-assessment may assist clients to rebuild connections or establish new healthy relationships. In summary, the use of experiential techniques in group work highlights the fact that authentically relating with the world is a proactive endeavor, requiring risk, intimacy and self-knowledge. It is within this context that we understand the power of curative relationships to help people come to terms with addictive disorders.

REFERENCES

Alcoholics Anonymous World Services, Inc. (1976). *Alcoholics Anonymous.* New York City: Alcoholics Anonymous World Services, Inc.

American Counseling Association. (2005). *ACA Code of Ethics,* Alexandria, VA: Author.

American Society of Group Psychotherapy and Psychodrama (2004). *Psychodrama.* Retrieved from http://www.asgpp.org/pdrama1.htm on February 7, 2004.

Barnard, M., & McKeganey, N. (2004). The impact of parental problem drug use on children: What is the problem and what can be done to help? *Addiction, 99,* 552-559.

Beecham, M. H., & Prewitt, J. (1996). Loss-grief addiction model. *Journal of Drug Education, 26,* 183-199.

Blatner, A. (2005). Psychodrama. In R. J. Corsini & D. Wedding (Eds.), *Current Psychotherapies* (7th ed.). Pacific Grove, CA: Wadsworth Press.

Blume, S. (1989). Treatment of the addictions in a psychiatric setting. *British Journal of Addiction, 84,* 727-729.

Brook, D. W., Brook, J. S., Richter, L., Whiteman, M., Arencibia-Mireles, O., & Masci, J. R., (2002). Marijuana use among the adolescent children of high-risk drug-abusing fathers. *The American Journal on Addictions, 11,* 95-110.

Collins, C. C., Grella, C. E., & Hser, Y. (2003). Effects of gender and parental involvement among parents in drug abuse treatment. *The American Journal of Drug and Alcohol Abuse, 29,* 237-261.

Corey, M. S. & Corey, G. (2006). *Groups: Process and practice (7th ed.).* Pacific Grove: CA: Brooks/Cole.

Covington, S. (1994). *A woman's way through the twelve steps.* Center City, MN: Hazleden.

Dayton, T. (2005). The use of psychodrama in dealing with grief and addiction-related trauma. *Journal of Group Psychotherapy, Psychodrama, & Sociometry, 58,* 15-34.

De Alba, I., Samet, J. H., & Saitz, R. (2004). Burden of medical illness in drug and alcohol dependent persons without primary care. *American Journal of Addiction, 13,* 33-45.

Duffey, T. (2005). The relational impact of addiction across the lifespan. In D. Comstock (Ed.), *Critical contexts in human development.* Pacific Grove, CA: Brooks/Cole–Thompson Learning.

Dushman, D. R., & Bressler, M. J. (1991). Psychodrama in an adolescent chemical dependency program. *Individual Psychology, 47,* 515-520.

Hanlon, T . E., O'Grady, K. E., Bennett-Sears, T., &. Callaman, J. (2005). Incarcerated drug-abusing mothers: Their characteristics and vulnerability. *The American Journal of Drug and Alcohol Abuse, 1,* 59-77.

Harwood, H. (2000). *Updating estimates of the economic costs of alcohol abuse in the United States: Estimates, update methods, and data.* (NIH Publication No. 98-4327). Rockville, MD.

Hillhouse, M. P., & Florentine, R. (2001). 12 step program participation and effectiveness: Do gender and ethnic differences exist? *Journal of Drug Issues, 31,* 767-780.

Jacobs, E. E. (1994). *Impact Therapy.* Odessa, FL: Psychological Assessment Resources.

Keane, H. (2004). Disorders of desire: Addiction and problems of intimacy. *Journal of Medical Humanities, 25,* 189-204.

Liddle, H. A. (2004). Family based therapies for adolescent drug use: Research contributions and future research needs. *Addiction, 99,* 76-92.

Markoff, L. S., Finkelstein, M., Kammerer, N., Kreiner, P., & Post, C. A. (2005). Relational systems change: Implementing a model of change in integrating services for women with substance abuse and mental health disorders and histories of trauma. *Journal of Behavioral Health Services and Research, 32,* 227-240.

McLachlan, S. (2003). Drifting. On *Afterglow* (CD). Beverly Hills, CA: Arista Records.

Miller, W. R., & Rollnick, S. (2002). *Motivational interviewing: Preparing people for change* (2nd ed.). New York: Guilford Press.

Miller, J., & Stiver, I. (1993). A relational approach to understanding women's lives and problems. *Psychiatric Annals, 23,* 424-431.

Millstein, R., & Spencer, T. J. (2002). A family study of the high-risk children of opioid- and alcohol-dependent parents. *The American Journal on Addictions, 11,* 41-51.

Nakken, C. (1996). *The Addictive personality: Understanding the addictive process and compulsive behavior.* Hazelden Publishing

Narcotics Anonymous World Service Office. (1988). *Narcotics Anonymous* (5th ed.), Van Nuys, CA: World Service Office.

Nerenburg, A. (2000). The value of group psychotherapy for addicts in a residential setting. *Sexual Addiction & Compulsivity, 7,* 197-209.

Orford, J. (2001). Addiction as excessive appetite. *Addiction, 96,* 15-31.

Phillips, S. D., Burns, B. J., Wagner, H. R., Kramer, T. L., & Robins, J. M. (2002). Parental incarceration among parents of adolescents receiving mental health services. *Journal of Child and Family Studies, 11,* 385-399.

Rohrbach, L. A., Sussman, S., Dent, C. W., & Sun, P. (2005). Tobacco, alcohol, and other drug use among high-risk young people: A five-year longitudinal study from adolescence to emerging adulthood. *Journal of Drug Issues, 35,* 333-355.

Schneider, J. P. (2000). Effects of cybersex addiction on the family: Results of a survey. *Sexual Addiction & Compulsivity, 7,* 31-58.

Skolnick, V. (1979). Addictions as pathological mourning: An attempt at restitution of early losses. *American Journal of Psychotherapy, 33,* 281-290.

Spanagel, R., & Heilig, M. (2005). Addiction and its brain science. *Addiction, 100,* 1813-1822.

Watkins, K. E., Hunter, S. B., Wenzel, S. L., Tu, W., Paddock, S. M., & Griffin, A. et al. (2004). Prevalence and characteristics of clients with co-occurring disorders in substance abuse treatment. *American Journal of Drug and Alcohol Abuse, 30,* 749-764.

Weiss, R. D., Jaffee, J. B., de Menil, V. P., & Cogley, C. B. (2004). Group therapy for substance use disorders: What do we know? *Harvard Review of Psychiatry, 12,* 339-350.

Wilson, M. (2000). Creativity and shame reduction in sex addiction treatment. *Sexual Addiction & Compulsivity, 7,* 229-248.

Yalom, I. D. (1995). *Theory and Practice of Group Psychotherapy* (4th ed.). New York: Basic Books.

Yontef, G., & Jacobs, L. (2005). Gestalt Therapy. In R. J. Corsini & D. Wedding (Eds.), *Current Psychotherapies (7th ed.).* Wadsworth Press.

doi:10.1300/J456v01n03_03

Chapter 4

Surviving and Thriving
After Trauma and Loss

June M. Williams
David A. Spruill

SUMMARY. Individuals and their communities experience trauma and loss during times of natural disaster. Using Hurricane Katrina as a context, the authors provide an overview of the phases of disaster coping and discuss the ambiguous losses that can occur during these traumatic and life-changing times. The use of rituals as a creative intervention is introduced to help individuals and families facilitate their grief processes. doi:10.1300/J456v01n03_04 *[Article copies available for a fee from The Haworth Document Delivery Service: 1-800-HAWORTH. E-mail address: <docdelivery@haworthpress.com> Website: <http://www.HaworthPress.com> © 2005 by The Haworth Press, Inc. All rights reserved.]*

KEYWORDS. Hurricane Katrina, creativity, counseling, mental health, trauma, grief

---

June M. Williams is affiliated with Southeastern Louisiana University.
David A. Spruill is affiliated with Louisiana State University.
Address correspondence to: June M. Williams, SLU 10863, Hammond, LA 70402 (E-mail: jwilliams@selv.edu).

[Haworth co-indexing entry note]: "Surviving and Thriving After Trauma and Loss." Williams, June M., and David A. Spruill. Co-published simultaneously in *Journal of Creativity in Mental Health* (The Haworth Press, Inc.) Vol. 1, No. 3/4, 2005, pp. 57-70; and: *Creative Interventions in Grief and Loss Therapy: When the Music Stops, a Dream Dies* (ed: Thelma Duffey) The Haworth Press, Inc., 2005, pp. 57-70. Single or multiple copies of this article are available for a fee from The Haworth Document Delivery Service [1-800-HAWORTH, 9:00 a.m. - 5:00 p.m. (EST). E-mail address: docdelivery@haworthpress.com].

Available online at http://jcmh.haworthpress.com
© 2005 by The Haworth Press, Inc. All rights reserved.
doi:10.1300/J456v01n03_04

And in the streets the children screamed
The lovers cried and the poets dreamed
But not a word was spoken
The church bells all were broken
The day the music died

(McClean, 1992)

Natural disasters vary in form but share one commonality. They are generally sudden, unexpected, and can bring with them experiences of serious devastation and loss. Indeed, the consequences of these disasters are far-reaching, generating life-changing losses and adjustments. Although weather forecasts attempt to forewarn communities of these potential disasters, forces of this kind tend to take on a life of their own, and by their very Nature can be unpredictable. Regardless of how much preparation people invest in anticipating these disasters, one thing remains clear: Natural disasters are uncontrollable forces of nature that can devastate and obliterate communities and the lives of individuals who live there.

In the aftermath of Hurricane Katrina, we were all inundated with media images of devastated neighborhoods, evacuees waiting in deplorable conditions to be rescued, individuals being airlifted to safety, and shelters overflowing with evacuees. The devastating losses of those affected by Katrina have been in the national, even international, spotlight: loss of homes, loss of jobs, loss of material possessions, and in some cases, loss of lives. Our purpose in this article is to provide an overview of the experiences of individuals affected by natural disasters, using Katrina as our context. Since we live and work in southeastern Louisiana, the examples we present will focus on the greater New Orleans area. Communities along the Mississippi Gulf Coast and experiences of those along the Mississippi Gulf Coast or in other regions of Louisiana suffered similiar losses. The trauma and loss that they experienced was extremely devastating. No doubt, the implications of these losses are far-reaching.

In this article, we will address the experience of natural disaster and the various forms of losses that come with this experience. In particular, we will describe how victims of natural disasters can suffer related ambiguous losses in addition to immediate trauma. As a creative intervention, we will share information about creating rituals to facilitate healing for individuals and families. Both authors have worked with issues of grief and loss professionally. In addition, we both personally experienced the effects of Hurricane Katrina in unique ways. Our families, students, and colleagues have been affected in various ways by Katrina. Certainly, members of our communities have been profoundly affected. Many have suffered tragedies; some have died. The familiarity and comfort of what we have known New Orleans to be no longer exists. These adjustments are shared by a collective.

We were scheduled to present a paper on ambiguous loss at the Louisiana Counseling Association Conference during Katrina's aftermath, but the conference was, of course, postponed. When we did present the material at the re-scheduled conference, we found the participant interest to be understandably overwhelming. Katrina had affected many of the participants in the workshop in a variety of ways. We would like to begin by sharing our personal experiences during and immediately following the storm.

PERSONAL PERSPECTIVES

When I (June) heard that Katrina was moving in the direction of my home, located in a suburb of New Orleans, I evacuated to my family's home, a couple of hours northwest of New Orleans. In the days following the storm, my only understanding of what would await me came from the images that I saw on television. Without access to telephones and with limited access to the Internet and e-mail, securing information was difficult. For almost a week, I was not sure of the state of my home, or the welfare of my neighbors. I was clear on the devastating impact that Katrina had on my community. I prepared myself for the possibility that I had lost my condominium and everything in it, and didn't know what other changes would face me upon my return. At the time of this writing, six months after Katrina hit, I remain displaced from home.

It was almost two weeks before I was able to return home and assess the damage to my personal property. Fortunately, the damage was minimal. No lives were lost. I needed to replace carpets, drywall, appliances and some furniture, clothing, and other possessions. Initially, I experienced survivor guilt and minimized my own losses. I was fortunate: I had a job at a university north of New Orleans and a safe place to stay with family. I had a home to return to, and my material losses were minimal. I found it difficult to acknowledge my own losses when so many others had lost so much. My friends lost homes, jobs, and almost everything they owned. Many of the students at our university had taken in family members and friends who had to evacuate, yet I was relatively comfortable in the home where I grew up, surrounded by family.

I teach a course in grief and loss counseling, and one of my mantras is "We cannot compare losses and grief reactions"; yet, I found myself doing so. It was not long, however, before I began to identify and experience some of my own losses. I am thankful for my family, friends, and colleagues who have been my support during this time. I have learned many lessons regarding patience, priorities, and self-care that will hopefully make me a better counselor and counselor educator.

In the hours before Hurricane Katrina made landfall in Louisiana and her effects began to be felt in Baton Rouge, I (Dave) surveyed the outside of our home and did my best to secure everything loose that could damage my home or those around me. Then we waited and watched. Despite the heavy winds and rain, we sustained no physical damage. Over twenty bags of debris were raked from our yard, including many large tree branches, but the trees still stood tall. Our neighbors were not as fortunate, with trees falling onto their homes, power outages for extended periods of time, and loss of communication with loved ones.

Cell phones didn't work because the cell towers were out of commission. Likewise, long distance phone service was stretched to capacity, and it was days before we could let loved ones around the country know we were fine. After a week of watching constant television storm coverage, I returned to work at the university, somewhat numb, but eager to embrace the expected deluge of displaced counseling graduate students from the many New Orleans area colleges and universities.

Counselor education students must be the greatest students in the world. While many had lost everything, they were resilient, polite, undemanding, and resolute. We did our best to accommodate their needs for shelter, registration, classes, use of the Internet, etc. It was both an honor to serve them as well as a humbling experience to witness their strength and to use their strength and positive attitudes to propel us to keep going.

We also were quickly asked to prepare workshops in handling stress and trauma and how to cope in the aftermath of Katrina. My colleagues and I delivered workshops to the university community, church clergy and parishioners, student teachers, librarians, and the Louisiana Supreme Court Justices and staff. We heard many horrific stories, many stories of courage and faith, stories with no end yet in sight as folks waited to get back home to survey their losses, and the widest range of emotions imaginable. Stressing that many of their responses were "normal reactions to abnormal events," it is my belief that we served as a source of stability and knowledge, comfort and hope, for people who had never anticipated such a life changing experience such as this. In the midst of all this, I also experienced a wide range of emotions, oscillating between happy and sad, laughing and crying at the drop of a hat, and at times feeling numb and dead inside. My colleagues and I agreed to monitor each others' emotions and behaviors, encouraging each other to say 'no' to opportunities to serve that might result in burning out and thus being of no use to anyone. I am grateful to my colleagues, family, friends, and those whose life situations touched me and changed my life forever.

COPING WITH DISASTER

Natural disasters can take many forms (e.g., hurricanes, tornadoes, floods, earthquakes), but one commonality of such events is that they affect entire communities as well as individuals (Collins & Collins, 2005). Numerous models have been created to explain the impact of such disaster trauma on individuals and communities. We have chosen to use Figley's (2006) four phases of disaster coping to present a picture of the trauma in the greater New Orleans area. Figley's phases include: (a) Phase 1: Anticipation and Preparation, (b) Phase 2: Disaster Impact, (c) Phase 3: Immediate Post-Disaster Impact and (d) Phase 4: Long term Post-Disaster Impact.

Figley refers to Phase 1, Anticipation and Preparation, as the "work of worry"–the time during which people are preparing for the impact of the event (2006). This stage begins with warning and ends at impact. Unlike earthquakes, tsunamis, or even tornadoes, hurricanes are typically preceded with a fair amount of warning. The exact path may not be possible to predict with adequate warning, but probable areas of impact can be identified with relative certainty. During this phase, Figley recommends that individuals maintain as much normalcy and routine as possible while simultaneously making plans to protect lives and property (2006). Such activity is an attempt to gain control over the stress.

Unfortunately, many in the New Orleans area were caught off guard by a hurricane whose track took a very quick and dramatic turn to the east. Katrina blew into the New Orleans area on Monday morning, but on Friday at noon, Louisiana was not even in the danger zone. By late afternoon Friday, the track had swung approximately 150 miles to the east, putting southeastern Louisiana in danger. By that time, many in the area had seen earlier forecasts and believed that they were safe. Many went about their normal routines, oblivious to the danger lurking in the Gulf. By the time that an evacuation was called, many decided not to evacuate. Although the majority evacuated, many thought, "We survived Betsy, so we certainly will be safe," or "We have never flooded before," or "Every time I evacuate for nothing; I'm not doing it again." For those who did evacuate, the hours leading up to the storm were a frenzy of activity–boarding up the windows, shopping for gas and other necessary supplies, finding a place to go, and mapping out a route to get there. But everyone, whether they stayed or left, was bracing for a probable impact from the storm.

The shortest, but perhaps most intense of Figley's phases, is Disaster Impact. This is a time that individuals are in immediate danger. Unfortunately, those who rode out the storm in the New Orleans area breathed a great sigh of relief when Katrina passed, apparently spared from her wrath. It was not until many hours after the storm passed that the levees broke and the waters rose rapidly, catching many off guard.

The period of disaster impact in the New Orleans area extended beyond what one might typically expect in such a disaster. For several days, survivors fought for their lives–huddled in attics, sitting on rooftops, perched in trees, and swimming to safety. Many were faced with gut-wrenching decisions and some had to leave behind friends and family in order to seek help. In some instances, survivors saw friends or family members drown, or perhaps they had to leave them behind to face a certain death. Those with pets struggled to save their beloved companions, but most who were rescued had to leave them behind. Even seemingly meaningless decisions took on larger than life proportions. I (David) have 3 special needs cats and 13 guitars. Although I was able to take all three cats, at one point I thought I may have to choose to leave one or more behind, creating a knot in my stomach. I also had to choose which few of my precious guitars to take with me. I was fortunate that our home was spared, but the intensity of that decision still weights heavily with me.

Following the impact, the third phase, Immediate Post-Disaster Impact, begins with return to sense of safety and ends with sense of normalcy (or "new normal"). Figley characterizes this stage as the most dangerous because people are inclined to want to return before it is safe (2006). After most of the survivors had been rescued or brought to safety, many returned to check on pets or property, often putting themselves in danger. Many residents who evacuated returned to check on their property, risking personal safety while maneuvering downed limbs, standing water, and downed live power lines. Figley uses the term "magical thinking" to describe coping behavior during this period as individuals desperately search for some sense of normalcy (2006). All along the Gulf Coast, the term "new normal" is one that is often used to describe what the residents hope one day to achieve.

Recovery from a disaster is ongoing, and Figley's final phases, Long term Post-Disaster Impact, starts after sense of normalcy returns and never ends (2006). For those affected by Katrina, the search for a "new normal" will be ongoing for many years to come. There are many signs of recovery: businesses are opening, schools are opening, people are rebuilding, and churches are holding services. Yet, not all businesses, schools, and churches are functional. Some of the survivors are in tremendous need of assistance, while others appear to be managing quite well. The community as a whole is simultaneously broken and healing. The recovery process is just beginning.

GRIEF AND LOSS IN TRAUMA'S WAKE

As one reads the descriptions of the various stages of a traumatic event, the many losses are evident. The most obvious of those losses include death, loss of homes and personal property, and loss of livelihood. Much like in the 9/11 disaster, these losses are very public losses, which add another layer to the grieving process. In the weeks and months following the disaster, the amount of national media coverage diminished, but local television stations and newspapers are still filled every day with stories related to Katrina. For many, the continuous nature of the trauma may interfere with the healing process.

In addition to the obvious losses, there are numerous losses that can be characterized as ambiguous losses, many resulting in disenfranchised grief. Pauline Boss' (1999) seminal work in the area of ambiguous loss provides a helpful lens through which to view many of the hurricane-related losses. In addition, an understanding of disenfranchised grief (Doka, 2002) can also help counselors to understand and have a deeper appreciation of the grief processes of the survivors.

According to Boss (1999), ambiguous loss is an unclear loss that defies closure. She describes two types of ambiguous loss: (a) psychologically present but physically absent and (b) physically present but psychologically absent or emotionally unavailable. The aftermath of Katrina, as well as other natural disasters, has resulted in a variety of ambiguous losses. Perhaps the most poignant of those losses are those whose friends and family members are unaccounted for. As the rescue and recovery efforts were underway, the bodies of those who died were taken to a makeshift morgue between Baton Rouge and New Orleans. In the majority of the cases, the bodies had decomposed to the point that identification was extremely difficult. Even now, several months later, some of the bodies still have not been identified, and many will never be recovered. In those cases, these individuals are psychologically present but physically absent. Their friends and family members think of them every day; they may hold out hope that somehow their loved one survived; they wonder if their loved one's body will ever be found and identified.

Such uncertainty often results in "frozen" grief (Boss, 1999). The usual rituals that society has for facilitating the grieving process are unavailable for the families of the missing because the loss is ongoing without any resolution. A further complicating factor is that different family members or friends may perceive the loss differently. The family system may also be "frozen" as some family members may consider the missing person dead while others may still be clinging to hope that the individual is still alive, or perhaps searching for proof of the death.

Even families who may not have experienced loss due to death may be dealing with separation. Many who work in the New Orleans area cannot find nearby housing for their families and may be commuting long distances or finding a place to stay during the week; returning "home" on weekends. We are friends with a family with two young children. They have relocated two hours from New Orleans, but the husband's job is still located in the New Orleans area. He is gone all week and returns on weekends. According to Boss (2006), ambiguous loss defies resolution and creates confusion over who is in or out of a particular family system. In this family, there is certainly ambiguity regarding the father's role in the system. He is both in and out–psychologically present but physically absent for much of the time.

Survivors of Katrina have also experienced numerous other ambiguous losses. Many residents whose homes were severely damaged are in limbo–uncertain as to whether they need to gut their homes and rebuild, renovate, or move. They are frozen in their decision-making as they wait for government officials to provide information and direction. Many were fortunate to still have jobs, but a cloud of uncertainly looms overhead as they constantly wonder whether or not their positions are secure. Entire neighborhoods have been affected. Some residents have returned while others have not. Those in the neighborhood are unsure about the future of their neighborhood. Will my neighbors return? Will I stay if my neighbors do not return? In every aspect of their lives, Katrina survivors are faced with uncertainty.

Our next section will present the use of rituals as an intervention in working with clients who have experienced trauma and loss.

USING RITUALS IN THE HEALING PROCESS

The Chinese describe "crises" as having two parts: danger and opportunity. Similarly, treatment of those who have experienced loss and trauma gives us opportunities to creatively help them to understand, process, and manage their experiences so they can move forward with their lives. In this section, the authors will provide an in depth look at the use of therapeutic rituals in the healing process.

Gladding (1998) describes counseling as a creative process in which the "healing arts" (e.g., music, dance, art, imagery, literature, play/humor, and drama) can be used effectively to enhance the counseling process (p. ix). Each of these creative mediums can assist clients in gaining unique perspectives on problem issues and result in the generation of options and possibilities previously unavailable. Boss (2006) has identified five characteristic symptoms of ambiguous loss: (a) immobilization and confusion, (b) physical and emotional exhaustion, (c) frozen grief, (d) denial of symbolic rituals, (e) loss of support. A theme that runs through each of these is the absence of the ability to move forward because the usual channels for expression and for finding meaning are absent and/or unavailable. Perhaps of greater importance is the new thinking about ambiguous loss which redefines it from a post-traumatic stress disorder treatment approach, (in which the loss is treated as a mental disorder), to a relational based approach in which the loss is treated as a "normal reaction to a complicated situation" (Boss, 1999, p. 10).

The treatment focus, thus, shifts from a mental disorder in an individual who has symptoms related to a past situation, to a situational ambiguity focus, one that recognizes the chronic trauma that seems to defy closure, and the paralysis that crosses generations and can last for decades. Treatment goals shift as well, with a focus on management, increased tolerance for ambiguity, and the development of dialectical thinking so that it becomes possible to hold two simultaneously opposing viewpoints. That is the seeming paradox of ambiguous loss, to replace searching for closure with finding meaning in the absence of clarity and closure.

Sadie was a nine-year-old girl who lost her mother and grandmother in the space of nine months and was now facing an unknown future as her grandfather sought to find placement for her with another relative. One of the things Sadie enjoyed doing with her mother was having her mother paint her fingernails. We made arrangements for an aunt to do this with her but their plans fell through. In our next counseling session, Sadie said her aunt had not been able to paint her nails. As I was expressing sadness that this had not occurred, Sadie spontaneously said "But *you* can!" So the next session we painted each other's nails with a bright, nine-year-old shade of red finger nail polish. I will always admire her spunk and ability to find meaning in unfamiliar situations and with her ability to connect with me in a creative way. This simple experience provided a way for her to link her past, present, and future in a meaningful way. Perhaps a new ritual had been created.

Therapists first became formally aware of rituals with the publication of Mara Selvini Palazzoli's book *Self-starvation: From the intra-psychic to the transpersonal approach to anorexia nervosa* in 1974. Rituals have actions and sometimes verbal messages, and are designed to produce rapid change through the creation of new sequences of interaction with new meanings attached to them. For rituals to be effective, they must also involve the participants and be understood from the participant's view point; that is, they must have symbolic meaning. Key components of rituals are symbolic acts, preparation and presentation, a guiding metaphor that holds the parts together, and a place for the integration of multiple meanings. These key components can serve as the building blocks for healing in grief and loss therapy.

How do you design rituals? Using a model developed by Richard Whiting (1988), the process begins with observation and is followed with creativity. Creativity does not occur in a vacuum; it is through the observation process that the themes, words, and symbols emerge that are incorporated into a ritual. In a case in which a father, Henry, had tragically lost his adult son, a ritual was created. In the ritual, Henry's sense of responsibility for raising and nurturing his son was connected with his grandchild's need for the same consistent and loving attention, now that his father was deceased. In the ritual, Henry would take his grandchild fishing (an activity Henry had enjoyed with his son). Henry expressed a fear that he would feel like crying as he mourned the loss of his son. He was asked to view this as good modeling and as another, deeper way to connect with his grandson, who also might benefit from openly grieving the loss of his father. A cross generational bond was created and this connection was to be repeated until such time as the grandchild had another father figure in his life.

Where do these creative ideas come from? Our clients "give" us the material we need to develop symbols for creative rituals. Design elements can include our client's language (e.g., "we felt the weight of the world," or "it was like here one moment and gone the next"), or can be therapist created symbols based on our client's words and/or model of the problem. When clients are unable to articulate symbols themselves, they can often relate to therapist developed symbols that facilitate a shift in beliefs and relationships.

When themes and symbols have been determined, the next step is to decide whether spontaneity or specificity will be emphasized in the ritual. In the previous example, specificity was emphasized because the client responded best to concrete directions and situations. In the case of Sadie, it was more open ended in that the only piece specified was where the fingernail polishing was to occur. How, who, what color, etc. was left open ended. What to emphasize depends on the clients' style, their model of the problem, approach to the therapeutic process, and ability to take risks and/or improvise. It is acceptable to incorporate both openness and closeness in the same ritual and asking for feedback from clients can be helpful in fine tuning therapeutic rituals.

Time and space are the next design elements. These are simply where and when the ritual will take place. Elements can include a prescribed time, a time limit, a specific place, etc. By prescribing these parameters, the ritual becomes something different and distinct from everyday activities and interactions. Rituals can be prescribed for both in-session and out-of-session and sometimes both. In-session rituals can be spontaneous, with a surprise element. They can also provide welcome relief from therapy that has become routine, as well as providing a witness to the ritual to add validity or confirmation, and allowing the ritual to take place in a safe environment. In-session rituals can be repeated outside of sessions once they have been successfully conducted in-session or alternated between in and out-of-session.

A ritual action that is especially well suited for grief and loss work is "letting go." In ambiguous loss, there is a tension between holding on and moving forward that results in client paralysis or being stuck. In a letting go ritual, clients might be asked to symbolically "let go" of items, memories, records, etc. that have interfered with their ability to live in the present and/or to move forward with their lives. Some "letting go" rituals also add the component of "holding on." In this type of ritual, clients can practice letting go without the fear of letting something go permanently. They can experiment with letting go and pulling it back again. Over time, as they become more comfortable with the idea of letting go, more and more can be let go without the accompanying fear, until they are able to move forward in more productive ways.

I have interviewed, read about, or seen as clients, numerous individuals who have been displaced by the destruction of hurricanes Katrina and Rita. Their experiences often result in ambiguous loss, a sense of paralysis, confusion, and denial. The use of rituals for this group can be particularly helpful to their ultimate adjustment, healing, and ability to move forward. A typical presenting problem might be an individual or family who has lost its home and possessions to flooding from the hurricane. They have now relocated, perhaps have found employment, enrolled their children in new schools and, to all outside appearances, made a good adjustment to a terrible situation.

Beneath the surface, however, these families must deal with ambiguities. These include whether or not to rebuild their former homes, without knowing if that will ever be possible. They are left to wonder when it might happen or how they could make it happen. They might question how long to hold out before making the decision and experience feelings of disloyalty to their former neighborhoods, friends, and family if they decide not to return; the sense of marginality, of having loyalties in both old and new locations, and many other complex issues. Some family members have not openly expressed their grief and loss because they are the "rock" of the family and must remain strong for the others. Families that used to live apart are now housed together, with the accompanying adjustment issues of rules, roles, hierarchies, and boundaries.

How can rituals be used to assist these individuals and families? The National Organization for Victim Assistance (NOVA), asserts that while rituals can be a source of reassuring routines as well as a way of integrating old traditions with new traditions, the encouragement of dialectical versus absolute ways of communication is the key to breaking the paralysis (NOVA, n.d.). Here is a case example that illustrates a possible use of a ritual to help a client go from "either/or" thinking to "both/and."

Joseph is a male in his fifties, head of his household, lifelong resident of a now flooded area in southwest Louisiana, and has relocated with his family to a safe city. His presenting problem is his perceived inability or desire to openly grieve (i.e., cry) and his immobility regarding the future plans of his family. After gathering intake information and getting a sense of his model of the problem, the next step is to validate his worldview, help him to view his situation as a normal response to a complicated situation, and encourage him to grieve openly or not grieve openly, whichever makes sense to *him*.

This family had purchased a new home in their new location, which they liked very much, but were struggling with the transition of saying good-bye to the old house in their old city. Complicating the issue was their struggle with accepting the reality of residing in the new house, and the likelihood of never returning to their old house. After carefully developing a sense of the struggle, a ritual was developed in which he and his family would go back to the old house, go from room to room, inside and out, and carefully select an object to take with them to their new home. They were to discuss it amongst themselves and explain why it was chosen and the meaning it had for them.

For example, the father had carefully maintained the garden, bushes, and yard. He selected a cutting from a tree that had been planted when their daughter was born. He planned to root it and plant it in the new home to symbolize a rebirth. In this way, he was honoring the past and simultaneously creating a future. Similar rituals for loss can include affirming memories, traditions, and stories (Imber-Black, 1988).

CONCLUSION

Our purpose in writing this article was to present a picture of some of the experiences of survivors of the worst natural disaster in our country's history in order to provide information for counselors who may work with survivors of natural disasters. Understanding how survivors of a disaster are affected at various points in the process and also recognizing the losses that they experience will help counselors effectively deal with individuals and families who have been impacted by disaster trauma.

By providing an overview of the use of rituals with such clients, we have hopefully provided the readers with a useful tool to use with their clients. Individuals and families who have lost loved ones, property, or a familiar way of life in a disaster are often deprived of the usual societal rituals for grieving their losses. Counselors who can work with clients in developing new rituals can help to facilitate clients' resiliency in the face of adversity.

REFERENCES

Boss, P. (1999). *Ambiguous loss: Learning to live with unresolved grief.* Cambridge, MA: Harvard University Press.

Boss, P. (2006). *Loss, trauma, and resilience: Therapeutic work with ambiguous loss.* NY: W.W. Norton & Company.

Collins, B. G., & Collins, T. M. (2005). *Crisis and trauma: Developmental-ecological intervention.* Boston, MA: Lahaska Press.

Doka, K. (2002). *Disenfranchised grief: New directions, challenges, and strategies for practice.* Champaign, IL: Research Press.

Figley, C. R. (2006). *Helping the traumatized in post-Katrina Louisiana.* Workshop presented at the Louisiana Association for Marriage and Family Therapy Conference, Baton Rouge, LA.

Gladding, S. T. (1998). *Counseling as an art: The creative arts in counseling* (2nd Ed.). Alexandria, VA: American Counseling Association.

Imber-Black, E. (1988). *Ritual themes in families and family therapy.* In E. Imber-Black, J. Roberts, & R. Whiting, (Eds.) *Rituals in families and family therapy* (pp. 47-83). NY: W.W. Norton.

McClean, D. (1992). American Pie. On *Legendary songs of Don McClean.* (CD). Seatlle: Curb Records.

National Organization for Victim Assistance (NOVA). (n.d.). *Grief and death and loss from hurricane Katrina.* Retrieved March 13, 2006, from http://www.trynova.org/crisis/katrina/reactions-griefafterdeath.html

Selvini-Palazzoli, M. (1974). *Self starvation: From the intrapsychic to the transpersonal approach to anorexia nervosa.* London: Human Context Books.

Whiting, R. A. (1988). *Guidelines to designing therapeutic rituals.* In E. Imber-Black, J. Roberts, & R. Whiting, R. (Eds.) *Rituals in families and family therapy* (pp. 84-109). NY: W.W. Norton.

doi:10.1300/J456v01n03_04

Chapter 5

The Loss of Innocence:
Emotional Costs to Serving as Gatekeepers
to the Counseling Profession

Stella Kerl
Margaret Eichler

SUMMARY. The practice of gatekeeping within the profession of counseling is well documented in the literature. Counselor educators are charged with the responsibility of serving as gatekeepers for the profession. However, a number of factors inhibit the practice of gatekeeping, including fears of retribution, loss, or damage. At the same time, failure to address student concerns contributes to damaging consequences to the profession and to the clients it serves. This manuscript addresses some experiences faced by counselor educators following their participation in a gatekeeping process and describes one method used by faculty to put words to name and creatively come to terms with their experiences. doi:10.1300/J456v01n03_05 *[Article copies available for a fee from The Haworth Document Delivery Service: 1-800-HAWORTH. E-mail address: <docdelivery@haworthpress.com> Website: <http://www.HaworthPress. com> © 2005 by The Haworth Press, Inc. All rights reserved.]*

KEYWORDS. Counselor Education, gatekeeping, creativity

Stella Kerl and Margaret Eichler are affiliated with Lewis and Clark College.

[Haworth co-indexing entry note]: "The Loss of Innocence: Emotional Costs to Serving as Gatekeepers to the Counseling Profession." Kerl, Stella, and Margaret Eichler. Co-published simultaneously in *Journal of Creativity in Mental Health* (The Haworth Press, Inc.) Vol. 1, No. 3/4, 2005, pp. 71-88; and: *Creative Interventions in Grief and Loss Therapy: When the Music Stops, a Dream Dies* (ed: Thelma Duffey) The Haworth Press, Inc., 2005, pp. 71-88. Single or multiple copies of this article are available for a fee from The Haworth Document Delivery Service [1-800-HAWORTH, 9:00 a.m. - 5:00 p.m. (EST). E-mail address: docdelivery@ haworthpress.com].

But "happily ever after" fails
And we've been poisoned by these fairy tales
The lawyers dwell on small details
This is the end of the innocence

(Hornsby & Henley, 1989)

Angela was a faculty member at a small liberal arts college in the mid-west. Her work in academia came after serving for several years in government work. Angela missed the environment of growth and the exploration of ideas she had so enjoyed as a graduate student. Consequently, when Angela learned about an opportunity to teach as an adjunct at a local college, she was quick to accept the position. She grew to love teaching and later accepted a tenure-track position at the college. Angela enjoyed the student questions, their desire to learn, and the excitement of helping them work with their first clients. She was a popular teacher who related well to students. Angela was eager, enthusiastic, and genuine. She often punctuated her lectures with stories: stories of client work, stories from popular media, and stories from her own life experience. She also held high standards regarding clinical work. Students who wanted to challenge their clinical work elected to receive supervision under her tutelage.

During the fall quarter of her sixth year, the chair of her department asked to schedule an appointment with her. It seemed that an angry student had written a complaint about her to the president of the university. This former student had chosen to take many of her classes but became angry with the fitness to practice report that Angela had filled out on her performance during her practicum course. The complaint against Angela, which came on the heels of the fitness to practice report, attempted to disparage her character and professionalism. Most hurtful to her were distorted details that, taken out of context, made her appear to be an irresponsible parent to her young children. She felt betrayed, angry, and humiliated. Angela knew there was ample evidence in her favor, and not long thereafter, the complaint against her was dismissed and the student did not return to the university. Still, the complaint was filed the year of her tenure review, which made the process much more difficult. The experience generated for Angela feelings of anxiety, self-consciousness, vulnerability, and loss.

Counselor educators, like Angela, assume the responsibility of providing guidance, direction, and assistance to students who will eventually serve clients in need. One of the roles they carry as counselor educators is the role of gatekeeper. That is, they must determine the fitness of their students to practice within the counseling profession (Vacha-Haase et al., 2004). This role becomes particularly challenging because they are vulnerable to attack and their work as counselor educators can be threatened. Some become "wounded in the line of duty" when they experience retribution for their efforts in the form of harassment, injuries to reputation, and legal charges.

However, when counselor educators ignore this role out of fear or apathy, other consequences exist. For one, they may begin to function as figureheads, or simply go through the motions of their job, and hide, even from themselves, the role that fear, apathy, or indifference play in their decision-making. In an effort to protect themselves or their universities, they may lose an important quality, energy, and sense of integrity. One counselor educator new to the field who, in her words, "maintained the party line" describes the impact of this incongruency between her actions and her beliefs. Denise, an assistant professor who, following instructions from a senior faculty member looked the other way when a student plagiarized a paper, later discussed the toll that her actions took on her own sense of integrity. She lamented:

> I am surprised at myself. I was so focused on getting tenure and did not want to make waves. When my mentor told me to let this go, I felt a mixture of relief and horror. He indicated that he was trying to protect me from what could be a messy situation and I did not want to deal with a messy situation. I realized later that I had made the wrong choice. (Denise, personal communication, February 12, 2006)

Ironically, others suffer when counselor educators ignore or minimize their gatekeeping responsibilities. Many students in the field of counselor education expect that professors will uphold their gatekeeping responsibilities and feel demoralized in cases where they see ethical infractions of their peers ignored. Students are trained on the need for gatekeeping and can be disappointed when professors do not take steps to secure the safety of clients or the standards of the profession.

This manuscript discusses the origins of gatekeeping and includes a literature review on legal and ethical issues related to maintaining standards to the profession. It also discusses some challenges that counselor educators may face in the gatekeeping process, including complaints, mediation, and lawsuits. Finally, the manuscript introduces creative dialogue as a means toward working through the disillusionment that these experiences can bring. It is our hope that in working through these experiences, counselor educators who are "hurt in the line of duty" can grow through the experience and find comfort and a newfound sense of professional inspiration.

GATEKEEPING

The origin of the term "gatekeeping" seems to have started from Lewin's (1947) use of the concept in the field of communication: The gatekeeper was the person who decided which pieces of communication would go forward and which pieces would not be allowed through the "gate." This field of study is still popular in journalism. The gatekeeper concept has evolved in other disciplines. In the field of counselor education, gatekeepers are the professionals whose responsibility it is to open or close the gates on the path towards becoming a counselor.

Becoming a gatekeeper is not typically the reason that counselor educators give for entering their profession. Much of the time, the motivation for entering academia can be somewhat idealistic. Myers (1997) and Csikszentmihalyi (1997) exalt the intrinsic rewards of being a university educator. Sorcinelli (1994), in her study of work satisfaction in new counseling faculty, wrote that "new faculty report high levels of satisfaction with the nature of academic work and the relative autonomy with which it is pursued, the opportunities for intellectual discovery and growth, the opportunity to have an impact on others, and the sense of accomplishment" (Sorcinelli, 1994, p. 474). Nelson, Englar-Carlson, Tierney, and Hau (2006) found that counseling academics decided to teach in counseling psychology and counselor educator programs when they realized that more visible careers did not offer them enough opportunity to make a difference. Other researchers found similar results, citing a sense of autonomy in work and making a significant contribution to the profession as being integral to the satisfaction of counselor educators (Hill, Leinbaugh, Bradley, Hazler, & Hill, 2005). Bronstein (1993) found that the rewards of academia were among the reasons that feminist and ethnic minority college professors chose their professions. Even medical doctors have identified the enjoyment of teaching as being a primary reason they taught in their field (Younghouse, 1987).

The Need for Gatekeeping

Admissions criteria are used in almost every counseling program, but even with careful screening of applicants, problems occur. Sometimes students who do not possess the necessary personal characteristics to become competent counselors, personal characteristics such as empathy, genuineness, acceptance, sharing feelings, giving and receiving feedback effectively, honesty, and establishing and maintaining relationships (Aponte, 1994; Sklare, Thomas, Williams, & Powers, 1996) become students. Undergraduate grade point average and verbal and quantitative G.R.E. scores, often used as admissions criteria for graduate programs, are unable to predict knowledge, personal development, and skills of counseling program graduates (Smaby, Maddux, Richmond, Lepkowski, & Packman, 2005). People drawn to counseling programs may also have psychological issues that impair their ability to practice effectively (Enochs, 2004).

The need for remediation and possibly for dismissal of students in the mental health professions is not always easily identifiable when measured using academic standards. Busseri, Tyler, and King (2005) looked at student dismissals in clinical psychology programs. They found that clinical psychology program directors surveyed reported a high degree of student dismissals due to ethical infractions or reasoning, failure to respond sufficiently to remediation plans, unprofessional demeanor, concerns raised by clinical supervisors, and emotional instability. Olkin and Gaughen (1991) indicated that about 3% of students each year are identified by counseling program faculty as "problem students." Rosenberg, Getzelman, Arcinue, and Oren (2005) found similar rates in their recent study of students in master's and doctoral programs in clinical and counseling psychology and their experiences of problematic peers. They also found that students looked to faculty members to take responsibility for dealing with the issue of problematic peers.

Ethical guidelines and standards of practice also point to the need for faculty members of counseling and therapy training programs to take seriously their role in the development of counseling students, especially in the need to address problematic issues. Section C.2.g. of the American Counseling Association (ACA) Code of Ethics (2005) urges counselors to refrain from offering or accepting professional services when their physical, mental, or emotional problems are likely to harm a client or others. Ethical standards for counselor educators and supervisors require that faculty and supervisors take care to assess and evaluate students' personal and professional development and ensure competence in both areas. Specifically, Section 10 directs counselor supervisors to demonstrate knowledge and competency in the evaluation of counseling performance. ACA Standard of Practice (2005) forty-one states that "counselors must assist students and supervisees in securing remedial assistance, when needed, and must dismiss from the training program students and supervisees who are unable to provide competent service due to academic or personal limitations" (ACA Code of Ethics and Standards of Practice, 2005).

The Council for Accreditation of Counseling and Related Educational Programs (CACREP) Standards, specifically Section II.F., states that faculty in counseling programs should assist in transitioning students who are not appropriate for the program into more appropriate areas of study (CACREP, 2001). However, this is most often done on an informal basis.

Gizara and Forrest (2004) explored the importance of the internship as a gatekeeper for quality control in clinical training experiences. Huprich and Rudd (2004) recommended that training programs pay better attention to the assessment and management of problem students. Gaubatz and Vera (2002) compared gatekeeping procedures among counseling programs as to the efficacy of more formalized procedures. The significance of this concern was evidenced more recently by a special section of *Professional Psychology: Research and Practice* that was devoted to addressing the issue of problematic students/trainees (see Elman & Forrest, 2004; Gizara & Forrest, 2004; Oliver, Bernstein, & Anderson, 2004; Vacha-Haase, Davenport, & Kerewsky, 2004). Miller and Koerin (2001) stressed the importance of gatekeeping functions in addition to teaching and mentoring functions of field instructors and supervisors.

Lumadue and Duffey (1999), in their important paper outlining the role of graduate programs in counseling as gatekeepers to the profession, write:

> Monitoring the competency of student counselors has always been an important component in counselor training programs . . . In addition to academic performance, counseling students are expected to possess personal qualities, characteristics, and evidence of readiness conducive to effective therapeutic practice. Given these expectations and the increasing awareness of the damage to clients that may be caused by counselors who do not possess these skills, faculty may be expected to serve as gatekeepers for the profession. (Lumadue & Duffey, 1999, p. 101)

Reluctance to Engage in Gatekeeping

This literature demonstrates the need for faculty in counseling programs to act as gatekeepers to the profession and to recognize when a student is unable to follow professionally accepted standards of practice. Olkin and Gaughen (1991) found that the majority of counseling and clinical programs relied on "problem" students to voluntarily leave or to be counseled out of the program. At times, dismissal from the counseling program might be necessary to uphold the standards of the profession and to protect clients from possible harm due to incompetent counselors (Grunebaum, 1986).

Many faculty members in counseling programs are reluctant to dismiss students, especially when the problematic issue is related to interpersonal or other non-academic problems. Kerl, Garcia, McCullough, and Maxwell (2002) wrote that "it is our observation that faculty of counseling may place too much responsibility on themselves to help or change students who experience interpersonal difficulties rather than dismissing them from counseling programs" (Kerl et al., 2002, p. 323). Since the majority of counseling faculty members are counselors/therapists themselves, they may focus more on empathy and helping than on evaluation and dismissal. Additionally, many counseling faculty believe that counselor education includes helping students to change attitudes and behaviors that are inconsistent with professional practice. They may spend many additional hours with problem students in an attempt to assist the students with interpersonal issues and worldviews that affect their counseling skills.

Vacha-Haase et al. (2004) sent a questionnaire to 281 training directors of American Psychological Association (APA) accredited clinical, counseling, and school psychology programs asking for experiences with impaired and problematic students. They write:

> Evaluating a student's work is a serious and sometimes nerve-wracking endeavor. In professional psychology, academic faculty generally serve as the profession's gatekeepers, responsible for protecting the public by identifying and intervening with graduate students exhibiting problematic behaviors . . . However, literature on the reporting of impaired psychologists may suggest that acting on concerns regarding problematic student behavior is difficult, to say the least, regardless of whether or not a program has written guidelines. (Vacha-Haase et al., 2004, p. 115)

They report several studies showing that psychologists would rather confront their colleagues informally or not at all about issues of concern, and that "this reluctance may understandably generalize to academic faculty, with the potential to discourage timely interventions with trainees, as well as model a hands-off approach to problematic behavior" (Vacha-Haase et al., 2004, p. 116).

Faculty members may also be reluctant to serve as gatekeepers due to the potential for conflict and negative attention, and may not want to make themselves vulnerable to complaints and legal challenges to their dismissals. Baldo, Softas-Nall, and Shaw (1997) warned of possible difficulties that a faculty member might experience when following the standards of practice regarding gatekeeping. They write:

> . . . faculty member(s) may become the focus of the student's feelings of aggression because of attributing their 'failure' in the program to the negative evaluation by the faculty member(s). In our experience, when a faculty member or members have been perceived by a student to be responsible for their negative review, those faculty members have been placed under unreasonable duress. (Baldo et al., 1997, p. 348)

Gaubatz and Vera (2002) wrote that counselor educators fear a number of consequences to investigating potentially deficient students, including concerns about being sued and concerns about receiving compromised teaching evaluations. Brown (1986) wrote about the fear of being sued that faculty members might feel when writing unfavorable letters of reference.

Frame and Stevens-Smith (1995) stated that faculty in counselor education programs may be reluctant to dismiss students due to "the combination of possible litigation and personal recrimination" (Frame & Stevens-Smith, 1995, p. 122). Baldo et al. (1997) stated that faculty in counseling programs may hesitate in dismissing students for reasons other than written academic wok due to a fear that the student may impose a lawsuit.

On the other hand, universities may also be sued if they fail to dismiss incompetent students. Custer (1994), in an article written for the APA Monitor (the monthly newspaper of the American Psychological Association), writes " . . . universities might be found legally liable for incompetent graduates" (Custer, 1994, p. 7). He cited a lawsuit filed against Louisiana Tech University (LTU) which argued that LTU had allowed the counselor to graduate without sufficient training. He remarks the prosecuting attorney stated, "A university has an obligation not only to the degree participants, but also to the public (to ensure) that a person who graduates from its program is competent in the area in which the degree is bestowed" (Custer, 1994, p. 7). Fortunately for the university, the case was settled for 1.7 million dollars prior to the inclusion of LTU as a defendant.

Emotional Consequences of Gatekeeping

Clearly, taking on the gatekeeping role in counseling programs causes increased stress due to its potential for conflict, in and out of the courtroom. Carli (1998), in her study on professional stress in women academics, discussed ways that participants respond to work-related stress. Responses included denial, lower feelings of entitlement, self-blame, and reduced feelings of control. Gizara and Forrest (2004) conducted interviews of internship supervisors and also found that gatekeeping functions caused emotional stress. They identified several conceptual themes in the experiences of supervisors. One description of a theme the researchers termed personal impact was particularly powerful. The researchers write:

> . . . within the participant group, the supervisors seemed to experience an especially heavy emotional price because of the close relationship that had already been established with the trainee. Being on the "front line" of the confrontation with the intern often resulted in painful return fire: "(The intern) was initially *extremely* angry with me," remembered one supervisor. "Even later (the intern) would call me at home to say to me once again, 'Why did you do this to me?'" Supervisors' descriptions also highlighted the fact that their long, intense involvement in an intern's growth made decisions to reduce or prevent client contact even more painful. This supervisor recalled a long, difficult process of explanation when the stance with the intern shifted from providing inordinate support and assistance to a decision that the intern could no longer see clients: It was very, very stressful. I spent many hours explaining why I had made the decision that I had made. Finally I said, "There are no more words to explain why this happened. I've told you everything I can tell you." (Gizara & Forrest, 2004, p. 137)

Sometimes angry students do more than calling their gatekeepers at home. The following stories reflect a compilation of experiences encountered by counseling education faculty who have experienced negative consequences as a result of gatekeeping functions. Like the experience discussed above (Angela), details of the succeeding events have been changed in order to maintain anonymity, while, at the same time, illustrating the emotional costs that gatekeeping roles can carry.

Mark: Falsely Accused of Sexual Harassment

Mark was an associate professor at a counseling psychology doctoral program at a large, research university on the west coast. He had always aspired to academia and had been very successful. Although Mark initially struggled as a teacher because of his introverted personality, he learned to energize his lectures with his own passion about research and found a niche in his department. Research was his true calling and he had a solid research agenda with many prominent publications. Mark had a large, federal grant that allowed him to hire a graduate student to assist in his research, and he had been a mentor to many students throughout the years.

Just before the end of the semester one year, Mark found an accounting discrepancy as he tallied the receipts for the grant. He discovered that his research assistant had withdrawn the funds. The student acknowledged having withdrawn the funds but insisted that the money was owed to her so that she could pay for her own dissertation research. She said she felt entitled to the money since she had done much of the work for the grant renewal. Mark explained that the federal guidelines for the grant were clear, and that the funds needed to be returned to the accounts and used for their original purpose.

Mark and the Department Chair asked the student to return the funds by the end of the week. The week passed and the funds were not returned. Additionally, the research assistant did not return to the university. The student was notified of due process. However, rather than entering the process or acknowledging her role in the accounting discrepancy, the student sued Mark for sexual harassment and included in the lawsuit various allegations, including one alleging that the research they worked on together had been her idea rather than his. Later, in depositions, Mark was challenged on issues of intellectual property and was also asked if he was gay.

Mark recalls the utter anguish he felt throughout this process. He could not reconcile the behaviors of this student with his long-standing impressions of her. He had worked closely with her. How could he have been so mistaken? How could he have trusted someone with his research; with his work; who could so rationalize, distort, and fabricate a situation? How could he have been mistaken about her character? Were there other problems with his research that he would also discover? What flaw in him kept him from seeing something that now looked so obvious? These questions haunted him.

Moreover, Mark was professionally wounded by the sexual harassment charge and the suggestion that his research was not his own. The experience was excruciatingly isolating. During the process, one member of the administration publicly questioned his sexual orientation. In an attempt to clear his name and defend his actions, Mark produced copious evidence of his innocence and spent weeks researching legal cases about sexual harassment. Ironically, he identified as a feminist and had worked to support gender equity in his field. He frequently discussed the importance of power issues in therapy to his students, and half-humorously wondered if the student accusing him had retrieved the idea to sue him from one of his lectures.

University administrators urged Mark to settle the case in order to avoid the negative publicity, but he was determined to have his day in court. Mark knew that he had not sexually harassed anyone; that his research was clearly and unequivocally his own, and he wanted the facts to speak for themselves. He also knew that the student had taken the grant money, and that the lawsuit against him was simply a smokescreen to detract from the very real evidence of wrongdoing on the student's part. After several months of on-going mediations, depositions, and meetings with attorneys, the charges against Mark were dismissed and he won the case. Uncharacteristically jubilant, Mark felt relief that justice had been served. The outcome reinforced his hope in the system and his belief that he would have compromised himself and everything he believed in if he had settled the case. However, the process was a debilitating one, in many respects. Still, in time, Mark also grew in respect for the part of him that would not cut his losses; the part that would not stand still and allow someone to attack, malign, and destroy him. The experience was painful at the same time that it was liberating. As difficult as the experience was, Mark became aware of the strength he gained. It was a life-changing experience for him; one that was as powerful as it was sobering.

Sophia: Isolated in Her Gatekeeping Role

Sophia had a successful private practice and was a well-known clinician in her community. She was active in the local professional association and had founded a non-profit organization dedicated to working with children with special needs. There was a nationally ranked counselor education program at the large university nearby, and Sophia frequently had contact with the faculty through her various activities, including serving as an on-site supervisor for their doctoral students. She enjoyed supervision and felt that it was one way of giving back to the community.

Soon thereafter, Sophia was invited to join the clinical faculty at the university. As a clinical faculty member, she would be employed by the university and would oversee the practicum as well as continuing to supervise interns. Although Sophia would have to cut down on private practice clients, she found her work with students rewarding, and enjoyed watching them develop into competent therapists. Sophia was also honored that she was asked to be a part of such a well-known program and looked forward to working with her colleagues, people whose work she admired and frequently used as a resource when she was a graduate student.

As Sophia moved into the role of practicum supervisor, she worked closely with Tim, an outwardly charming and charismatic doctoral student. During her first semester in the practicum, she noticed that many of Tim's logs of client contact hours seemed odd. When she asked Tim about them, he gave a vague response and couldn't explain the problems. She initially attributed the problems to sloppy recordkeeping, but then began to notice other issues with Tim that concerned her. He became defensive during supervision and made excuses about his lack of videotaped sessions. As Sophia investigated further, she found that Tim had encountered other similar problems, but that he had managed to sidestep them.

Sophia took her concerns to the faculty but they were reluctant to address these gatekeeping issues. Sophia was uncertain of what to do–her best clinical judgment told her that Tim needed serious help. Tim failed her practicum course and she tried to counsel with him on her concerns. He became angry and urged her to change the grade. Other faculty members also pressured her to pass him. They were concerned that Tim would be problematic and wanted him to graduate and move on. This was very confusing for her. Additionally, she began to notice a change in the way that several of the other students interacted with her. What was once a friendly and easy-going environment became a decidedly cold one. She felt alienated, disillusioned, and alone.

CREATIVE DIALOGUE AND PROFESSIONAL INTEGRITY

For Angela, Mark, and Sophia, serving in the role of gatekeeper had personal and professional costs. Because so much of their time during the gatekeeping process was predominantly spent on professional outcomes and/or legal processes, their emotional experiences were not identified, validated or even recognized. Fortunately, emotions have a life of their own and provide us with essential information about ourselves that transcend intellect and courtrooms. Our purpose in developing the following intervention was to explore creative ways of attending to the emotional impact that followed the gatekeeping events so that counselor educators, like Angela, Mark, and Sophia, can work through their experiences and regain their professional vigor and passion.

The creative process began by simply exploring and trying to understand these experiences with our colleagues, and together with them, looking for creative ways of coping. As colleagues, it was important to respect and honor their experiences. We were co-therapists investigating the phenomena of experience. In dialogue, we discovered that the emotional experience of being attacked was commonly shared. Recognizing that commonality afforded us a unique opportunity to explore ways of healing and personal discovery; searching for movement towards an emotional space that would allow the professional to once again engage in the passion of her/his work.

Many questions surfaced while trying to psychologically frame the type of attack and understand the experience using clinical perspectives. Did the experience feel like a traumatic assault? Was it a loss similar to a death and dying model? Was it metaphorically like being raped or like Post-Traumatic Stress Disorder (PTSD)? Was there a dissociative component, elements of depersonalization, or was it more like the experience of an Adjustment Disorder? Not surprisingly, the experiences of traumatic assault and loss were consistently reported. However, conceptualizing the experience from that frame alone did not seem to help. Instead, we found that by adding to that conceptualization a "loss of innocence," we were better able to capture the experience, and simply naming it seemed to help.

Without emotional exploration, emotional expression, and ways for new meaning making, we remain stuck in a place that can hold on to us with powerful and overwhelming emotions. The perception of being assaulted generates a primal need for survival; we become defensive and move into a "fight or flight" mode in order to protect ourselves. We believe that creative dialogue can help us to move away from a protective, defensive worldview and discover elements of self that were hidden or buried during the attack. Fox (2002) states, " . . . to allow creativity its appropriate place in our lives and our culture, our education, and our family relationships, is to allow healing to happen at a profound level" (Fox, 2002, p. 9).

Emotional expression thrives through creative venues where symbolic elements are key to bringing into awareness elements of an experience previously disguised. Creativity evokes the idea of fun or play with a sense of the possibility of hope and change. Movement is generated by using the more oblique approach of the creative process instead of focusing on the problem. Nachmanovitch (1990) writes " . . . the power of creative spontaneity develops into an explosion that that liberates us from outmoded frames of reference and from memory that is clogged with old facts and old feelings" (Nchamanovitch, 1990, p. 192).

With no other discussion, our colleagues were assigned the task of generating a list of at least fifty single words that "described the experience." The words became expressive symbols, revealing their experience without limiting it with intellectual rhetoric. Sharing the words became a welcomed validation.

Most of the words were emotion-based: betrayal, vulnerability, fear, outrage, shock, disbelief, and bitterness. Also present, however, were hope, eagerness, and trust. Many were action words: distancing, caution, avoidance, learning, strategy, and connecting. Others were descriptive words: lies, gall, district attorney, who cares, I can't do it, and what now? This process was a way to communicate without "explaining" and a way to listen without needing to respond. Greenspan (2003) states:

> So it is with the emotions that make us feel most vulnerable: grief, fear, and despair. These dark emotions are in-the-body energies mediated by beliefs we have gathered from the culture of family and society around us. Their purpose is not to make us miserable, drive us crazy, or shame, weaken, or defeat us, but to teach us about ourselves, others, and the world, to open our hearts to compassion, to help us heal and to change our lives. (Greenspan, 2003, p. 12)

The trust in a person's ability to organically move towards healing and balance has great power. To bring awareness and understanding amidst the seemingly endless chaotic emotions and frustration of the experience allowed our colleagues movement toward resolutions. By engaging in this creative dialogue, we established an intriguing venue for collegial work and established a relationship that diminished a possible sense of isolation.

Emotional expression can generate opportunities for new meaning, allowing for a reconnection with ourselves in a more authentic, integrated way. Connection with our self is the portal to connect with others. As professionals in the fields of Counselor Education and Psychology, we are the trained "instruments" that enlist our authentic emotional and intellectual selves in the job of educating and training future counselors. It not only commands our presence and abilities to engage with others, but establishes our right to feel excited and passionate about the profession we have chosen.

As Angela, Mark, and Sophia engaged in the creative dialogue to process the negative emotional effects of their experiences, they also were able to identify something else: a deep sense of self-respect. While the disillusionment and loss were certainly difficult, processing the experience also revealed a shared commitment to professional integrity. It is our wish that they continue the journey, remain connected with trusted professional colleagues, inspire those who remain ambivalent about their roles as gatekeepers, and once again find their professional passion.

The work referenced in this manuscript illustrates the need for counselor educators to find connection, safety, and authentic expression when they suffer this form of "on the job injury." Indeed, Gizara and Forrest (2004) found isolation to be a compelling description of the gatekeeping experience for supervisors undergoing this process. Using the words of a participant in their study, they described how the lack of professional literature on the topic contributed to feelings of isolation:

> I think the emotional elements of this experience don't get validated because there's not enough out there on the topic. So knowing people's affective reactions to working with these situations. To get the validation. I think I'd like that for myself personally. I would find that helpful. (p. 137)

The purpose of this manuscript is to give voice to this loss and to address and further discuss this important need.

REFERENCES

American Counseling Association. (2005). 2005 ACA Code of Ethics. Retrieved February 2, 2006 from http://www.counseling.org/Resources/CodeOfEthics/TP/Home/CT2.aspx

American Counseling Association. (2005). ACA Standard of Practice. Retrieved February 2, 2006 from http://www.counseling.org/Resources/CodeOfEthics/TP/Home/CT2.aspx

Aponte, H. J. (1994). How personal can training get? *The Journal of Marital and Family Therapy, 20*(1), 3-15.

Baldo, T. D., Softas-Nall, B. C., & Shaw, S. F. (1997). Student review and retention in counselor education: An alternative to frame and Stevens-Smith. *Counselor Education and Supervision, 36*(3), 245-253.

Bronstein, P. (1993). Challenges, rewards, and costs for feminists and ethnic minority scholars. In J. Gainen & R. Boice (Eds.), *Building a diverse faculty* (pp. 61-70). San Franciso, CA: Jossey-Bass.

Brown, R. S. (1986). Can they sue me? Liability risks from unfavorable letters of Reference, *Academe, 72*(5), 31-32.

Busseri, M. A., Tyler, J. D., & King, A. R. (2005). An exploratory examination of student dismissals and unprompted resignations from clinical psychology PhD. training programs: Does clinical competency matter? *Professional Psychology: Research and Practice, 36*(4), 441-445.

Carli, L. (1998). Coping with adversity. In L. H. Collins, J. C. Chrisler, & K. Quina (Eds.), *Career strategies for women in academe: Arming athena* (pp. 275-302). Thousand Oaks, CA: Sage Publications, Inc.

Council for Accreditation of Counseling and Related Educational Programs (CACREP) Standards. (2001). Retrieved on February 2, 2006 http://www.cacrep.org/Standards RevisionText.html

Csikszentmihalyi, M. (1997). Intrinsic motivation and effective teaching: A flow analysis. In J. L. Bess (Ed.), *Teaching well and liking it: Motivating faculty to teach.* Baltimore, MD: Johns Hopkins University Press.

Custer, G. (1994). Psychology and society: Can universities be liable for incompetent grads? *Monitor on Psychology, 25*(11), 7.

Elman, N., & Forrest, L. (2004). Psychotherapy in the remediation of psychology trainees: Exploratory interviews with training directors. *Professional Psychology: Research and Practice, 35*(2), 123-130.

Enochs, W. K. (2004). Impaired student counselors: Ethical and legal considerations for the family. *Family Journal: Counseling and Therapy for Couples and Families, 12*(4), 396-400.

Fox, M. (2002). *Creativity: Where the divine and the human meet.* NY: Jeremy P. Tarcher Putnam.

Frame, M. W., & Stevens-Smith, P. (1995). Out of harms's way: Enhancing monitoring and dismissal processes in counselor education programs. *Counselor Education & Supervision, 35*(2), 118-130.

Gizara, S. S., & Forrest, L. (2004). Supervisors' experiences of trainee impairment and incompetence at APA-accredited internship sites. *Professional Psychology: Research and Practice, 35*(2), 131-140.

Gaubatz, M. D., & Vera, E. M. (2002). Do formalized gatekeeping procedures increase programs' follow-up with deficient trainees? *Counselor Education and Supervision, 41*(4), 294-305.

Greenspan, M. (2003). *Healing through the dark emotions: The wisdom of grief, fear, and despair.* Boston: Shambala.

Grunebaum, H. (1986). Harmful psychotherapy experience. *American Journal of Psychotherapy, 40*, 165-176.

Hill, N. R., Leinbaugh, T., Bradley, C., Hazler, R., & Hill, N. R. (2005). Female counselor, educators: Encouraging and discouraging factors in academia. *Journal of Counseling & Development, 83*(3), 374-380.

Hornsby, B., & Henley, D. (1989). The end of the innocence. On *The End of the Innocence* (CD). New York: Geffen Records.

Huprich, S. K., & Rudd, M. D. (2004). A national survey of trainee impairment in clinical, counseling, and school psychology doctoral programs and internships. *Journal of Clinical Psychology, 60*(1), 43-52.

Kerl, S. B., Garcia, J. L., McCullough, C. S., & Maxwell, M. E. (2002). Systematic evaluation of professional performance: Legally supported procedure and process. *Counselor Education and Supervision, 41*(4), 321-334.

Lewin, K. (1947). Frontiers in group dynamics. *Human Relations, 1*(2), 145.

Lumadue, C., & Duffey, T. (1999). The role of graduate programs as gatekeepers: A model for evaluating student counselor competence. *Counselor Education and Supervision, 39*(2), 101-109.

Miller, J., & Koerin, B. B. (2001). Gatekeeping in the practicum: What field instructors need to know. *Clinical Supervisor, 20*(2), 1-18.

Myers, D. G. (1997). Professing psychology with passion. In R. J. Sternberg (Ed.), *Teaching introductory psychology: Survival tips from the experts* (pp. 155-163). Washington, DC: American Psychological Association.

Nachmanovitch, S. (1990). *Free play: The power of improvisation in life and in the arts.* NY: Jeremy P. Tarcher Putnam.

Nelson, M. L., Englar-Carlson, M., Teirney, S. C., & Hau, J. M. (2006). Class jumping into academia: Multiple identities for counseling academics. *Journal of Counseling Psychology, 53*(1), 1-14.

Oliver, M., Bernstein, J., & Anderson, K. (2004). An exploratory examination of student attitudes toward 'Impaired' peers in clinical psychology training programs. *Professional Psychology: Research and Practice, 35*(2), 141-147.

Olkin, R., & Gaughen, S. (1991). Evaluation of dismissal of students in masters level programs. *Counselor Education and Supervision, 30*(4), 276-283.

Rosenberg, J. I., Getzelman, M. A., Arcinue, F., & Oren, C. Z. (2005). An exploratory look at students' experiences of problematic peers in academic professional psychology programs. *Professional Psychology: Research and Practice, 36*(6), 665-673.

Sklare, G., Thomas, D., Williams, E., & Powers, K. (1996). Ethics and an experiential "Here and Now" group: A blend that works. *Journal for Specialists in Group Work, 21*(4), 263-273.

Smaby, M. H., Maddux, C. D., Richmond, A. S., Lepkowski, W. J., & Packman, J. (2005). Academic admission requirements as predictors of counseling knowledge, personal development, and counseling skills. *Counselor Education and Supervision, 45*(1), 43-57.

Sorcinelli, M. D. (1994). Effective approaches to new faculty development. *Journal of Counseling & Development, 72*(5), 474-479.

Vacha-Haase, T., Davenport, D. S., & Kerewsky, S. D. (2004). Problematic students: Gatekeeping practices of academic professional psychology programs. *Professional Psychology: Research and Practice, 35*(2), 115-122.

Younghouse, R. H. (1987). Factors that motivate physician faculty members in a medical school to teach CME courses. *Journal of Medical Education, 2*(1), 63-65.

doi:10.1300/J456v01n03_05

Chapter 6

Healing into Life After Sport: Dealing with Student-Athlete Loss, Grief, and Transition with EFT

H. Ray Wooten

SUMMARY. Student athletes are some of the most highly trained and celebrated groups in our society. However, for as highly prepared as they are for athletic competition, they are often unprepared for life after sport. The goal of this manuscript is to present a brief overview of the context and developmental anomalies experienced by many athletes, difficulties in dealing with loss and grief, and the alternative therapy Emotional Freedom Technique (EFT) as an approach to effectively deal with student athletes experience of loss. doi:10.1300/J456v01n03_06 *[Article copies available for a fee from The Haworth Document Delivery Service: 1-800-HAWORTH. E-mail address: <docdelivery@haworthpress.com> Website: <http://www.HaworthPress.com> © 2005 by The Haworth Press, Inc. All rights reserved.]*

KEYWORDS. Athletes, grief, loss, creativity, counseling, Emotional Freedom Technique

---

H. Ray Wooten is affiliated with St. Mary's University.

Address correspondence to: H. Ray Wooten, St. Mary's University, Department of Counseling & Human Services, One Camino Santa Maria, San Antonio, TX 78228-8527 (E-mail: hwooten@stmarytx.edu).

[Haworth co-indexing entry note]: "Healing into Life After Sport: Dealing with Student-Athlete Loss, Grief, and Transition with EFT." Wooten, H. Ray. Co-published simultaneously in *Journal of Creativity in Mental Health* (The Haworth Press, Inc.) Vol. 1, No. 3/4, 2005, pp. 89-102; and: *Creative Interventions in Grief and Loss Therapy: When the Music Stops, a Dream Dies* (ed: Thelma Duffey) The Haworth Press, Inc., 2005, pp. 89-102. Single or multiple copies of this article are available for a fee from The Haworth Document Delivery Service [1-800-HAWORTH. 9:00 a.m. - 5:00 p.m. (EST). E-mail address: docdelivery@haworthpress.com].

Available online at http://jcmh.haworthpress.com
© 2005 by The Haworth Press, Inc. All rights reserved.
doi:10.1300/J456v01n03_06

A 23-year-old man sits with his hands folded on the top of head as if he just finished running and reflects on the end of sports career:

> People have been telling me to let it go. "Let the dream go" they tell me . . . but they don't get it . . . the dream has been my entire life, the dream is my bones . . . the dream is my blood. The dream is me. How could anyone understand . . . when I don't understand what's happening to me myself.

INTRODUCTION

Personal adversity is something we have all encountered and negotiated, at some level, in our lives and relationships. Adversity elicits a variety of personal coping responses that attempt to create an experience of equilibrium or homeostasis. Thus, change can be experienced as extremely threatening. The threat is often to one's sense of inner certainty and predictability of how the world works. This is often the experience communicated from student athletes that have discovered that the "game is over."

Furthermore, we have come to understand that an individual's development creates a set of cognitive and behavioral templates that help shape and organize the world. These templates or scripts are continually revised and elaborated over time creating a set of knowledge structures and comfort zone of experience. The comfort zone is created out of a need for safety and predictability yet may impede information that may help in adjusting to adversity or change.

In the case of many athletes any information contrary to "the dream" of taking their sport to the next level is seen as discordant and a potential threat to self-identity. Mariss (1986) states that the identification with "hopes about the future . . . what we will become" is often more meaningful than self-identity in the present (p. 108). So when the sports career is over and athletic identity is now in questions what were once focused goals and benchmarks for athletic success are now experienced as threats when they have been the only reality that has supported the athlete's identity. This is often the result of some individuals (i.e., athletes) that have been raised developmentally with an aura of entitlement or being "special" that has underpinned the development of their sense of self. The self has been created dependent on athletic skill that has been deemed "special." However, "specialness" is contingent to the individual athlete being able to play and continuing to be competitive.

Parkes (1971) suggests that any negative difference from one's expectations constitutes a loss. The life of the athlete is scripted for eventual loss. This loss is based on the internalized expectations and subsequent reluctance to allow one's identity to be based on anything other than athletics. Unfortunately, the athletic script does not address the end of the dream leaving many athletes unable to acknowledge their loss and space to grieve. The goals of this chapter is to present a brief overview of the context and developmental anomalies experienced by many student-athletes that may hinder their ability to deal with loss and grief. A case study is presented and Emotional Freedom Technique (EFT) an alternative therapy is outlined to illuminate the efficacy of the approach in dealing with loss and grief

DEVELOPMENT AND THE ATHLETE

Student-athletes are some of the most highly trained and celebrated groups in our society. Thousands of fans and sport enthusiast follow games and contests closely while elevating many teams and athletes to celebrity status. Sports are often revered as the benchmark for teamwork, discipline, goal setting, preparedness, and leadership. However, for as highly trained and prepared as these athletes are in their sport they are often as equally unprepared for life after sport.

Issues and concerns plaguing the student-athlete have been well documented (Chratrand & Lent, 1987; Danish, Petitpas, & Hale, 1993; Frauenknecht & Brylinsky, 1996; Murphy, Petitpas, & Brewer, 1996; Parham, 1993). These issues are developmental in nature and include identity, personal competence, role conflict, and career and life planning (Jordan & Denson, 1990; Pearson & Petitpas, 1990; Wooten, 1994). Coleman (1961) initially identified potential developmental difficulties when he investigated the centrality of athletics in developing adolescent peer groups. Subsequent research (Denson, 1994; Goldberg, 1991; Pearson & Petitpas, 1990) has described transitional, academic, and developmental threats that result from over-identification with sports. Potential threats of distress include identity issues, perception of control, social support, and transitioning out of sports. The extent of these threats dictates the severity as a student-athlete is eventually transitioned from sports.

Researchers (Greendorfer & Blinde, 1985; Ogilvie & Howe, 1982; Svoboda & Vanek, 1982) discussed how identity issues for athletes are influenced by the degree to which they define their self-worth as related to their participation and achievement in sports. Athletes who focus solely on sport activities to the exclusion of involvement in other activities develop a self-identity that can be characterized as unidimensional or foreclosed. Pearson and Jones (1992) suggest that without input from their sport these athletes have little to support their sense of self-worth. Furthermore, Gorbett (1985) suggests that social identity can be affected as athletes have reported a loss of status and importance upon transitioning from sports. Ogilve and Howe (1986) coined the phrase "role restricted" to characterize athletes whose socialization process occurs primarily in the sports environment. As a result, alternative role taking due to termination from sports context can be inhibited or limited (Greendorfer & Blinde, 1985).

Student-athletes that have foreclosed on an athletic identity are at risk of losing their primary social support system when athletic involvement ends. Social support for athletes revolves around a ready made system that include friends and colleagues but also coaches, mentors, athletic trainers, and a variety of athletic support services that has been ready to serve. Jordan and Denson (1990) suggest that a support system based entirely in the sports setting constricts the athlete's ability to acquire alternative roles and assume a non-sport identity.

Klieber and Brock (1992) suggest that a profound lack of control also exacerbates the distress experienced in transitioning from sports. The causes of termination from sports are found most frequently to be a function of aging out, getting "cut," ending eligibility, and injury. These factors are clearly out of the control of the athlete and create a potentially negative and threatening situation in terms of self identity, self efficacy, and helplessness.

With the aforementioned information on the potential pitfalls, one would think that athletes would sensitize themselves to the stressors and proactively involve themselves in preventative activities. However, a common theme in the research literature concerning athletes is their denial of their inevitable termination from sports. Substantial research supports the notion that a significant number of athletes do not acknowledge the reality that their sports career will end (Blinde & Stratta, 1992; Haerle, 1975; Lerch, 1981; Svododa & Vanek, 1982). As a result athletes are often plagued with issues concerning reconstructing an identity outside athletics, developing personal competencies, and developing life-career plans and strategies for when the "game is over" (Wooten & Hinkle, 1992).

WHEN THE INEVITABLE HAPPENS
AND THE GAME ENDS

Athletes are inundated with a variety of messages that instill the old adage "when the going gets tough the tough get going." In some cases this is sage advice. However in cases of loss, as in the ending of one's sports career, this is often interpreted as a message to silently bear the pain. Many athletes become confused, angry and despondent when they perceive themselves incapable of "training" through or "toughing out" such an experience of loss and grief. As a result many athletes have manifested emotional disturbances and poor adjustment when faced with loss. Danish, Petitpas and Hale (1993) identified key characteristics of athletes that experienced difficulties in adjusting. These include: feelings of anger, confusion, rapid mood swings, fatalistic thinking, withdrawal from significant others and exaggerated bragging about accomplishments.

In general, athletes have had experiences where they negotiated obstacles and hurdles in their life and on the field with hard work and perseverance. Loss of their sport's identity and career however presents a totally new experience. Bruce and Shultz (2001) describe this as nonfinite loss, which is characterized as enduring and evolutionary in nature. They describe those that might experience nonfinite loss as "anyone who experiences an irrevocable loss of something that plays a central role in who they perceive themselves to be" (Bruce & Shultz, 2001, p. 7). Athletes experiencing difficulties in transitioning from sports often comment on being immobilized, lost, confused and perplexed about their situation and their feelings. There is no frame of reference for their experience as many athletes are inadequately prepared for this event.

Suggestions to help alleviate transitional difficulties for athletes have been primarily centered around career life planning (i.e., Chartrand & Lent, 1987; Danish, Petitpas, & Hale, 1993; Wooten, 1994). The programs have been well intentioned and implemented in many colleges and universities. However, little has been discussed in the literature when it comes to the actual grief and loss of the athlete. The rehabilitative literature (Gordon, Milios, & Grove, 1991; Hardy & Crace, 1990; Kolt, 2000) describes stages (e.g., denial, anger, bargaining) that athletes may go through when dealing with injuries but do not address rehabilitation of personal identity. Pearson and Jones (1992) reported that injured athletes felt that physiotherapists and other healthcare members of the team had not consciously considered the psychological impact of injuries on athletes.

Much has been written about athletic identity and its correlates to career development and vocational maturity (i.e., Haerle, 1975; Murphy, Petitpas, & Brewer, 1996) however a dearth of literature exists concerning the actual grief and loss process for the athlete.

In the case study below an athlete is incapacitated following his termination from sports. An alternative therapy, Emotional Freedom Technique (EFT), is utilized to help release stuck emotions and stubborn emotional patterns. EFT is gentle, quick, and versatile in relinquishing fears, unresolved emotions and limitations.

THE CASE OF BILL

Bill was a very successful college student athlete. He had been a three-year starter on a winning major college football team. He was competitive in the classroom and was named to the all-conference scholar athlete team. In the spring semester of which he was to graduate he decided to focus on his football skills and position in the upcoming NFL draft. He told himself that he needed time to train, as well as travel to the scouting combines to give him the best opportunity to succeed. He stated that he could always come back in the off-season once he made a professional team and finish the remaining classes for graduation. Bill worked hard, traveled to tryouts and worked out for the professional scouts. Nonetheless, he was chosen very low in the draft. Not to be discouraged, Bill used this setback as a motivator to work even harder. He was "cut" from the NFL team that drafted him after several weeks and was picked up by another franchise. Bill played in several preseason games, however was released before the season began.

Over the next two years Bill trained hard, stayed motivated and tried out for several Canadian football teams, European football teams, and finally the Arena Football League. He managed to hang around for a week or so at each place but was always released. Bill eventually came back to his parents and his childhood home. His parents reported that he went to his room, closed the door and did not come out. Bill was reported to be a recluse, depressed and increasingly more agitated. Bill's parents stated they became frightened that he was having a heart attack that was later diagnosed as a panic attack by the emergency room physician. After some discussion, Bill agreed to see a counselor.

When Bill came for his first session he was clearly a shell of his previous self. He was slouched, gaunt, had poor hygiene, with dark circles around his eyes. During the initial session he had little energy but seemed to build momentum as the session progressed. He was oriented, made eye contact, and progressively became more talkative. He discussed his past athletic history, his need to finish his last semester of college, letting his parents and community down by not having a professional sports career, and fear of the future. He stated that he wanted to finish school but felt shame when he thought about going back to his alma mater. He felt that everyone would think he was a failure and he stated that he did know how to handle that. Subsequent sessions were filled with nihilistic thinking and musings about how could this happen to him and that he could not bear the loss of all his hopes and dreams. Bill continuously wondered how he could have worked harder, run faster, and played better. Bill appeared to be caught in a dream. The content of the dream was of "almost," "maybe" and "what ifs." This continuous rumination that had been going on for almost a year and appeared to have no end in sight . . . Bill was insistent on maintaining the illusion of the world of sport for himself while not adapting to what was his current reality. Bill was hanging onto his sport identity, the dreams, and fantasy lifestyle afforded by a professional football career. Bill would recall nostalgically the games and cheers from his childhood and adolescence. He recalled feelings and thoughts that accompanied those moments and the subsequent decisions he made about himself and his life. Many of his thoughts and decisions created a rather distorted view of himself. The erroneous parts of Bill's personal narrative centered on being worthless without football. He held thoughts that his parents love was contingent on how well he did in sports and this he was sure was also true of the community. He wondered if his parents still loved him and lamented about how he was a burden to them. Bill was convinced that a sport identity was all he had and was terrified at the thought of relinquishing any part of it. It would take some time to help Bill differentiate the myriad parts of him that he had historically repressed or denied.

This differentiation became increasingly more difficult as Bill continued to dissociate any strong feelings that he would experience. Bill apparently had strong feelings when discussing situations that elicited anger, hurt, fear, and sadness. We discussed from the initial sessions that an embodied experience was one of the aims of therapy. Bill had complied when asked to do some anger release work (e.g., scream in pillow, twist a towel). However, Bill stated that he felt numb when he started to experience strong feelings of loss, sadness, and shame. The numbing appeared to be instantaneous when Bill would begin to experience the loss. This was the developmental edge where the grief work would need to begin and where Bill would encounter other parts of himself that had been repressed or ignored. It became clear that talk therapy was beneficial as we moved towards adaptive functioning but ineffective when numbness and dissociation was the dominant feature in therapy. We worked towards an embodied process that proved to be fruitful for some time. However, we were faced with what appeared to be an insurmountable wall of numbness and dissociation when it came to experiencing or discussing loss and grief. After a couple of sessions of working with the numbness and unable to get a breakthrough Bill reported that he was frustrated and felt like he was banging his head against a wall. I asked him if he would like to try an alternative that I believed might provide the breakthrough he was looking for. He stated in the affirmative and we proceeded immediately.

An alternative therapy that had proven helpful with other clients working with dissociation, as well as other feelings and issues was the Emotional Freedom Technique (EFT). Gary Craig developed EFT after training with Roger Callahan who developed Thought Field Therapy (TFT) a meridian based energetic therapy (Look, 2005). Craig transformed and simplified the TFT procedure. EFT is a meridian based technique that works by tapping on a series of points on the body that correspond to acupuncture points in the energy meridian system. The meridian system is the conduit between the energy field and the physical body (Craig, 2006). When there are blockages in the energy field there are corresponding disruptions in flow of energy through the meridian system. Mountrose and Mountrose (2000) states "these blockages are in turn, reflected in the unconscious patterns (thoughts and emotions) in the mind and in the functioning of the physical body (p. 26)." Blockages in the meridian system are a result of the inability or difficulty in releasing emotions and traumatic situations. The difficulty or inability to release emotions can come initially from a variety of sources (e.g., parents, environment). Nonetheless, these unreleased experiences take on a life of their own in your own unconscious and eventually begin to run your life in the form of limiting beliefs and judgment.

From an energy based meridian system it follows that the emotional shock of the loss is "stuck" in the subtle energy system of the human body (meridian system). EFT releases blockages in the meridian system, mind, body, and in more subtle levels of the energy field by tapping on specific acupuncture points. The result is a new awareness, expansion of new possibilities, and creation of a joy filled life.

EFT SEQUENCE

The basic EFT short sequence was employed to help Bill release the numbness he saw as inhibiting his therapeutic process. Bill had a sincere desire to clear the pattern and became even more focused when I explained EFT and his part in the process. The EFT sequence was explained as a five-step sequence. In the first step Bill was informed that EFT works best with a specific emotion. In his case he chose the feeling of numbness and was instructed that he would focus on bringing that feeling or issue into the present moment.

In step two, Bill was instructed to stay with the emotion and feel it as intensely as he could or to the level he felt comfortable. He was also given the instruction to give a subjective measure of the feeling intensity. This is often referred to as "subjective unit of distress" (SUD). The SUD is given on a scale from 0-10, zero meaning no feeling and ten being the most intense. Bill gave his SUD a ten.

Step three addressed the unconscious blockages that may have deterred Bill from experiencing the full effect of EFT. The phenomenon has been coined "psychological reversal" (PR). PR has been described as having a disruption securely implanted in the meridian system. This results in someone being motivated to change but their unconscious subverting attempts towards that change. Craig (2006) likens PR as to having a battery in backwards in a portable radio. The radio will have enough power but will never play. Before success can be achieved PR has to be inverted to the correct polarity. This is accomplished by an affirmation that usurps limiting beliefs and judgments that are the root of many of our difficulties. EFT incorporates a generalized affirmation and an acupuncture point in the sequence that clears most forms of PR. Bill was asked to rub the "Sore Spot" on his chest in a circular fashion while repeating the affirmation "Even though I have this _____, I deeply and completely accept myself" three times with conviction The Sore Spot is located by starting at the inside edge of the collarbone, then moving your fingers down approximately three inches and away from the center of your chest approximately three inches. Feel around in this general area with your fingers until you feel a tender spot. Bill filled in the blank with his specific emotion, rubbed the sore spot in a circular fashion and repeated the affirmation three time, "Even though I have this numbness, I deeply and completely accepts myself." Bill was reluctant at first to say the affirmation but was reminded that he did not have to believe the affirmation but be willing to say it. He complied with the instructions stating that he was a team player and ready to play his part in saying the affirmation

Step four then requires that you begin the tapping sequence. The tapping sequence is seven acupuncture points located on the face and body. As you tap each spot approximately seven times with moderate pressure you repeat a reminder phrase (i.e., "This _____") once at each point. In Bill's case he used the reminder phrase "This numbness." Bill was instructed to use his index and middle finger together as his tapping device and was instructed that since the points were bilateral he could tap on either side of the body. Furthermore, Bill was relieved when I told him that he did not have to do the tapping precisely. EFT has proven to be successful even when tapping in close approximation to the acuppuncture points (see Appendix).

The acupuncture tapping points are as follows:

1. Eyebrow: This point is at the inside edge of the eyebrow, above the inside corner of the eye.
2. Side of the eye: This point is on the temple, the point next to the outside of the eye.
3. Under the eye: This point is located just below the middle of the eye near the edge of the bone.
4. Under the nose: This point is the indention just below the nose and the middle of the upper lip.
5. Chin: This point is on the middle of the chin just below the crease.
6. Collarbone: This point is next to the U-shaped indention below the neck at the edge and just under the collarbone.
7. Under the arm: This point is on the side of your chest approximately four inches below your armpit.

The fifth step is one of evaluation. At the end of the tapping sequence the client takes a deep breath and allows time for the energy to settle. The client is asked to then focus on the disturbing feeling or issue that was to be cleared and asked for another measure of intensity (SUD). The SUD level is compared to the original measure and a determination is made as to whether the feeling or issue has been cleared. If there continues to be emotional intensity then repeat the sequence to clear the remaining intensity.

Bill reported that he felt some tingling and heat in his body. Bill was asked to evaluate the numbness and to notice if there was a shift in emotion or issue. Bill remarked that he continued to feel numbness and gave himself a SUD level of six. He felt motivated that there had been some movement and proceeded with the second round of EFT. In this case of partial relief we continued with the feeling of numbness. We slightly changed the reminder phrase to "This *remaining* numbness" to distinguish this round from what had been previously cleared. Bill worked the round tapping intently and repeating his reminder phrase. He reported a shift in the second round and stated that he was feeling a profound sense of loss. We began to process the feeling of loss however Bill appeared disconnected from the experience. Bill indicated that he wanted to continue but felt the experience of loss was to enormous. I realized that talking about it was futile. With little discussion Bill agreed to another EFT sequence. Bill gave the feeling of loss a SUD level of ten. He began the process of rubbing his Sore Spot in a circular fashion and repeating his new affirmation "Even though I have this loss, I deeply and completely accept myself" three times. Bill barely completed the tapping sequence when the feeling of loss manifested in an emotional yet welcomed manner. Bill reported that he wanted and needed a release of all that was blocked in his life. Bill wept, cursed, howled and continued to process all that had transpired the past few years. When any type of dissociation would occur Bill would automatically begin the EFT sequence and process to release the block in order to transform the pattern.

EFT was a therapeutic technique that Bill felt he was in charge of. He could quickly discern an issue or feeling that needed attention and could respond accordingly. EFT helped Bill break up into smaller pieces what often felt like an insurmountable or overwhelming experience. For example, Bill was concerned that people would "pity" him. He instantly would be overcome with anger and rage and had on occasion accosted friends when he perceived a pity response from them. In therapy sessions Bill could begin to break down the anger and rage using EFT in order to get to the underlying feelings and issues. The EFT process helped increase resilience and flexibility for Bill by reducing the potency of outdated messages about his self, the old expectations and ideals, and the safety to re-explore the world.

Bill continued in therapy using a combination of talk therapy and EFT. He likened EFT to a "blocking back" that helped to reduce some of the stumbling blocks that deterred him from true acceptance of who he is while adapting to the world. Bill worked and "tapped" his way to integration and wholeness. Bill progressively worked his way back into the world, relationships, and an expanded view of himself.

CONCLUSION

In this chapter we have examined and outlined an alternative therapy technique that focuses on releasing stuck emotions that can prevent the ability to move forward in life. The success of EFT lies in the simplicity and power to clear emotional blockages from the meridian and energy body of the individual. In the case of grief and loss for athletes EFT can help to assuage troubling emotions allowing space to work on the ultimate goal of adapting to change and the acceptance of self. In the case of Bill, the pain was buried so deep that he was incapacitated. EFT helped Bill to create a space for the feelings to surface, the ability to transform them, and increased insight to integrate the experience.

REFERENCES

Blinde, E. M., & Strata, T. M. (1992). The "sport career death" of college athletes: Involuntary and unanticipated sport exits. *Journal of Sport Behavior, 15*, 3-20.

Bruce, E. J., & Schultz, C. L. (2001). *Nonfinite loss and grief: A psychoeducational approach*. Baltimore, MD: Brookes Publishing.

Chartrand, J., & Lent, R. (1987). Sport counseling: Enhancing the development of the student-athlete. *Journal of Counseling and Development, 66*, 164-167.

Coleman, J. S. (1961). *The adolescent society: The social life of the teenager and its impact on education*. NY: Free Press.

Craig, G. (2006). *Thriving now: Transforming pain into optimal health*. Retrieved from http://www.thrivingnow.com/for/Health/gary-craig/ on February 7, 2006.

Danish, S., Petitpas, A., & Hale, B. (1993). Life development interventions for athletes. *The Counseling Psychologist, 21*, 352-358.

Denson, E. L. (1994). Developing a freshman seminar for student-athletes. *Journal of College Student Development, 35*, 303-304.

Frauenknecht, M., & Brylinsky, J. (1996). The relationship between social problem-solving and high risk health behaviors among collegiate athletes. *Journal of Health Education, 27*, 217-227.

Goldberg, A. D. (1991). Counseling the high school student-athlete. *The School Counselor, 38*, 332-340.

Gordon, S., Milios, D., & Grove, J. (1991). Psychological aspects of the recovery process of sport injury: The perspective of sport physiotherapists. *Australian Journal of Science and Medicine in Sport, 23*, 53-60.

Greendorfer, S. L., & Blinde, E. M. (1985). Retirement from intercollegiate sports: Theoretical and empirical considerations. *Sociology of Sport Journal, 2*, 101-110.

Haerle, R. K. (1975). Career patterns and career contingencies of professional baseball players: An occupational analysis. In D. Ball & J. Loy (Eds.), *Sport and social order* (pp. 461-519). Reading, MA: Addison-Wesley.

Hardy, C. J., & Crace, R. K. (1990). Dealing with injury. *Sport Psychology Training Bulletin, 1,* 1-8.

Jordan, J., & Denson, E. (1990). Student services for athletes: A model for enhancing the student-athlete experience. *Journal of Counseling and Development, 69,* 95-97.

Klieber, D. A., & Brock, S. C. (1992). The effect of career ending injuries on the subsequent well being of elite college athletes. *Sociology of Sport Journal, 9,* 70-75.

Kolt, G. S. (2000). Doing sport psychology with injured athletes. In M. Anderson (Ed.), *Doing sport psychology* (pp. 223-236). Champaign, IL: Human Kinetics.

Lerch, S. H. (1981). The adjustment of retirement of professional baseball players. In S. L. Greendorfer & A. Yiannakis (Eds.), *Sociology of sport perspectives* (pp. 138-148). West Point, NY: Leisure Press.

Look, C. (2005). *Abundance with EFT: Emotional Freedom Techniques.* California: Authorhouse.

Mariss, P. (1986). *Loss and change.* London: Routledge & Kegan Paul.

Mountrose, P., & Mountrose, J. (2000). *Getting thru to your emotions with EFT.* Sacramento, CA: Holistic Communications.

Murphy, G. M., Petitpas, A. J., & Brewer, B. W. (1996). Identity foreclosure, athletic identity, and career maturity in intercollegiate athletics. *Sport Psychologist, 10,* 239-246.

Parham, W. D. (1993). The intercollegiate athlete: A 1900s profile. *Counseling Psychologist, 21,* 411-429.

Parkes, C. M. (1971). Psychosocial transitions: A field for study. *Social Science and Medicine, 5,* 101-115.

Pearson, R., & Jones, G. (1992). Emotional effects of sport injuries: Implications for physiotherapists. *Physiotherapy, 78,* 762-770.

Pearson, R., & Petitpas, A. (1990). Transitions of athletes: Pitfalls and prevention. *Journal of Counseling and Development, 69,* 7-10.

Svoboda, B., & Vanek, M. (1982). Retirement from high level competition. In T. Orlick, J. T. Parrington, & J. H. Salmela (Eds.), *Procedures in Fifth World Congress of Sport Psychology* (pp. 166-175). Ottawa, Canada: Coaching Association of Canada.

Wooten, H. R. (1994). Cutting losses for student-athletes in transition: An integrative transition model. *Journal of Employment Counseling, 31,* 2-10.

Wooten, H. R., & Hinkle, J. S. (1992). Career life planning with college student-athletes. *TCA Journal, 20,* 41-46.

doi:10.1300/J456v01n03_06

APPENDIX

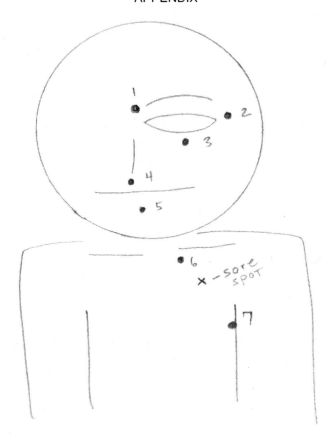

Printed with permission.

Chapter 7

A Novel Approach:
Using Literary Writing
and Creative Interventions
for Working Toward Forgiveness
After Relationship Dissolution and Divorce

Albert A. Valadez
Marcheta Evans

SUMMARY. The relationship between empathy and forgiveness is explored through the painful experience of divorce and relationship loss. Authors propose a literary exercise, the Novel Approach, to help clients discover the power of empathy and find resolution to past pains. Included is a case study used to describe the Novel Approach and to highlight its facilitative power for creating a deeper empathic understanding. doi:10.1300/J456v01n03_07 *[Article copies available for a fee from The Haworth Document Delivery Service: 1-800-HAWORTH. E-mail address: <docdelivery@haworthpress.com> Website: <http://www.HaworthPress.com> © 2005 by The Haworth Press, Inc. All rights reserved.]*

Albert A. Valadez and Marcheta Evans are afflilated with the University of Texas at San Antonio.
Address correspondence to: Albert A. Valadez, PhD, University of Texas at San Antonio, 501 West Durango Boulevard, San Antonio, TX 78207.

[Haworth co-indexing entry note]: "A Novel Approach: Using Literary Writing and Creative Interventions for Working Toward Forgiveness After Relationship Dissolution and Divorce." Valadez, Albert A., and Marcheta Evans. Co-published simultaneously in *Journal of Creativity in Mental Health* (The Haworth Press, Inc.) Vol. 1, No. 3/4, 2005, pp. 103-121; and: *Creative Interventions in Grief and Loss Therapy: When the Music Stops, a Dream Dies* (ed: Thelma Duffey) The Haworth Press, Inc., 2005, pp. 103-121. Single or multiple copies of this article are available for a fee from The Haworth Document Delivery Service [1-800-HAWORTH, 9:00 a.m. - 5:00 p.m. (EST). E-mail address: docdelivery@haworthpress.com].

Available online at http://jcmh.haworthpress.com
doi:10.1300/J456v01n03_07

KEYWORDS. Divorce, creativity, counseling, literary exercise, empathy, forgiveness

> And so she woke up
> Woke up from where she was lying still
> Said I got to do something
> About where we're going

(U2, 1990)

Most of us marry with the dream of sharing our lifetimes with the partners who pledge to spend the rest of their days co-creating life with us. We, in turn, also pledge to love, support, and share the joys, sorrows, challenges and triumphs that life brings with them. Few of us marry with expectations that this dream will end. Still, our dreams are shattered when either we or our spouses decide to abort the dream. Making a decision to divorce or end a meaningful relationship can shake our very foundation and create surreal feelings of loss, emptiness, confusion, and abandonment. Recovering from these lost dreams becomes a challenge.

Indeed, divorce, or the loss of a significant relationship, aside from the death of a loved one, is among the most traumatic interpersonal losses that we can experience. Conservative estimates show the divorce rate in the United States to be at almost fifty percent (Rodgers & Rose, 2002). Consequently, more and more children are finding themselves in single parent or blended family households (Jones, 2003).

The ending of a relationship and the divorce within a family carry with them many issues. Partners may feel rejected, unwanted, humiliated, and duped, at the same time that they may experience feelings of longing, despair, hope, and fear (Ellison, 2002). People who initiate the ending of a relationship may feel very different feelings from their partners and may be more prepared for the loss than their counterparts, who may have been caught off guard by what they perceive to be a unilateral decision to end the relationship. In other cases, couples collaboratively reach the decision to terminate a relationship or divorce. Regardless of the circumstances, managing the diverse feelings that divorce and lost relationships create is a challenge and becomes a critical issue in the success of future relational and emotional development.

Social norms associated with the dissolution of a relationship or divorce further complicate matters. Although divorces are as commonly experienced as life-long intact marriages, negative social stigmas continue to exist. Clients often report immense pressures from family members to maintain their marriages and are challenged by religious expectations. Terminating what had been anticipated as a life-long commitment can cause enormous emotional and relational consequences. In addition, individuals experience upheaval with respect to their home, credit, and health care, contributing to what can seem like an endless sea of insecurity (Richardson & McCabe, 2001).

DISENFRANCHISED LOSS
AND RELATIONSHIP DISSOLUTION

Although this manuscript addresses the needs of divorcing couples and families, it is important to also address the needs of people involved in long term relationships who never marry because their partnerships are not socially or legally sanctioned (Doka, 1989; Glaser & Borduin, 1986). They, too, suffer experiences not unlike those of divorcing couples when their relationships end. However, in addition to the issues that many divorcing couples face, they also face issues that disenfranchised losses can bring (Doka, 1989; Kamerman, 1993).

For example, couples in gay and lesbian relationships undergo experiences of disenfranchised grief when their committed relationship ends (Doka, 1987, 1989; Kamerman, 1993). In one example, Carol and Elizabeth had been partners for over 10 years. During that time, they invested in numerous ways into each other's lives. They were supportive of each other and saw each other through many difficult life circumstances. They also enjoyed each other in innumerable ways. As a result, it was shocking for Carol when Elizabeth chose to leave the relationship. And given that their relationship was not legally sanctioned, Carol was left to recover without benefit of the rituals commonly afforded to legally married couples. This loss triggered feelings about other losses, including her unrequited desire to bear children. With her childbearing years beyond her and without a loving life partner, she felt even more isolated, marginalized, and alone. For Carol, the dissolution of her partnership was every bit as powerful as a divorce. And given the disenfranchised nature of her loss, she suffered unique issues in the process.

Other couples in untraditional, long-term relationships outside of marriage also suffer losses akin to the divorce experience. Their losses, too, can be experienced as disenfranchised (Deck & Folta, 1989; Doka, 1989). For example, Tess and Randy sustained a long-term relationship that lasted 15 years. Although their relationship was unconventional, in that both Tess and Randy maintained their own homes and lead independent lives, the relationship was loving and exclusive. When they were not able to negotiate their differences, it became easy for Tess to leave the relationship, leaving Randy devastated. Because the relationship was not legally recognized, the ending was abrupt and without ritual. Randy was left to question what he had done with the last 15 years of his life. There was no formalized context to dignify his experience or his loss. With a sense of isolation and surrealism, Randy was forced to come to terms with his unrealized dream.

Indeed, when relationships outside of legally sanctioned marriages dissolve, they carry unique forms of pain. Like divorce, the dissolution of these relationships results in suffering; and because of the disenfranchised nature of the loss, it can exacerbate feelings of confusion, loneliness, and acute sorrow. These feelings are frequently experienced by the children of parents whose relationships are disrupted. However, the loss that children experience can be overlooked in these circumstances. When children live with parents who are cohabiting with partners and not married, their loss, too, can be disenfranchised (Doka, 1987). Children may be forced to sever relationships with people who have carried significant roles in their lives but who hold no legal connection to them. This form of loss can impact children profoundly at the same time that it remains socially and legally ambiguous.

THE IMPACT OF DIVORCE ON CHILDREN

Children can be hurt whenever there is dissolution to a family system. The literature describes how threats to security, self-blame, and general anxiety about the future are common themes described by children of divorce (Richardson & McCabe, 2001). Some children feel responsible for the divorce or experience guilt over feelings they carry about one or both of their parents. They may feel a need to take care of their parents' emotional needs and leave their own needs aside. Other times, children act out their feelings and experience difficulties in school or at home (Wood, Repetti, & Roesch, 2004).

In addition, children often assume spoken or unspoken roles within the family system. As a result, the experience of divorce has an impact on the current roles they carry. For example, in many cases, the oldest child in the family assumes a role of responsibility within the family and may be called upon to assist in the care of younger siblings (Thompson & Rudolph, 2000). In addition, the oldest child may develop a peer relationship with a parent and lose the developmental place children hold within the family. Youngest children, on the other hand, run the risk of remaining childlike far beyond what is developmentally appropriate for them (Thompson & Rudolph, 2000). For this reason, younger children may not have an opportunity to put to words their thoughts or feelings about the dissolution of the family. In contrast, the second-born or middle child may feel left out of the family (Thompson & Rudolph, 2000).

Difficulties generated by a divorce can exacerbate these experiences for children. In some cases, children fill the role of partner to one or both parents by meeting their emotional needs (Thompson & Rudolph, 2000). In addition, children run the risk of becoming the messenger between one parent and the other, and in some cases, are quizzed on the actions of one parent or the other, creating feelings of discomfort and disloyalty.

Children must also adjust to changes such as a new family structure, and in some cases, relocation, socioeconomic shifts, and new friends (Thompson & Rudolph, 2000). In addition, many divorcing parents are absorbed in their own feelings of animosity and anger that they lose sight of the need to establish an amicable and nurturing co-parenting relationship. When parents are unsuccessful at establishing the foundations for co-parenting, the child's self-concept and sense of well being are greatly compromised (Richardson & McCabe, 2001).

POWER AND CULTURE

Another consideration that families undergoing divorce face is the shift in power that can come during a divorce process. In most instances, family members hold varying degrees of power within their family system. The power can shift when crises such as divorce occur. Given that, it is important to consider how each member of the family assumes power during the course of divorce. For example, children who serve as confidantes to one or both parents may feel power that is beyond their developmental capacity to manage. On the other hand, other children go unnoticed during a divorce and experience very little power within the family. Additionally, parents negotiate power as they consider issues of finances, possessions, and child custody.

In addition to issues of power, therapists working with families undergoing divorce must consider the cultural influences that families face. Certainly, understanding the perception of divorce for families from various cultures is an important therapeutic consideration. Hall (1977) described members of high-context cultures as people who emphasize the collective while those from low-context orientations tend to value individualism and autonomy.

Because members of a family from high-context cultures emphasize a collective order, divorcing family members may feel pressure to avoid what can be seen as a collective failure. In addition, clients from high-context cultures may be influenced by their extended family members with respect to their divorce issues and run the risk of having therapists pathologize their experiences as dependencies. No doubt, undergoing divorce is a significant stressor for most individuals and understanding the role that culture plays in the experience is an important therapeutic need.

DIVORCE WITHIN THE BLENDED FAMILY

Families that experience divorce where one or both partners have had previous marriages also suffer unique losses. These losses potentially include relational challenges with step-children and other members of the extended family. In these cases, what had appeared to be a new dream for a stable life is, again, shattered. Divorce impacts all members of a blended family. The degree of impact is influenced by a number of issues, including the quality of the relationships within the blended family, the shared connections, relocation issues, and financial considerations.

For example, Maggie was married for 25 years and helped raise her husband's four children. Her husband, Jack, was the custodial parent, and together they cared for the children since adolescence. When Maggie and Jack later divorced, their children were grown with families of their own. The children from Jack's first marriage faced another loss involving a mother figure and expressed their ambivalence and anger toward Maggie. It appears they felt forced to make a choice between the two parents, like children often do. The children felt a need to support their biological parent, Jack, while continuing to love and care for their step-mother.

This dynamic created tension, particularly during holidays and family celebrations. This tension became particularly painful for Maggie, as she felt isolated and disenfranchised. She felt completely disposable, which was in stark contrast to the central role she had long assumed in their lives. Maggie and Jack's biological children also felt the tension and carried the burden of negotiating loyalties, while also trying to protect each parent. Jack, too, suffered unique feelings of grief and failure because of his previous divorce and the impact this new experience would have on his children. Divorce, in this family, brought with it losses on a number of levels along many fronts. Certainly, in a time where partners re-marry and create new blended families, unique issues arise when these families are disrupted by divorce.

A CONCEPTUALIZATION OF THE DIVORCE PROCESS

As counselors work with divorcing couples, it is important for them to understand how the divorce process unfolds. Kressel (1997) proposes that divorcing families undergo four stages. In the first stage, the *pre-decision period*, partners become dissatisfied with the relationship and find themselves arguing or withdrawing from one another. During this stage, some couples realize that the relationship is in jeopardy and may take constructive steps to save the marriage. If they are not able to productively negotiate their needs together, they reach the second stage, or the *decision period*, where the couple decides what the immediate future for the family will look like. Generally, they consider decisions about whether to end the relationship or whether to seek outside assistance. If outside assistance is chosen, they enter the *negotiation period* and the partners seek the help of a therapist. Alternatively, when couples decide to terminate the marriage, the negotiation stage can include mediation or legal counsel to negotiate property division and co-parenting arrangements. A period of *reconciliation* is the next stage in the process. This stage can be marked with feelings of guilt, anger, and loneliness (Kressel, 1997). These feelings can be so intense that clients find it difficult to "move on" and enter into other trusting relationships. This manuscript will address some means by which we reconcile or process these residual feelings and experiences.

No doubt, the experience of divorce can have far-reaching relational and psychological implications for all members of a family. Divorce is a disconnecting experience; and as a result, can lead us into a deeper sense of shame and isolation (see Jordan, 2001). In addition, divorce can be seen as a psychological dragnet that is thrown over our pasts, bringing to the surface other previously unresolved losses. These losses can generate feelings of failure, anger, guilt, betrayal, disappointment, and embarrassment. As a result, some divorcing couples find it difficult to process their own feelings, to find context for the experiences of their former spouses, and to create new growth-fostering experiences (see Jordan, 2001).

Having context for how another person may feel is a relationally based quality. Indeed, it is a skill taught in many counselor education and mental health programs. For example, Carl Rogers (1959) described core conditions necessary for therapeutic change which are commonly taught in clinical programs. These skills include experiences of empathy, congruence, genuineness, positive regard, and psychological presence (Miller, 1989; Rogers, 1959). Although these qualities are generally considered valuable in the context of the client-therapist relationship, we contend that they are also necessary for success in personal relationships. A premise of this manuscript is that just as we teach students to apply these principles in counseling practice, we can also facilitate empathy development with clients undergoing painful divorce. One goal of this manuscript is to illustrate how relationships are strengthened when we are connected with our empathic potentials. These potentials are experienced in the client/counselor relationship and creatively addressed through The Novel Approach, an intervention designed to help individuals undergoing relationship loss or divorce experience increased empathy towards themselves and toward their former partners.

JOURNAL WRITING AND THE NOVEL APPROACH:
WORKING TOWARD FORGIVENESS

The healing properties of journal writing are well documented in the literature (Brouwers, 1994; Caldwell, 2005; Riordan, 1996). The Novel Approach, which is predicated on narrative therapy (Payne, 2006; White & Epston, 1990), is a teaching tool that uses journaling and literary writing to facilitate a process of reconciliation and forgiveness by helping clients to develop empathic responses to their situations. However, distinctions between journal writing and The Novel Approach exist. For example, while journal writing encourages writers to express and document their feelings regarding the day or a given problem, the Novel Approach encourages them to write from the perspective of other characters in their story, as well as their own. The purpose of this work is to assist clients to forge through their path toward forgiveness.

Counselors and theologians alike have long appreciated the healing qualities of forgiveness (Konstam et al., 2000). However, empirical studies on the efficacy of forgiveness as a therapeutic intervention are scarce (Butler, Dahlin, & Fife, 2002). Some argue that counselors underutilize forgiveness as a therapeutic intervention because clients associate the act of forgiveness with pardoning painful grievances, reconciling with offenders and condoning offenses (Butler et al., 2002). Indeed, a common concern reported in the forgiveness literature is that people who have been hurt or violated fear the need to condone the act perpetrated against them (Enright & the Human Development Group, 1999). Others have found that while empathy-based interventions resulted in increased communication among troubled couples, forgiveness was not found to be a significant by-product when compared to hope-based intervention programs (Ripley & Worthington, 2002).

The confusion surrounding forgiveness may be found in the diversity of its definitions (Konstam et al., 2000) since operationalizing the process of forgiveness can be difficult. For purposes of this article, forgiveness will be defined by the authors as an intrapersonal process whereby we examine past pain through an empathic lens. As a result, we emerge from the experience with a keen awareness of contributing contextual factors. The goal of this process is to transcend pain and achieve a greater understanding of the experience and a deepened sense of peace.

Forgiveness models vary in process. Some models require clients to engage in an intense information-gathering quest that requires them to process *the hurt*. Hargrave (1994) emphasizes the process of reconciliation with the offender so the client can relearn how to trust others and themselves. For example, one of Hargrave's stages includes understanding; specifically, the understanding of limitations and weaknesses of the offender, so that clients can begin to relate to their fallible nature (Murray, 2002). Overall, the literature indicates that in having a clear rationale for forgiveness, therapists familiar with forgiveness models facilitate client receptivity (Butler et al., 2002).

While laypersons and counselors suggest that embarking on the path to forgiveness has potential to create emotional healing, the commitment and energy needed to invest in the process can prove too cumbersome and painful for many people to undergo (Simon & Simon, 1990). In many cases, forgiveness, then, remains elusive as we maintain feelings of resentment, anger, and frustration over painful situations as a natural default. As a result, when we peel back the bandage we often refer to as time, we expose a wound that comes in the guise of unresolved pain. This becomes problematic when our anger and disappointment find their way into our current relationships.

After experiencing a painful relationship loss or divorce, even with the passage of time, clients experience mistrust. How many of us, following painful separations and divorces, fear future hurt and disappointment? Many push away the potential for great love to avoid what is believed to be the ultimate and inevitable disappointment from infidelity or abandonment (Ellison, 2002). This atmosphere of suspicion and cynicism creates a context for clients to experience new relationships, even those with great potential, with guardedness, distance, and a lack of intimacy. No doubt, the consequences of unresolved pain following divorce or other relational injuries can be exhaustive. The challenge for many clients in these authors' experiences has been to balance the "hard knock" lessons gained from past failed relationships with openness for authentic connection and intimacy with new partners.

To heal from past pains, contemporary counseling encourages individuals to forgive people who are perceived wrongdoers. "Forgive and forget," "bury the hatchet," and "live and let live" are common phrases we encounter (Simon & Simon, 1990). Taking this step toward forgiveness is difficult. Sometimes, it is as difficult for us to forgive ourselves for our perceived transgressions as it is for us to forgive a person who we feel has hurt us. At the same time, we know that by harboring resentments, we keep ourselves from fulfilling our full emotional potential. As a result, the issue of forgiveness remains as alive as it can be elusive.

We believe that forgiveness is an affective transformative process that includes the cognitive component of insight coupled with an empathic compassion for self and the people we with whom we have shared our lives. This process is one of many challenges faced by couples recovering from relationship loss or divorce. The Novel Approach is one of several creative ways in which the relationally empathic understanding of self and others can be achieved. This intervention involves identifying a contextual event in which pain occurs, creating a cast of key characters, and assigning each character his/her own chapter with a title and first person accounting that captures the experience.

THE NOVEL APPROACH

The Novel approach is a technique used to help people transform painful experiences into opportunities for deepened understanding and connection. It is based on the premise that while we are involved in a painful situation, it is difficult for us to connect with our own pain and the pain of others in an authentic manner. By working with interventions that allow us to gain perspective into the experience of others, we develop the capacity for empathy and have an opportunity to move out of emotionally disconnected positions to more flexible ones. In doing so, we are able to achieve greater appreciation for our pain, courage, strength, and resolve, in addition to the challenges and experiences of others. Using Linda as an example, we illustrate how The Novel Approach can be used to facilitate forgiveness through empathy in a divorce situation.

Linda is a 47-year-old African-American woman and mother of three girls. She expressed having a strong religious background and strong commitment to higher education and family. She presented for therapy because she was struggling with issues surrounding the divorce she initiated several years ago. Although Linda appears to thrive and has achieved many successes, she carries with her feelings of pain, confusion, and regret regarding her part in the divorce experience. One of Linda's greatest challenges seems to be reconciling her moral and spiritual beliefs with the actions that preceded her divorce and her choice to leave her husband and begin a new life.

Many people who choose to divorce experience a range of feelings, including guilt, remorse, defensiveness, fear, and relief (Ellison, 2002). Linda was no exception. She described feelings of guilt and frustration after her first marriage ended. She also discussed how her first marriage was devoid of conflict and how she found her ex-husband, Brandon, to be an "easy going" person who was not willing to address differences in the relationship. According to Linda, Brandon rarely expressed affect and seemed oblivious to Linda's dissatisfaction.

Linda's thirteen-year marriage ended after she engaged in an extramarital affair with her former high school boyfriend, Stewart. Stewart and Linda rekindled a relationship that had ended precipitously, when Janet, Linda's mother, moved the family to another state. Ironically, Janet initiated the idea of reconciliation between Linda and Stewart. She thought that if they were to see each other, Linda could come to terms with the loss and invest in her marriage.

Linda's Experience

There are many reasons given by people who choose to divorce. There are times when people end relationships because they do not feel like they matter to their partners or because they do not feel heard or represented in the relationship. Other times, people leave relationships because they never emotionally invested in the relationship or because they were developmentally unprepared for the experience. Sometimes, people divorce because they feel their partners exert too much control and they become lost in the relationship. Their hopes and dreams are disconnected from their own needs, and instead, revolve around their partner's needs, wants, and desires. Whatever the case, the experience of divorce brings pain, confusion, and the need for reconciliation of the experience.

In Linda's case, she described the anger and guilt feelings she experienced toward herself and her ex-husband, Brandon. She felt especially angry because she did not perceive him to be an active participant in the marriage. Although she experienced him to be a "good person to her and to the children," she described him as disconnected from her and emotionally absent. As her feelings of loneliness deepened, her experience of isolation and disconnection in the relationship grew. With them came feelings of resentment and dissatisfaction she did not know how to manage. When a man she had perceived to be "the true love of her life" reentered the picture, she agreed to meet him. This reconnection impacted her marriage and family life, and Linda's choice to leave the marriage became clear.

Although theory would posit that her unresolved feelings toward the ending of her aborted relationship with Stewart influenced her perception of Brandon and her investment in that relationship, Linda's therapeutic work ultimately revolved around two distinct needs. These included helping her connect with her authentic experience following the dissolution of the marriage and coming to terms with feelings toward herself and Brandon. For Linda, this involved undergoing a process of forgiveness.

Linda, however, did not feel she deserved to forgive herself for the pain she caused her family and saw her own pain and lack of forgiveness as a penance she must bear. Further, Linda felt unworthy of experiencing happiness and perceived herself to be a disappointment to God. Clearly, she felt like a source of hurt for her ex-husband, children, and family. Although Linda knew that forgiving herself and others is vital to her well-being, she was unaware of how to accomplish this task. Because Linda enjoyed writing and was committed to working through her pain, she was eager to start the process.

THE PROCESS

Linda agreed to participate in an exercise that is a variation of a genogram. To begin the exercise, she laid out a large 3' × 3' piece of butcher paper. She entitled the exercise *The Divorce*. At the center of the paper, she drew a circle with her name in the middle. She then drew other circles representing the various people who were involved in her story. These included Brandon, her ex-husband; Stewart, Linda's high school sweetheart; Janet, Linda's mother; Mary, Linda and Brandon's oldest daughter; Maricela, their middle daughter; and JoAnn, Linda's youngest sister. Linda then drew three lines on the left and right side of each circle and wrote positive (left side) and negative (right side) personality characteristics of each person in the novel.

Linda described herself as a driven, hard-working, and loyal person, on the one hand. On the other hand, she perceived herself as an emotional martyr, uncompromising, and easily angered. She then drew a line from her circle to each of the characters to illustrate a connection. She also wrote a sentence that described the relationship on each connecting line. For example, on the line that extended from Brandon to her, she described the relationship as, "Good, but emotionally unfulfilling." She drew a counter line from character to character, describing the relationship from what she perceived the other person's perspective of the relationship to be.

In succeeding sessions, Linda outlined her chapters and assigned titles to the chapters. She considered her rationale for structuring the book as she did and wrote rather than typed her chapters. Perhaps the greatest challenge for Linda came in writing each chapter in the first person, as if she were the character telling the story. The following outlines the chapters of her novel.

A Novel: The Divorce

In processing excerpts from the chapters, she discovered the projective qualities of the exercise. There were words she wished her mother and other characters could say to her.
From *Brandon's* perspective, she wrote:

> I love this woman so much. I don't understand how this happened. Sure there are times I felt frustrated—what man doesn't in a marriage? I put my faith in God and tried my best to be a model for my family. I did everything she asked—perhaps I did too much. But nonetheless, I didn't share my feelings because I wanted harmony. I did it for her and for the children. I will ask the Lord to help me be strong. I'm angry but it might just be too late. I know the people at the church will be disappointed. I don't know what I could have done differently.

And from Janet's perspective, she added:

> When I called Linda and encouraged her to contact Stewart, I honestly thought she would just close that chapter of her life and that the contact would help her move on with her marriage to Brandon. My track record with men has not been great. I was in a marriage because I felt it was what society thought was the right thing to do and I did not want to raise a child alone. I ended up not taking care of the child anyway and was still unhappy. Perhaps my greatest gift to Linda was an unintentional one—perhaps I inadvertently gave her a chance at the happiness I never had—the happiness I was not able to give her as a mom. I want you to know Linda, if I had known how to give you the gifts you deserved, I would have.

One of Linda's greatest struggles came when she wrote the chapter entitled, "Don't Disappoint Me, Linda." This chapter spoke from the perspective of JoAnn, her youngest sister. JoAnn was fourteen years younger than Linda and looked to her as a mother figure. In fact, she had lived with Brandon and Linda for several years. Linda expressed anger toward her because she had aligned with Brandon. JoAnn even encouraged him to report to the court that the marriage ended because of infidelity rather than the agreed upon reason of "irreconcilable differences." Linda believed that JoAnn's attempt was to shame her into changing her mind. She imagined JoAnn to say:

> Linda simply does not understand me. Mom never showed love to me or any of my sisters. Linda is the only person who cared and I think she is making the biggest mistake of her life. She has the perfect marriage with the perfect man. Church, children and a house– they have everything. If Linda doesn't stay in this marriage, how will any of us ever have faith in love? You are the only stable person in my life. If you go down this road you are going to end up like mom and will likely go to hell. You have to stay together because I'm so scared.

Linda realized how immersed she had been in her own pain and how she forgot about JoAnn's pain. Their mother, Janet, had married and divorced five times. When Linda wrote the words "I'm so scared" to describe JoAnn's experience, she realized that JoAnn was terrified of losing the only reliable and consistent parental figure she had in her life.

In reflecting on her role as parent and discussing the impact of her divorce on her own children, Linda described how Mary, the oldest child, held the most power in the family during the time of the divorce; and was quick to clarify that Mary's power came from her awareness of the details of the problems. Linda felt guilty for disrupting the stability of her daughter's life as she entered her teen years. Linda's perspective on Mary's experience as a 12-year-old follows:

> Hello, my name is Mary and this is MY story. I love my mom and dad. They are the world to me. I can't even imagine them not living in the same house. Sometimes at night I stare at the moon and pray to God to help me find a way to keep them together. One day God sent me a message to put family pictures of us being happy all around the house so that my mom could see them. It did not work. It is easier to talk to God than my mom because I know he loves me. I wonder if mom loves me. I am scared about what me and my sisters are going to do–where we are going to live. Right now I know I have to take care of my sisters and make sure they are o.k.

She discovered parallels between JoAnn's story and Mary's character and saw how they both wanted to preserve the marriage for similar reasons. Linda also saw how Mary had adopted the same role with her sisters that Linda had adopted with JoAnn. Relating to this pressure and responsibility, she discussed the experience of the divorce with Mary, and asked her forgiveness.

REFLECTIONS ON THE PROCESS

Reflecting on this case provides us with an appreciation for how difficult it can be to achieve empathy in painful situations. In Linda's case, the more intensity and resentment she felt toward the characters, the harder it seemed for her to empathize with their experiences. Her anger could be seen in passages that excused her behavior and defended her decisions. Linda also discovered that she failed to have empathy for herself. As a result, she felt shame; and in her shame, avoided responsibility. Having this awareness gave her an opportunity to become more accountable and to generate an even deeper empathic experience. Linda's own excerpt reflects this challenge:

> I have failed to mention one other person that needs to be forgiven in this process: Me. How do I forgive myself? How do I look at myself in the mirror and know I am going to be okay? I was supposed to be Ms. Perfect. I did all the right things: I got the good grades. I took care of my grandparents. I didn't have sex until I was married. I never used drugs or alcohol. I was active in the Church. I took care of the youth and the Seniors. I went as far as I possibly could in school. I lived in a beautiful home and had a wonderful husband and fantastic children. I played all kinds of sports and helped my daughters grow into the independent, loving people they are. Yet, after my divorce, I felt like a failure to everyone by my shallow standards. How could I have betrayed myself, my value system, my beliefs, my family, my God?

This intervention can elicit empathy for a number of reasons. First, it challenges the client to write, preferably in a free associative manner, in the first person of each character. Additionally, by engaging in an authentic experience with the counselor, clients are able to move past feelings of shame and isolation and enter into a place of deepened connection with self and others (see Jordan, 2001).

Like any creative intervention, A Novel Approach requires flexibility and spontaneity. Linda found that processing the chapters was, at times, more powerful than writing them. The text gave context for everyone involved. By becoming more self-aware and investing in her happiness and well being, she became more responsible and compassionate in her roles as wife, daughter, mother, and sister. And, by experiencing authenticity in her relationships, she was able to heal the feelings of shame that had haunted her. The reconciliation process is ongoing, one that requires her to commit more energy to developing empathy and deepened levels of forgiveness, as reflected in Linda's final excerpt:

> One of the main questions I ask myself is, "would you do it again knowing what you know now?" I honestly don't know. I know that I would do some things differently. I grieve the losses we have all experienced and I am aware of the many consequences that this decision created for me and for my family. I am also aware of my role in the pain that my loved ones carry. Reconciling my responsibility with my life choices has been a challenge. Ask me again when I am taking my last breath. I hope the answer will be "YES" . . . that in the end, when we look back, we will be able to say we were blessed through this tragedy. Perhaps we grew through some experiences that life may not have offered otherwise. That would be forgiveness.

CONCLUSION

Much like the characters that come alive in a good book, the characters created by clients evoke a moving experience. At times, I (first author) became emotionally caught up with some of the characters as I processed my own experiences of being a child from a divorced family. Although there is caution against the potential misuse of countertransferential feelings, an alternative frame would welcome the counselor's productive use of deepened empathy.

Losing a meaningful relationship characterizes the loss of a dream. The opening lyric of U2's *Running to Stand Still* (1990) speaks to this loss following the ending of a relationship: "And so she woke up, woke up where she was, lying still" and reminds us of how individuals, like Linda, awaken from the dream of spending the rest of their lives with their partners following the dissolution of a relationship. And, like

Linda, people seek therapy with an awareness that they "have to do something" to process their residual feelings of grief and loss. During these times, people experience feelings of rejection, hurt, guilt, and remorse. A Novel Approach is one of many creative means for facilitating the growth-fostering process involved in working through these feelings and gaining empathy and forgiveness following the death of their relational dream.

REFERENCES

Brouwers, M. (1994). Bulimia and the relationship with food: A letters-to-food technique. *Journal of Counseling and Development, 73*(2), 220-223.

Butler, M. H., Dahlin, S. K., & Fife, S. T. (2002). "Languaging" factors affecting clients' acceptance of forgiveness intervention in marital therapy. *Journal of Marital Therapy, 28*(3), 285-299.

Caldwell, R. L. (2005). Literature Review–Theory: At the confluence of memory and Meaning–Life review with older adults and families: Using narrative and the re-author stories of resilience. *Family Journal, 13*(2), 172-175.

Deck, E. S., & Folta, J. R. (1989). The Friend Griever. In K. J. Doka (Ed.) *Disenfranchised grief: Recognizing hidden sorrow* (pp. 77-89). Lexington, MA: Lexington, Books.

Doka, K. (1987). Silent Sorrow: Grief and the loss of a significant other. *Death Studies, 11*, 441-449.

Doka, K. (Ed.). (1989). *Disenfranchised grief: Recognizing hidden sorrow.* Lexington, MA: Lexington Books.

Ellison, S. (2002). *The courage to love again: Creating happy, healthy relationships after divorce.* New York: Harper Collins.

Enright, R. D., & The Human Development Study Group (1999). The moral development forgiveness. In W. Kurtines & J. Gewirtz (Eds.), *Handbook of moral behavior and development* (pp. 123-152). Hillsdale, NJ: Erlbaum.

Glaser, R. D., & Borduin, C. M. (1986). Models of divorce therapy: An overview. *American Journal of Psychotherapy, 40*(2), 233-243.

Hall, E. T. (1977). *Beyond Culture.* NY: Doubleday.

Hargrave, T. (1994). *Families and forgiveness: Healing wounds in the intergenerational Family.* New York, NY: Brunner/Mazel.

Jones, A. C. (2003). Reconstructing the stepfamily: Old myths, new stories. *Social Work, 48*(2), 228-237.

Jordan, J. (2001). A relational-cultural model: Healing through mutual empathy. *Bulletin of the Menninger Clinic, 65*(1), 92-103.

Konstam, V., Marx, F., Schurer, J., Harrington, A., Lombardo, N. E., & Deveney, S. (2000). Forgiving: What mental health counselors are telling us. *Journal of Mental Health Counseling, 22*(3), 253-268.

Kressel, K. (1997). *The process of divorce: How professionals and couples negotiate settlement.* Lanham, MD: Jason Aronson Inc.

Miller, M. J. (1989). A few thoughts on the relationship between counseling techniques and empathy. *Journal of Counseling and Development, 67*(6), 350.

Murray, R. J. (2002). The therapeutic use of forgiveness in healing intergenerational pain. *Counseling and Values, 46*(3), 188-199.

Payne, M. (2006). *Narrative Therapy.* Thousand Oaks, CA: Sage Publication.

Richardson, S., & McCabe, M. P. (2001). Parental divorce during adolescence and adjustment in early adulthood. *Adolescence, 36,* 467-490.

Riordan, R. (1996). Scriptotherapy: Therapeutic writing as a counseling adjunct *Journal of Counseling and Development, 74*(3), 263-270.

Ripley, J., & Worthington, J. (2002). Hope-focused and forgiveness-based group interventions to promote marital enrichment. *Journal of Counseling and Development, 80,* 452-464.

Rodgers, K. B., & Rose, H. A. (2002). Risk and resiliency factors among adolescents who experience marital transition. *Journal of Marriage and Family, 64,* 1024-1037.

Rogers, C. (1959). A theory of therapy, personality and interpersonal relationships as developed in the client-centered framework. In S. Koch (Ed.), *Psychology: The Study of a Science: Vol. III Formulations of the Person in the Social Context* (pp. 184-256). New York, NY: McGraw-Hill.

Thompson, C. L., & Rudolph, L. B. (2000). *Counseling Children* (5th ed.). Belmont, CA: Wadsworth.

Simon, S. B., & Simon, S. (1990). *Forgiveness: How to make peace with your past and and get on with your life.* New York, NY: Warner Books.

U2. (1990). Running to stand still. On *The Joshua Tree* [CD] New York, NY: Island.

White, M., & Epston, D. (1990). *Narrative means to therapeutic ends.* New York, NY: W.W. Norton & Company, Inc.

Wood, J., Repetti, R., & Roesch, S. C. (2004). Divorce and children's adjustment problems at home and school: The role of depressive/withdrawn parenting. *Child Psychiatry & Human Development, 35*(2), 121-142.

doi:10.1300/J456v01n03_07

Chapter 8

Soup, Stitches, and Song:
Helping Parents Grieve
When Their Adolescent Dies

Jane Bissler

SUMMARY. This article discusses ways that clinical practitioners can utilize creative strategies in working with clients who are experiencing grief following the death of their adolescent child. It presents a brief literature review regarding this specific type of parental grief as well as practical and helpful ways to utilize books, songs, and tangible projects in the grieving process. doi:10.1300/J456v01n03_08 *[Article copies available for a fee from The Haworth Document Delivery Service: 1-800-HAWORTH. E-mail address: <docdelivery@haworthpress.com> Website: <http://www.HaworthPress. com> © 2005 by The Haworth Press, Inc. All rights reserved.]*

Jane Bissler is a licensed professional clinical counselor and recognized as a Fellow in Thanatology by the Association of Death Educators and Counselors. She owns and is the clinical director of Counseling for Wellness, LLP. She is also an adjunct instructor at Kent State University.

Address correspondence to: Jane Bissler, Counseling for Wellness, LLP, 420 West Main Street, Kent, OH 44240 (E-mail: jbissler@counselingforwellness.com).

[Haworth co-indexing entry note]: "Soup, Stitches, and Song: Helping Parents Grieve When Their Adolescent Dies." Bissler, Jane. Co-published simultaneously in *Journal of Creativity in Mental Health* (The Haworth Press, Inc.) Vol. 1, No. 3/4, 2005, pp. 123-134; and: *Creative Interventions in Grief and Loss Therapy: When the Music Stops, a Dream Dies* (ed: Thelma Duffey) The Haworth Press, Inc., 2005, pp. 123-134. Single or multiple copies of this article are available for a fee from The Haworth Document Delivery Service [1-800-HAWORTH, 9:00 a.m. - 5:00 p.m. (EST). E-mail address: docdelivery@haworthpress.com].

Available online at http://jcmh.haworthpress.com
© 2005 by The Haworth Press, Inc. All rights reserved.
doi:10.1300/J456v01n03_08

KEYWORDS. Creativity, child/adolescent death, parental bereavement, grief counseling

> Your eyes have died
> But you see more than I
> Daniel you're a star
> In the face of the sky

(John, 1973)

I was ill-prepared for the sheer number of grieving parents of adolescents that presented for counseling when I began my practice. The traumatic and heart wrenching stories were not, however, the surprising part. Astonishingly, many parents said at least one other counselor told them that while the death of their child was a terrible tragedy, they must find closure and move on with their lives. When I consulted with other professionals, some reported finding this work to be unfulfilling as they felt helpless to make a difference. Being with another person's pain following the death of their dream is a challenge for counselors. It becomes a particular challenge when the loss involves the death of a child.

PARENTAL GRIEF

Billy was fifteen years old when he traveled over the Christmas holidays to visit Mark, his best friend since second grade. Mark had moved to another city earlier that summer, and Billy was adjusting to life without his constant companion. An only child, Billy was easy going, reserved and friendly. His parents were significantly older than many of the parents of his peers. The three shared a close bond and were working together to adjust to the growing autonomy that adolescence brings.

When Mark invited Billy to visit his new home during the holidays, Billy's parents initially hesitated. However, at seeing the excitement that the invitation brought Billy, and in knowing that Billy had seemed lonely since Mark's move, they agreed. They trusted Billy and cautioned him on safety measures. As he boarded the plane, they gave him their blessing.

Several days into the trip, Billy and Mark were driving in a car with one of Mark's new friends. The driver had been drinking and was driving recklessly. Reports indicate that Billy asked to be dropped off; he did not want to be in the car once he understood the circumstances. His pleas went unheeded. Minutes later, the car crashed into a tree. Although the driver and all passengers were injured, only one person was killed. Tragically, Billy did not survive the crash. Within hours his mother received the phone call that would change her life.

Although grief is defined as intense emotional suffering caused by loss (Webster's New World Dictionary of the American Language, 1988), Moules' (1998) perspective on grief is a more appropriate fit when describing parental grief for an adolescent. He sees grief as a life-changing experience that not only has elements of suffering and pain, but, one that carries a constant reminder of an ongoing relationship with the deceased.

We feel untold grief in the experience of losing a child we have known and cared for even before birth; a child we have loved and nurtured throughout their lives. As parents, we never believe that our children could or would die before us. Rando (1986) discusses how the special hardships faced by parents whose children die include the derailment of generativity strivings, the longest of Ericksonian stages. This stage defines what we have done to leave our mark by producing something that will outlive us in some way. Many of us leave our mark through parenthood.

Gamino, Sewell, and Easterling (2000) also report how the death of a child does not fit with the natural order of life. When parents lose their children, they lose their perceived sense of what the future will bring and their trust that life will continue as they have known it. They also join a minority of parents who have difficulties continuing with life in a meaningful way. Neugarten (1979) discusses that death, however catastrophic, is much more tragic when it happens off-time in the life cycle. Other authors (Budman & Gurman, 1988; Wortman & Silver, 1990) report that "dysynchrony" between when a developmental occurrence is anticipated and when it truly occurs creates difficulties with coping. Therefore, the death of an adolescent is seen as a death that "should not have happened." It causes a mystifying difficulty for the griever and reconciling such an arresting occurrence with beliefs in a reasonable, methodical world of predictable outcomes can become unmanageable. This type of grief can manifest in intrusive, distressing preoccupation; with experiences of yearning, longing, or searching (Jacobs, 1993; Jacobs & Prigerson, 2000; Rando, 1993; Worden, 1991).

The parental/child relationship is also discussed by Raphael and Middleton (1987). They discuss how the child becomes many things to parents, including a part of themselves and each other; descendents of their ancestors, and more. They also report that the loss of a child will always be agonizing, for it is in some ways a destruction of that part of the self. Further, death at this age is not anticipated in Western civilization and is even denied. In all societies, the death of an adolescent represents some downfall of family or community, some loss of optimism and the loss of a dream.

According to Klass and Marwit (1989), children are thought to personify the future for their parents. This is especially true in adolescence, as they begin to talk about their focus for high school and college. When children follow in their parents' footsteps, parents see their influence, which allows them to continue to be a part of their adolescent's lives. When an adolescent child dies, parents often believe the major component of their future died with them. Parents mourn the future developmental stages of their children's lives, a grief that is exacerbated when friends and relatives of their children attain these goals. These are most evident during high school and college graduations, marriages, and the birth of a new generation. This experience of loss is identified as the "amputation metaphor" (Klass & Marwit, 1989). The basis of the metaphor of amputation that parents so often report is reflected in a sense of unspeakable hurt and the loss of their dream.

Indeed, Raphael and Middleton (1987) report on the reworking of the parents' own adolescent issues as their children reach adolescence. When a family has an adolescent child, the parents strongly represent the relationship by their musing of their personal adolescence; thus, generating transferred aspects, projections, and fears. Not only does the adolescent carry parental projections, but they carry those of society. These researchers discuss the ambivalence that is characteristic of these years. As a result, experiencing loss at this time becomes especially difficult to resolve.

Sanders (1980) reports that parents who experience the death of a child reveal more intense grief reactions of somatic types, greater depression, as well as anger and guilt, with accompanying feelings of despair than parents who experience the death of either a spouse or parent. She further reports that the death of a child results in loss of control, "which exposes those survivors to greater vulnerability of external influences" (p. 310). Sanders states, "most of the parents gave the appearance of individuals who had just suffered a physical blow and which left them with no strength or will to fight, hence totally vulnerable" (p. 317). The greatest task for parents, according to Sanders, is to make sense of the circumstances and the death of their child. This task can create an obsessive questioning of "why" which can also manifest in a number of somatic experiences.

Rando (1993) describes child loss as one of the most devastating losses in adulthood. Gamino, Sewell, and Easterling (1998) show a strong inverse relationship between age at time of death and reported level of grief. This effect is consistent with developmental theory, which posits that the death of a young person defies the natural order of life and is more difficult for the survivors to sanction. Klass and Marwit (1989) report in a literature review of parental models of grief, "When we examine the grief of parents after the death of a child, neither the attachment model nor the psychoanalytic model seems to adequately account for many of the phenomena observed" (p. 31). They found that the death of a child creates "two disequilibria" (p. 39); disequilibrium in the social environment and in the ongoing relationship with the inner representation of the child. These authors also suggest that bereaved parents and other family members experience marginalization in their social roles as a result of their loss.

Additionally, Rubin (1992) finds that bereaved parents of adolescents remembered the first year following the death as more catastrophic than parents of younger children. He reports that parents of deceased adolescent children start out more preoccupied with the loss and there is little change in these feelings over a three year period. Subsequently, Murphy's (2000) eight-year study of bereaved parents whose 12- to 28-year-old children died by accident, homicide, or suicide began with several a priori hypotheses that the experience of sudden, violent death interferes with parental cognition, perception, and expression of emotion. She found that the ages of both parents and children at the time of death impede the meaning making process. Further, insufficient social support can lead to a sense of alienation for the parents. It is interesting to note that 33% of the parents met PTSD criteria defined by DSM-III-R (American Psychiatric Association, 1986). The results further demonstrate the likelihood of multiple negative outcomes if a parent meets PTSD diagnostic criteria. In virtually all studies of the outcome of child loss, clear indications of continuing distress are routinely present. Counselors working with bereaved parents find the use of rituals to be a healing factor in their work.

RITUALS

Therese Rando (1985), a major researcher in the field of bereavement, defines ritual as a " . . . specific behavior or activity which gives symbolic expression to certain feelings and thoughts of the actor(s) individually or as a group. It may be a habitually repetitive behavior or a one-time occurrence" (p. 236). Many times, rituals are created to satisfy the needs of the mourner. These are ways to commemorate, memorialize and give meaning to a life that was lived and shared with the grieving person. One goal in creating and participating in rituals is to transform the possibly maladaptive meaning clients attach to their experience of the death. This is done by creating a link between the experience of living with the loved one and the experience that the client now has of living without that loved one. When clients act out their rituals with their counselors or with their bereavement groups, they are supported in externalizing the meaning they have placed on this experience, which then legitimizes and validates their experience. In so doing, they can work toward finding a new way of being and create a new family dream.

Soup

  Tear Soup is a book that can be used by some people who suffer experiences of loss (Schwiebert & DeKlyen, 2003). It serves as a ritual that parents can use to remember their child, to connect with other people who also loved their child, and to honor their memory. The story begins by showing some helpful ingredients that Grandy, the main character in the book, keeps in her kitchen. Grandy shares her recipe, which contains a pot full of tears, one heart willing to be broken open, a dash of bitters, a bunch of good friends, many handfuls of comfort food, a lot of patience, buckets of water to replace the tears, plenty of exercise, a variety of helpful reading material, and enough self care. Grandy's recipe suggests seasoning the soup with memories. She includes the option of one good therapist and/or support group and provides directions for her soup. For example, first, we choose the size of pot that fits our loss. We can increase the pot size if we miscalculate the measurements. Next we combine ingredients and set the temperature for a moderate heat. Cooking times will vary depending on the ingredients needed. Strong flavors will mellow over time. We stir often and cook no longer than we need to.

  She adds suggestions for the soup. Among these are that we be creative, trust our instincts, cry when we want to, laugh when we can, freeze some soup to use as a starter for next time and keep our own soup-making journal so we won't forget. This book and video can be incorporated into clinical practice to normalize feelings of grief (Schwiebert & DeKlyen, 2003).

  An important aspect of rituals is the socialization process of reconfirming relational ties. Bereaved parents are reminded that they are not alone in their grief when rituals are created with others. Additionally, Gowensmith (2000) discusses that it is important to carefully choose the people with whom we share these experiences. Our support system helps us to assimilate the loss. Further, post funeral rituals allow parents to continue emotional connection with their children (Rando, 1985).

In one example, Mary's only son, Bill, was killed in a motorcycle accident. Mary used the soup ritual to assist her to work through his death. In her soup, she included Bill's favorite vegetables and culinary flavors. She made it a touch too salty to reflect her tears. Mary shared the soup in therapy, with friends, neighbors, and family members, and invited Bill's friends to her home to enjoy the soup. To ritualize this experience, Mary explained why she made the soup, why each element of the soup was included, and why Bill would have loved the soup. She told stories about Bill and encouraged others to share their tales of him, as well. .

In time, Mary moved to a different emotional place. She began to connect with others through her loss and together they supported each other during the difficult times. The soup was used in her community as a shared ritual. In fact, several of her friends, who later grieved their own losses, shared their soup, as well. In this case, each time that Mary shared the soup, she joined with others, further assimilated her loss, and advocated to preserve Bill's memory. She is now oriented to the future and works to help others create their own rituals.

In another case, Marian created a ritual as she grieved the loss of her daughter, Susie. Susie's death was tragically experienced by all members of her family. Marian used the soup ritual to help her grieve her unspeakable loss. Each week for several months, she brought a recipe card to her therapy session. These cards contained a special memory of Susie. As she read them during the counseling session, she was able to attribute a flavor to a memory. For instance, one card described the family's trip to Pike's Peak and how they rode the cog railway to the top of the mountain. She talked of the way Susie and her other children played while they bumped into each other, melding their flavors together. Marian remembered the feeling of the cold air on their faces and how this experience added depth to the soup. She described the look of joy in their shared experience. She added how this sweet element to her soup was like "candy for the eyes" and for their soup life together.

One day, Marian brought in a card that was crumbled and torn. With difficulty, she read the card and told a memory of when she and her husband placed their daughter, Susie, in a drug and alcohol rehabilitation center. She said the card was going to add some bitter flavor to the soup, but it was part of their life together and therefore needed to be included.

She reported that all tear soup has a bit of bitterness if it is depicting a true life.

At the end of her work in therapy, Marian brought her soup recipe box. The box not only contained all the recipe cards for her soup, but also pictures that went with the cards and trinkets that Susie had collected throughout her life. Marian keeps the recipe box on the coffee table in her family room and has a stack of unwritten recipe cards that Susie's friends can use to share a memory or current life experience. Marian has expanded the box three times; and each time, the recipe continues to gain depth and reality.

Recipes can also be used to commemorate children during special days and holidays. For example, some clients create rituals by writing recipe cards for their Thanksgiving celebration and asking their guests to do the same. Many cards contain memories of how their adolescent used to spend the holiday, the child's favorite food, or other endearing moments. By using food in the form of a recipe, clients identify and express their feelings and ritualize the grief process. And by creating ritual, they work toward assimilating the loss of their dream.

Music

Another useful tool for helping parents work through the loss of their child is music. This tool is particularly helpful for bereaved parents who find it difficult to put their feelings into words (Nelson & Weathers, 1998). Many bereaved parents describe how songs bring forth special meanings. At times, the tunes represent the loss of a person, other times they reflect the life of the person they have lost. Either way, songs seem to bring comfort to the grievers.

Sarah's 15-year-old son, Brian, was killed in an accident. The loss has, naturally, been a tragic one for her. Unfortunately, Sarah perceives her family to be unsupportive of her experience. It could be that in struggling with their own feelings, they cannot manage hers. Sarah brings the music to therapy where she explores the meaning of the songs and how the words connect her to her son and her loss. In the beginning, her choice of music reflected themes of pining and depression, with themes of riding away into the sunset, never to be heard from again. Sarah's music has more recently included a spiritual message. She has identified a particular country song, *I Believe*, written by Skip Ewing and Donny Kees (2002) to be particularly comforting:

I don't have to hear or see,
I've got all the proof I need,
there are more than angels watching over me
I believe, I believe.

(Ewing & Kees, 2002)

The song gives voice to her belief that she and Brian are close, even now, and provides her with support when it appears that her family cannot.

In another case, after Miranda's seventeen-year-old daughter, Angela, died, Miranda, wrote a love song for her. Angela and Miranda had enjoyed a close bond, and her death was devastating to her. Miranda performs this song on her tours and considers the song to be a special prayer of thanksgiving for her daughter. She takes Angela with her to each performance, and through song, Miranda has created a new healing ritual.

Stitches

Bobby, Anne Marie's 16-year-old son from a previous marriage, died suddenly of cardiac death. Members of the family were horrified when he collapsed after walking the family dog. Apparently, Bobby suffered from a condition that had gone undiagnosed. His death was sudden, tragic, and devastating.

Bobby's younger siblings were three, five, and eight years old at the time of his death. Adjusting to the loss has been difficult for everyone. Using quilt making as a ritual for working through grief, five quilts were made from Bobby's clothing for each member of the family. One of Bobby's shirt pockets was sewn into each quilt, on the upper right quadrant. At seeing the quilts, the oldest child commented that the pocket looked as if it was actually on Bobby's chest. As part of the ritual, each child places a note into Bobby's pocket every night. The note, which is confidential and not read by others, addresses any issue, thought, or feeling that come to mind. Even the three-year-old participates by drawing a picture of what she would want to tell Bobby or by scribbling "the words" on her paper. This ritual allows the children to share their day with Bobby.

Bobby's mother and step-father also utilize these quilts as they work through their own grief. For example, Bobby's mother wraps herself in her quilt. Bobby's step-father uses it as a wall hanging. Both parents find their quilts to be tangible symbols of Bobby's life, hopes, and dreams and have helped the children feel a continuing bond with their oldest brother.

Another family who lost their adolescent son/brother, Stephen, has used his clothing in a different way. In this case, his favorite saying "always remember" is embroidered on jackets and shirts. Because clothes wear out in time, they decided to make pillows of his sweatshirts. The bottom of the shirt and sleeves are sewn closed and the neck is used as an opening for stuffing. Each family member stuffs his or her own shirt about half way and writes a letter to Stephen. Family members share their letters before folding them into very small packages and placing them into the center of the pillow. When the pillows are filled, the neck is sewn shut. As part of the ritual, they share a story about Stephen. These stories are generally funny, poignant and important to the family.

CONCLUSION

The death of an adolescent child brings untold grief to surviving family members. Parents lose connections with their children and can feel alienated and isolated from each other in the process. They also lose connection with their hopes and dreams for their child, and in some ways, with aspects of themselves. Parents in grief must share their grief with someone who will listen; with someone who can be with their pain and who is moved by their experience. Therapists working with parents can use creative interventions to facilitate this connection. Nonphysical symbolic objects, such as prayers, poetry and music may help hurting parents connect with feelings that might otherwise be difficult to access (e.g., Bright, 1999). They can also be used to facilitate connections with each other. However unsolicited and unwarranted, these experiences become opportunities for personal change (Gamino, Sewell, & Easterling, 2000; Hogan, Morse, & Tason, 1996; Stroebe & Schut, 1999).

Few nightmares exist that could parallel a parent's loss of a child. Many times, when families face this tragedy, they seek ways to honor the relationship and their own grief. Soup, stitches, and songs serve as vehicles for meeting these important needs. Many families find that by using rituals creatively, they can work toward reconciling their heartbreaking loss of this dream and find new, mutually supportive and connected ways to live.

REFERENCES

American Psychiatric Association. (1986). Diagnostic and statistical manual of mental disorders (3rd Ed. Rev.). Washington, DC: American Psychiatric Association Press.

Bright, R. (1999). Music therapy in grief resolution. *Bulletin of the Menninger Clinic, 63,* 481-499.

Budman, S. H., & Gurman, A. S. (1988). *Theory and practice of brief therapy.* New York: Guilford Press.

Ewing, S., & Kees, D. (2002). I believe. On *Diamond Rio Completely* (CD). Nashville: Arista.

Gamino, L. A., Sewell, K. W., & Easterling, L. W. (1998). Scott & White grief study: An empirical test of predictors of intensified mourning. *Death Studies, 22,* 333-355.

Gamino, L. A., Sewell, K. W., & Easterling, L. W. (2000). Scott and White study phase 2: Toward an adaptive model of grief. *Death Studies, 24,* 633-661.

Gowensmith, W. (2000). The effects of postfuneral rituals on adjustment to bereavement. *Dissertation Abstracts International: Section B: The Sciences and Engineering, 60,* 10-B. (UMI No. 419-4217).

Hogan, N., Morse, J. M., & Tason, M. C. (1996). Toward an experiential theory of bereavement. *Omega: Journal of Death and Dying, 33,* 43-65.

Jacobs, S. (1993). *Pathological grief: Maladaptation to loss.* Washington, DC: American Psychiatric Press.

Jacobs, S., & Prigerson, H. (2000). Psychotherapy of traumatic grief: A review of evidence for psychotherapeutic treatments. *Death Studies, 24,* 479-495.

John, E. (1973). Daniel. On *Don't Shoot Me, I'm Only The Piano Player* (Record). New York: Island.

Klass, D., & Marwit, S. J. (1989). Toward a model of parental grief. *Omega: Journal of Death and Dying, 19,* 31-50.

Levav, I. (1982). Mortality and psychopathology following the death of an adult child: An epidemiological review. *The Israel Journal of Psychiatry and Related Sciences, 19,* 23-38.

Moules, N. (1998). Legitimizing grief: Challenging beliefs that constrain. *Journal of Family Nursing, 4,* 142-167.

Murphy, S. A. (2000). The use of research findings in bereavement programs: A case study. *Death Studies, 24,* 585-602.

Nelson, D., & Weathers, R. (1998). Necessary angels: Music and healing in psychotherapy. *Journal of Humanistic Psychology, 38,* 101-109.

Neugarten, B. (1979). Time, age, and the life cycle. *American Journal of Psychiatry, 135,* 887-894.

Rando, T. A. (1985). Creating therapeutic rituals in the psychotherapy of the bereaved. *Psychotherapy, 22,* 236-240.

Rando, T. A. (Ed.). (1986). *Parental loss of a child.* Champaign, IL: Research Press.

Rando, T. A. (1993). *Treatment of complicated mourning.* Champaign, IL: Research Press.

Raphael, B., & Middleton, W. (1987). Current state of research in the field of bereavement. *The Israel Journal of Psychiatry and Related Sciences, 24,* 5-32.

Raphael, B. (1983). *The anatomy of bereavement*. New York: Basic Books.
Rubin, S. (1992). Adult child loss and the two-track model of bereavement. Omega: *Journal of Death and Dying, 24*(3), 203-215.
Rubin, S. (1985). The resolution of bereavement: A clinical focus on the relationship to the deceased. *Psychotherapy, 22*, 231-235.
Sanders, C. M. (1980). A comparison of adult bereavement in the death of a spouse, child and parent. *Omega: Journal of Death and Dying, 10*(4), 303-21.
Schwiebert, P., & DeKlyen, C. (2003). *Tear soup*. Portland, Oregon: Grief Watch.
Stroebe, M., & Schut, H. (1999). The dual process model of coping with bereavement: Rationale and description. *Death Studies, 23*, 197-224.
Videka-Sherman, L. (1982). Coping with the death of a child: A study over time. *American Journal of Orthopsychiatry, 52*, 688-698.
Webster's new world dictionary of the American language (3rd College Edition). (1988). New York: Simon & Shuster.
Worden, J. W. (1991). *Grief counseling and grief therapy*. New York: Springer Publishing Company.
Wortman, C. B., & Silver, R. D. (1990). Successful mastery of bereavement and widowhood: A life course perspective. In P. B. Baltes & M. M. Baltes (Eds.), *Successful aging: Perspectives from the social sciences* (pp. 35-71). New York: Cambridge University Press.

doi:10.1300/J456v01n03_08

Chapter 9

Overcoming Heartbreak:
Learning to Make Music Again

Joanne Elise Vogel

SUMMARY. As a universal theme, love touches each of our lives in different and unique ways. This manuscript addresses the often overlooked sense of grief and loss that occurs when our dreams of love are shattered. It also addresses how addiction and commitment conflicts impede intimacy and loving relationships. While movies, music, and books offer many commentaries on this phenomenon, this article provides clinicians with some creative strategies for aiding clients in letting go and loving again. doi:10.1300/J456v01n03_09 *[Article copies available for a fee from The Haworth Document Delivery Service: 1-800-HAWORTH. E-mail address: <docdelivery@haworthpress.com> Website: <http://www.HaworthPress. com> © 2005 by The Haworth Press, Inc. All rights reserved.]*

KEYWORDS. Love, heartbreak, grief and loss, creativity, counseling, commitmentphobia, addiction, Relational-Cultural Theory

Joanne Elise Vogel is affiliated with the University of Central Florida and serves as Proj-ect Director for the Stronger Marriages, Stronger Families Program, a federal grant designed to strengthen couple relationships.

Address correspondence to: Joanne Elise Vogel, College of Education at the University of Central Florida, P.O. Box 161250, Orlando, FL 32816-1250 (E-mail: jovogel@mail.ucf.edu).

[Haworth co-indexing entry note]: "Overcoming Heartbreak: Learning to Make Music Again." Vogel, Joanne Elise. Co-published simultaneously in *Journal of Creativity in Mental Health* (The Haworth Press, Inc.) Vol. 1, No. 3/4, 2005, pp. 135-153; and: *Creative Interventions in Grief and Loss Therapy: When the Music Stops, a Dream Dies* (ed: Thelma Duffey) The Haworth Press, Inc., 2005, pp. 135-153. Single or multiple copies of this article are available for a fee from The Haworth Document Delivery Service [1-800-HAWORTH, 9:00 a.m. - 5:00 p.m. (EST). E-mail address: docdelivery@haworthpress.com].

> Last night I dreamed I held you in my arms
> The music was never-ending

(Springsteen, 1987)

When our love relationships go well, we enjoy the friendship, laughter, passion, and all the good things that loving experiences can bring. The music is not only never-ending, but also melodious. Other times, when love moves from euphony to cacophony, our dreams seem farther away, and perhaps, out of reach. It is during these times that we must form a more realistic appraisal of our situation. And when it appears that our relationships must end, we have the choice to grieve our loss, make sense of its impact, and determine when and how to love again.

Releasing relationships where we have invested care, time, and love remains among the most difficult experiences many of us will face. Not only does it take time to work through the heartache of a lost relationship, but memories of a certain song, favorite place, and shared experiences can create a flashback to our associated dreams. Chung et al. (2003) offer that relationship dissolution can have similar presentations to post-traumatic stress symptoms with intrusive thoughts and avoidant behavior. However, rather than nightmares, dreams of the person may act as bittersweet reminders of the lost love.

While research more clearly establishes the emotional difficulties, traumatic impact, and stress of relationship dissolution that married/ divorcing couples experience (e.g., Bloom, Asher, & White, 1978; Menaghan & Lieberman, 1986; Stack, 1990), less has been written about these challenges for dating, cohabiting, or other romantically-involved couples. In many cases, these losses are experienced as disenfranchised. Doka (1987) and Kammerman (1993) posit that because disenfranchised losses do not have social recognition or legitimacy, they do not easily carry social or relational support. However, these losses are particularly painful and carry with them unique issues.

Whether married or not, most people feel grief when estranged from a person they love and care for (Barbara & Dion, 2000). Lagrand (1988) discusses the grief reactions that manifest as a result of relationship dissolution. Unlike the feelings of grief and loss associated with death, for- mer partners live in our world, and we are reminded of the life we hoped to enjoy with them. In some cases, they may inhabit our physical space in the community where we live, work, or play. At times, we hear of their personal and professional accomplishments: graduations, promotions, engagements, marriages, and pregnancies. It may be difficult for many of us to avoid being haunted by the things that we could have said or done differently while the relationship was "alive."

Additionally, some of the difficulties that come with relationship loss are exacerbated when we carry complicating myths about love, or alternatively, when our relationships appear to have unrealized promise. Similarly, when we read books and watch movies that describe how a lover's persistence pays off in winning the heart of their beloved (Baumeister et al., 1993), we may hold out hope for a similar outcome. These factors influence our thinking about whether to try harder or whether to release a valued relationship. In cases where at least one person in the relationship suffers from addiction or commitment conflicts, this process becomes even more complicated. These dynamics will be discussed later in the manuscript.

In this manuscript, we will discuss some common barriers and challenges to our love relationships, such as substance abuse (Nakken, 1996), addiction (Covington, 1994; Covington & Beckett, 1988), and commitment conflicts (Carter & Sokol, 1995; 2004). Further, we will discuss some creative interventions that can be used to help people undergoing relationship loss. Whether these losses result because of a unilateral decision made by one partner or because of a mutual decision, these interventions can be incorporated into the counseling process. They can also be adapted to situations where relationships end because of conflicts related to addiction, intimacy, or commitment.

THE PROCESS OF LETTING GO

Even the most confident person can experience feelings of helplessness, confusion and a decrease in self-worth following the loss of an important relationship. People second guess what went wrong; lament what they might have done differently or feel anger and disappointment toward the person they, in fact, love. Many times, at the close of an important relationship we become angry with ourselves. Fortunately, when we have relationships available that are supportive and authentic, when we are willing to take the time to grieve our losses and make sense of our experiences, and when we learn more about ourselves and our contributions to these experiences, we gain confidence in our ability to create a compassionate context for the experience, and perhaps, to free our hearts to love again.

However, letting go of a relationship is difficult, particularly if we sustain hope for reconciliation. It becomes particularly difficult for us to release relationships colored by addiction (Covington, 1994; Covington & Beckett, 1988; Peabody, 2005), commitment conflicts (Carter & Sokol, 1995; 2004), or other sources of ambivalence. Still, the process is facilitated when we normalize some of the vastly fluctuating and painful emotions we feel. For example, following the ending of a romantic relationship, people who invested in the relationship commonly suffer depression (Mearns, 1991). Some individuals exhibit post-traumatic symptoms and intrusive thoughts (Chung et al., 2003). Others experience sleeplessness, weight loss, and increased substance use or abuse. When relationships have been intermittently reinforced, such as those bridled with addiction and commitment conflicts, these symptoms become even more heightened (Cater & Sokol, 2004; 1995). In these cases, as Lagrand (1988) observed, many reactions following the dissolution of a relationship manifest as grief reactions. Below we find the experiences of two people facing this difficult issue.

Lauren and Derrick; Rosa and Martin

Lauren presented for therapy because she was confused about what to do with her feelings about her relationship. Although she loved Derrick very much, she felt his interest wane and was grieving what appeared to be the end of what was once a very dynamic, caring, and passionate bond. She recalls how Derrick initiated the relationship and how they seemed to enjoy each other and share similar interests. And, although Lauren was the first to say so, Derrick professed to love her and behaved in loving ways. Still, as time went on, Derrick appeared to be confused, and in time, so was she.

Lauren presented for therapy bewildered and hurt. In her words, she could not "wrap her head around" what was happening and could not reconcile Derrick's intermittent hostility, given the warm and endearing words and behaviors he commonly expressed. She did not know what had "tripped the switch" and felt responsible for having said or done something that would distress him enough to turn away. This confusion, coupled with her investment, kept her hooked into "doing it better."

In another example, Rosa and Martin, who had been married for fifteen years, experienced problems in their relationship. After many years of attempting to have children, they decided to adopt a child. Finally, Martin had the family that he hoped for and dreamed of. After their son entered elementary school, things seemed to change in Rosa and Martin's relationship. Although Martin felt something was amiss, he was unsure of how to address the problem. One evening Rosa disclosed that she was having an affair with an old friend and had spoken to an attorney about divorcing Martin. When Martin presented for counseling, he was devastated, depressed, angry, lonely, and anxious. He had begun drinking to ease some of the pain. Martin shared that he had been married once before, although he and his ex-wife parted amicably. He thought that his current marriage would last forever and believed they would grow old together.

Counselors working with Lauren and Martin can help them work toward reconciling their experiences and ideas about love and loving by creatively working with their thoughts, feelings, and beliefs. Indeed, creative interventions can be employed to help clients realistically appraise their relationship, and when necessary, grieve their dream. Below, we find a three part creative intervention process that uses storytelling/writing, pictures, and music. Although the process can be followed systematically, like with all therapies, we must be flexible in our implementation of the interventions and take the needs of our clients into account. Also, as therapists, it is particularly important that we help clients feel empowered and authentically connected to their experience and to us. By using creative interventions in a relationally therapeutic context, and by co-creating a relationship where authentic expression is possible, clients are better able to distinguish relationships that empower them from those that do not. Examples of these interventions will follow. First, however, we will discuss some qualities that support loving relationships and then describe some common dynamics that interfere with our ability to sustain them. Perhaps this information can serve as a resource for counselors working with clients in their practices.

LOVE AND ADDICTION

Empowering love relationships support the well being of both persons; taking into account their respective needs, wants, and feelings. Relationships are also empowered when partners share intimacy. One relationship quality identified in the literature as a component of love (Sternberg, 1997) is, indeed, intimacy. Timmerman (1991) identified four qualities characteristic of intimacy. She purports that both people must trust each other; perceive feelings of emotional closeness; openly communicate; and enjoy reciprocity or mutuality in the relationship. Buhrmeter and Furman (1987) discuss how maintaining trust is a significant factor in sustaining intimacy. Trust grows when we believe our partner has our best interest at heart; when we are able to say what we need to say without fear of retribution or indifference. Emotional closeness comes when two people are interdependent, connected, and committed. Sternberg (1997) purports that for consummate love to exist, intimacy, passion, and decision/commitment must be in place. Although all romantic relationships experience ebbs and flows with respect to these qualities, and although some relationships are sustained without these in place, relationships, at best, find balance when all three qualities are present.

There are many reasons for why relationships end. In some cases, we are not psychologically, financially, or emotionally ready to take our relationships to the next level. One person in a relationship may not feel the investment or care that the other person feels. Some relationships end because of the death of our partner. Other times, our relationships end because one or both partners have unfinished business related to previous hurts or feelings of rejection or abandonment, or because they do not have the psychological and relational capacities to sustain them (Carter & Sokol, 1995; 2004).

Our capacity to be authentic and genuine impacts our ability to engage in and enjoy relationships of depth. However, several factors challenge these efforts. Substance abuse and addiction are among these factors. In these cases, we become distanced from others with whom we could enjoy a growth-fostering romantic relationship and from our relational potentials. Indeed, one of the central tenets of substance abuse and addiction literature is that when we abuse substances and suffer from addictions, our relationships also suffer (Covington, 1994; Jampolsky, 1991; Nakken, 1996; Peabody, 2005). The literature discusses how addictions breed fears that make intimacy and commitment problematic (Beattie, 1996; Wegscheider-Cruse, 1987). Further, common addictive behaviors, like rationalization and denial, keep us from understanding our contributions to our relational difficulties.

Sometimes, seeing the impact that our behaviors have on others can be painful. During these times, we may rationalize our experiences to protect ourselves from seeing how our behaviors and choices damage relationships and hurt people we care for. Covington (1994) provides a compassionate and realistic accounting of these challenges in her book, *A Woman's Way Through the Twelve Steps*. Using the Twelve Steps as a base and providing language and a perspective that women can relate to, she speaks to the relational challenges that women face in the addictive process; challenges that create a threat to our relational connections.

According to Relational-Cultural Theory (Miller, 1976; Miller & Stiver, 1993; Stiver, 1990), we all have a desire to form connections with others. Through these connections, we engage in relationships that are mutually rewarding; relationships where we are able to safely represent our thoughts, feelings, and needs to one another. However, when we do not have relationships based in authentic and mutual relating, or when our relationships are clouded by power differentials, some of us hide aspects of ourselves to avoid rejection or other negative consequences. In doing so, we create patterns of disconnection that can be isolating and painful (Jordan, 2001). Although disconnections occur in relationships at one time or another, these disconnections characterize relational dynamics involving addictions (Duffey, 2005) and impede our capacity for intimacy and commitment. As a result, sustaining a love relationship when substance abuse or addiction is present becomes a challenge.

The literature discusses addictive qualities that interfere with our capacity to form connections. Peabody (2005) describes some common addictive patterns that sabotage relationships. These include the following:

> . . . fears of losing his or her identity; fears of dependency/avoids bonding; creates rigid personality boundaries (won't let people in); is sensitive to everything that leads to bonding; seduces and withholds to avoid bonding; minimizes feelings that lead to bonding; gets nervous when things go well or bonding occurs; wants more space or has to run; can't make commitment; is indifferent to others; feels entitled to be taken care of (his or her way); won't put up with discomfort; has complete control of the schedule; says to partner "just stay put and let me come and go." (p. 129)

We cannot enjoy and sustain loving relationships within these margins. Moreover, when we love someone who professes to love us, at the same time that these limitations are present, we experience a very hurtful and often misunderstood form of disenfranchised grief. The literature on addiction, codependency, and intimacy has been replete with information describing this relational dynamic (Covington, 1994; Ingram, 1986; Peabody, 2005; Wegscheider-Cruse, 1987). This dynamic is elucidated in Ingram's (1986) discussion on how we unconsciously transfer our fears of intimacy into "an affirmation: an insistence on freedom" (p. 76). The literature examines how individuals with unusual needs for external freedom also have a difficult time self-regulating their internal sense of freedom or comfort. Freedom then becomes an illusion, and in a relational sense, remains elusive.

FREEDOM

Freedom is an interesting and often misunderstood concept. While some people would suggest that freedom comes to those who are able to do anything they would like to do at whim, others suggest that freedom involves a different form of choice (Ingram, 1986; Wegscheider-Cruse, 1987). From a relational perspective, freedom comes when we feel free to remain in relationships that involve other people's needs and feelings. In contrast, lack of freedom comes to us when we feel forced to run from our uncomfortable feelings or from relationships that trigger them. Ingram discusses this dynamic: "One experiences not the threat of intimacy, but that one needs space, can't stand coercion, loves freedom, isn't ready yet, and so forth. In its easiest formulation the quest for freedom and the avoidance of anything that compromises it" (Ingram, 1986, p. 76).

Ingram suggests that as we develop our capacity to emotionally negotiate life, we increase our capacity to experience and enjoy intimacy and commitment. However, when we have limiting or restrictive needs that impede this challenge, we lack the inner freedom that intimacy and loving relationships require. He adds, "Intimacy with another or caring for another mobilizes anxiety that is attenuated through denial, detachment, contempt, rationalization, and the sabotage of trust" (Ingram, 1986, p. 77). Leaders in the addiction field concur (Covington, 1994; Peabody, 2005; Wegscheider-Cruse, 1987). What then, do we do when these issues surface in a relationship we value?

Steven Carter and Julia Sokol speak to this issue in their groundbreaking books, *He's Scared She's Scared: Understanding the Hidden Fears that Sabotage Your Relationships* (1995) and *Men Who Can't Love: How to Spot the Commitment Phobic Man Before He Breaks Your Heart* (2004). The authors discuss a relational dynamic that involves a person's unusual needs for boundaries, space, and distance within a relationship and present diverse examples of how this dynamic is experienced. Carter and Sokol identify this dynamic as *commitment phobia*, and explain its correlation to claustrophobia: " . . . men and women with commitment conflicts need distance. They don't like feeling as though someone is closing in on them and limiting them in any way" (Carter & Sokol, 1995, p. 29). There are a number of reasons for why people experience conflicts related to commitment or intimacy. Childhood experiences, later experiences with abandonment, such as divorce, betrayal, or rejection, immaturity, or characterological problems can all impede the flow necessary for relationships to thrive.

When commitment conflicts are present, relationships are power-fully regulated (Carter & Sokol, 1995). More specifically, by establish-ing unreasonable boundaries, people maintain control of the shared closeness and of the pace at which romantic relationships develop. In short, commitment conflicts arise when a motivating factor involves maintaining options to sustain a perceived sense of freedom.

Restrictive Boundaries and Commitment

When commitment conflicts are active and profound, boundaries are set to serve as a source of warning to love partners that they should not have any expectations of the relationship. These messages become espe-cially confusing to them in light of the charming, supportive, and loving affection that are also communicated. Ironically, some partners accom-modate these confusing expectations when they are delivered in the form of mixed messages. When people feel compelled to avoid closeness while participating in a relationship, they invite partners into their lives and then manage the distance:

- By setting up limits in terms of time and availability
- By denying access to parts of his or her world (not inviting a part-ner to family or work related functions, not introducing a partner to friends)
- By refusing to participate fully in a partner's world (turning down invitations to special events, avoiding a partner's family and friends)
- By not sharing holidays, birthdays, and special occasions
- By not sharing special interests
- By placing peculiar restriction on exchanges of money or gifts so that there will be no expectations
- By establishing a lifestyle that clearly says, "I want to be alone."
- By making it clear that you perceive all expectations such as inti-macy and/or exclusivity as unwelcome demands (Carter & Sokol, 1995, p. 21).

These authors explain how people may genuinely care about the per-son with whom they have a relationship, while establishing patterns of intermittent avoidance. They add the following observation:

The need to create distance and shake these unpleasant feelings is frequently intense enough to overlook any feelings of love one may hold for a partner. Getting away becomes the only priority. The fear may be real or imagined, reasonable or unreasonable. The key lies in perception. (Carter & Sokol, 1995, p. 38)

Marriage and Commitment Phobia

In spite of the terror that the prospect of marriage or commitment can bring, people with commitment conflicts, indeed, marry. For example, they may marry a person or close personal friend to escape from feelings of love/phobia for someone else. They may attempt to prove the inappropriateness of the original relationship by purportedly committing to another relationship. Sometimes they express their ambivalence by attempting to maintain a relationship with two people.

Frederico owned and operated a small company. As part of his work, he traveled regularly to Mexico. Sometimes, he would take his girlfriend of 10 years, Ana, with him. More often, Ana, a graduate student, would stay home to tend to her job and her studies. Although Frederico and Ana shared many happy, fun times during their relationship; and although they appeared to have an intimate connection, she discovered that he married someone else from Mexico. Ana was naturally devastated. She confronted Frederico, who was shocked that she had discovered his secret. Although they ceased contact for a period of time, Frederico called her on her birthday and attempted to rekindle communication. He could not explain what he had done, and professed to still love her. Ana talked to him in an attempt to make sense of what had happened, but was unsuccessful. Interestingly, Frederico was not suggesting that they resume their relationship as it had been. Still, he was not able to commit to his marriage, either. In time, Ana requested that he no longer call her. She decided that she would never be able to make sense of the situation and gave up her effort to do so.

Other times, people with active commitment conflicts marry and then create distance in the relationship by ignoring the needs of their spouse or by being unavailable to the spouse and available to others. When the spouse chooses to leave the relationship, the partner with the active conflict can become devastated, and sees the dissolution of the marriage as "proof " that commitments are not to be trusted. This wound can become like a battle scar that is worn when subsequent relationships appear to deepen. In this case, the scar serves as a barrier to a new relationship; a strategy for disconnection (Jordan, 2001), or a form of rationalization (Carter & Sokol, 1995), for why the relationship is untenable.

Conflictual Characteristics

Coming to terms with these relationships can take time because of the ambivalent and mixed messages that characterize them (Carter & Sokol, 2004). For example, when we carry commitment conflicts, we express and feel sorrow for our behaviors in one breath and continue to enact hurtful behaviors in another. Our touch says one thing and our words say another. We seduce at the same time that we find fault in our partner. Fault finding and citing vague excuses are common ways for us to end our relationships when we have commitment conflicts. Ironically, as we do so, we can be completely unaware of how irrational our behaviors are, and in fact, pride ourselves on our capacity for empathy and sensitivity (Carter & Sokol, 1995; 2004).

Citing one of many examples in their text where this dynamic is expressed, Carter and Sokol (1995) write "Even though Brad acknowledges that he manipulates his relationships according to his whims, he prides himself on his sensitivity to women's issues" (p. 68). Certainly, these ambivalent conflicts are expressed in unique ways. These include being very "seductive/rejective; intimate/withdrawn; accepting/critical; tender/hostile . . . very romantic/distant" (Carter & Sokol, 1995, p. 59).

As partners in these situations, we may feel safe in the acceptance, tenderness, and perceived intimacy we experience. Then, in the face of rejection, withdrawal, hostility or callousness, the experience becomes increasingly painful and difficult for us to release (Carter & Sokol, 1995). Like the lyrics by Coldplay (2002), "Come up to meet you, tell you I'm sorry. You don't know how lovely you are," the words can be eerily confusing. It is at those times that we begin to wrestle with reality. Unfortunately, we must pass through a hall of mirrors as we come to terms with this reality, since the relationship assumes different faces depending on whether the reflection centers on the beginning of the relationship, the middle, or the end.

According to Carter and Sokol (1995; 2004), these relationships follow predictable stages and carry their own predictable patterns. In the beginning stages, as a partner with commitment conflicts, we are enthusiastically captivating and inviting; charming, and somewhat solicitous. Later, as anxieties begin to rise and become intense, we are unable to think about anyone else's welfare but our own. At this point, we can appear angry or hostile; refuse to take phone calls; and may even flaunt what can look like a new investment in another relationship (Carter & Sokol, 1995; 2004). When it appears that our partners are no longer available, we make what Carter and Sokol refer to as "curtain calls."

Again, Coldplay (2002) lyrics come to mind: "Tell me your secrets, and ask me your questions, Oh let's go back to the start." Because our behaviors seem inconceivable to our partners, given the person they saw us to be at the beginning of the relationship and the depth of feeling that these relationships can trigger, they may find it increasingly difficult to recover. Still, some former partners seek counseling and wrestle with releasing the relationship and the dreams that go with them.

CREATIVE APPROACHES FOR RECOVERING FROM BROKEN HEARTS AND BROKEN DREAMS

When clients seek a counselor's help because their relationships are ending, they present for therapy expressing a number of feelings. Although many feel pain, hurt, and bewilderment, some also express feelings of shame, humiliation, and regret. They often blame themselves for the break-up and feel relationally disconnected and disempowered. Their relational competence is often challenged (Jordan, 1999). By developing an empathic, growth-fostering relationship (Jordan, 2001; Jordon, Miller, Stiver, & Surrey, 1997; Miller & Stiver, 1997) with clients, counselors can help them connect with their vulnerabilities and experience these vulnerabilities compassionately. Within this connection, counselors can employ a number of creative activities to facilitate their work together.

These creative activities may take varying lengths of time to process, based upon the client's stage of grief. For example, creative interventions that combine storytelling with writing allow clients to reflect upon their deepest, most intimate and compelling relational questions (Dickerman, 1992). These interventions assist clients to reconsider their dreams and increase self-awareness. In the examples listed above, Lauren may wonder why Derrick would delay becoming involved in a committed relationship, given that he professes to love her; they mutually support each others' professional aspirations; and they each have freedom within the relationship to maintain their respective friendships and other important values. Martin may question how so many shared experiences and years together would lead his wife to seek divorce. He may also question whether he is to blame for the marriage's demise.

In these cases, creative interventions can help clients to work through these thoughts, feelings, self-perceptions, and doubts. They can consider the cultural context of their grief and the ways their loss can feel disenfranchised. This can be seen in Lauren's situation because of her unmarried status. No doubt, the experience of divorce can be traumatic. But what of the pain involved in the dissolution of a relationship not legally sanctioned? The challenge for people suffering the loss of a relationship within this context can be misunderstood, minimized, and marginalized, leaving a person to feel uniquely alone and disconnected. Along the same vein, Martin, too, may feel shame, isolation, and unsupported because of the stigma associated with a second divorce. Societal expectations, coupled with our own hopes and dreams for our relational successes affect our resilience as we navigate through painful periods of relational loss. Creative interventions, then, must be employed with the goal of helping clients connect with their authentic experience and vulnerabilities in ways that foster growth, empowerment, and resilience. It is within that context that the creative interventions described below can best be facilitated.

Expressive Writing

Losing an important relationship is an exceedingly painful experience. Writing is one avenue for working through this experience. The literature purports that by freely expressing stressful thoughts and feelings, we reduce the negative mental and physical effects of challenging life events (Pennebaker, 1997; Smyth, 1998). In one example, Pennebaker and Beall (1986) propose writing for twenty minutes per day, for three days, about a self-selected or specified stressful event. In this activity, therapists can also guide clients to consider how they perceive their former partner and to reflect on their feelings toward him or her. Through their writing, they can describe what aspects of the relationship seemed to work for them, the parts of themselves they most appreciated while in the relationship, and the parts of themselves they did not like while in the relationship. Finally, they can reflect upon their perspective of how the relationship ended. When clients access enough objective perspective that would warrant claiming some personal responsibility for the situation, they are better able to negotiate some resolution.

By writing, clients express emotions at the same time that they make sense of their experience. This is particularly helpful when the relationship was ambivalent or confusing, as it can be when addiction or commitment issues are involved, or in cases where individuals do not feel the freedom to disclose their pain to friends and members of their social network (Lepore & Greenberg, 2002). Because anniversaries may pose particularly difficult times for some clients, they may also feel especially wounded while traveling, listening to music, or seeing photographs of the former partner. At these times, writing exercises can be used to help ground them in reality. As Lepore (1997) notes, expressive writing may not affect the frequency of intrusive thoughts but moderates the impact of intrusive thoughts on depressive symptoms.

In addition, expressive writing exercises may offer a more supportive or productive alternative for clients working toward making sense of the loss. It can serve as an adjunct to therapy by having the client process the experience out of session and later share these writings with their counselor. In either case, the client will likely gain a clearer understanding of various aspects of the relationship and better come to terms with the pain surrounding its loss. After completing the expressive writing activity, clients and counselors will have spent some time looking at the hopes, dreams, and desires of the relationship, in addition to some of the more troubling and problematic aspects or memories of the relationship.

Photographs

The next activity addresses the vivid memories of the past relationship (see Harvey, Flanary, & Morgan, 1986). These vivid memories often include the beginning of the relationship, special occasions, and the ending. When working with relationships that involve commitment conflicts, these can be particularly disturbing, because the beginning of the relationship can appear very promising, while the middle part of the relationship is by nature profoundly confusing, making the end of the relationship particularly devastating (Carter & Sokol,1995; 2004). Also, given that people with active commitment conflicts tend to avoid special occasions with their partners, these can be especially difficult memories for partners to bear. In these cases, they are grieving "what could have been" or "what didn't happen." Given the flashbulb quality of these memories and events, clients can engage in activities designed to "take" more realistic pictures of the relationship and of their memories.

Pictures speak to the visual part of our memory bank and can be especially powerful for people releasing a love relationship. Interestingly, when we review photo albums and look at the pictures we select for picture frames, most relationships are depicted in staged and posed moments, complete with smiles and what appear to be happy memories. However, these pictures fail to capture many of the actual dynamics of the relationship since they rarely include average or even conflicted moments. For this reason, we can expand our repertoire of vivid relationship memories by adding other "snapshots." In this activity, clients find a picture, draw a picture, or take a picture that would typically represent the relationship at its worst. After discussing client images, they can bring actual photos or representations of their relationship to prepare for the next activity, which focuses on developing a coherent story of the connection by creating a relational scrapbook.

Storybook

The construction of narratives has been shown to assist individuals to make sense of and come to terms with the ending of a relationship (Kellas & Manusov, 2003). Since we not only grieve the relationship but also the loss of our dreams associated with our relationship, constructing a cohesive story and understanding its relevance can be particularly helpful. Weiss (1975) contends that assigning characters, roles, and plots creates an organizational schema for making sense of the loss. As a result, this activity focuses on joining the expressive writing and photograph activities into a storybook or scrapbook format with cohesive and chronological movement. This work includes the introduction/ meeting, main characters, plot, special occasions, possible plot twists and turns, the unwinding, and the termination/ending.

Again, the therapist will optimally exercise creativity and flexibility in adapting the format to meet the client's needs. Some clients may opt to create a scrapbook or photo album to include pictures and/or drawings while others may wish to write out the events similar to a journal, screenplay, or song. This activity focuses on the progression and cohesion of the story or narrative rather than a specific mode of expression. Some evidence suggests that complete narratives improve understanding and adjustment to relationship dissolution (Sorenson, Russell, Harkness, & Harvey, 1993; Weber, Harvey, & Stanley, 1987; Weiss, 1975). For those who have struggled to understand the unraveling of the relationship and its termination, this activity should include hunches, possible explanations, or the most probable explanation for its ending. At times, coping strategies such as narratives offer the only available means of closure for the relationship (Kellas & Manusov, 2003; Weber, Harvey, & Stanley, 1987).

It is especially important for therapists and clients to process these stories, so that through the process, clients are able to consider their own relational images, dynamics, fears, personalities, and world worldviews. This process allows them to focus on the story as they see it, consider how it affects them, and reflect on how it may affect their future relational goals.

Future Relationship Activity

These creative activities may take varying lengths of time to process, depending on the client's stage of grief. Some clients may also wish to engage in an activity with the goal of looking toward the future and loving again. To point them in this direction, they can complete the Realistic Relationship Activity. This activity focuses on having a client describe what the desired relationship would look like. Therapists may provide the client with a silhouette of two people together as the background upon which to write the various aspects desired in the next relationship. That is, clients can use words that illustrate the dynamics they would like to see in their next relationship. For example, they may include how they like to share recreational time together. They can describe the banter or playfulness they hope to have. They can also describe how they would express love and how they would like to receive love. Clients can also describe how they can resolve conflicts, what freedom will look like in the relationship, the degree of comfort they see in sustaining intimacy and connection, and what commitment would look like. The client can use this model as a baseline or benchmark as they enter future relationships; keeping in mind the difference between idealistic and realistic depictions. This benchmark would allow them to take into account how the wants, needs, and feelings of both partners can be considered.

CONCLUSION

Love can be one of the most rewarding experiences in life. When lost, it can be among our most hurtful of experiences. Relationships where one or both partners suffer from addictions or where intimacy and commitment conflicts exist exacerbate the pain involved in losing a relationship we love. Some people avoid their experiences, and in self-protection, become callous to love and to the feelings of others they invite into relationship. This form of disconnection leads to relational isolation and pain of a different form. Alternatively, some people invest in healing through the growth-fostering relationships available to them. When we make such an investment, we have an opportunity to deepen our relational capacities, rebuild our self-esteem, trust, and hope for the future. Moreover, when we reflect on our experiences and engage authentically with others, we have an opportunity to understand, integrate, and move beyond the hurt. As we use a mixture of writing, expressive arts, and storytelling, we have an opportunity to gain self-awareness, understanding, and compassion.

And in doing so, we broaden our options for consciously constructing our possibilities for enjoying a new dream.

My heart is that much harder now.
I thought that it would stay that way, before today.

(Watt, 1996)

REFERENCES

Barbara, A. M., & Dion, K. L. (2000). Breaking up is hard to do, especially for strongly "preoccupied" lovers. *Journal of Personal and Interpersonal Loss, 5,* 315-342.

Baumeister, R. F., Wotman, S. R., & Stillwell, A. M. (1993). Unrequited love: On heartbreak, anger, guilt, scriptlessness, and humiliation. *Journal of Personality and Social Psychology, 64*(3), 377-394.

Beattie, M. (1996). *Codependent no more: How to stop controlling others and start caring for yourself.* Center City, MN: Hazelden.

Bloom, B., Asher, S. J., & White, S. W. (1978). Marital disruption as a stressor: A review and analysis. *Psychological Bulletin, 85,* 867-894.

Brooks, J. L., Mark, L., & Sakai, R. (Producers), Graf, A., & Crowe, C. (Directors). (1996). *Jerry Maguire* [Motion Picture]. United States: TriStar Pictures.

Buhrmeter, D. N., & Furman, P. (1987). The development of companionship and intimacy. *Child Development, 58,* 1101-1113.

Carter, S., & Sokol, J. (1995). *He's scared she's scared: Understanding the hidden fears that sabotage your relationships.* New York: Dell Publishing.

Carter, S., & Sokol, J. (2004). *Men who can't love: How to recognize a commitment-phobic man before he breaks your heart.* New York, NY: M. Evans.

Chung, M. C., Farmer, S., Grant, K., Newton, R., Payne, S., & Perry, M. et al. (2003). Coping with post-traumatic stress symptoms following relationship dissolution. *Stress and Health, 19,* 27-36.

Covington, S. (1994). *A woman's way through the twelve steps.* Center City, MN: Hazelden.

Covington, S., & Beckett, L. (1988). *Leaving the enchanted forest: The path from relationship addiction to intimacy.* Boston, MA: Harper Collins Publishers.

Dickerman, A. C. (1992). *Following your path: Using myths, symbols and images to explore your inner life.* Los Angeles: Tarcher.

Doka, K. (1989). Disenfranchised grief: Recognizing hidden sorrow. Lexington, MA: Lexington Books.

Duffey, T. (2005). The relational impact of addiction across the life span. In D. Comstock (Ed.), *Diversity and Development: Critical Contexts that Shape Our Lives and Relationships* (pp. 299-317). Belmont, CA: Brooks/Cole.

Harvey, J. H., Flanary, R., & Morgan, M. (1986). Vivid memories of vivid loves gone by. *Journal of Social and Personal Relationships, 3,* 359-373.

Ingram, D. H. (1986). Remarks on intimacy and the fear of commitment. *The American Journal of Psychoanalysis, 46*(1), 76-79.

Jampolsky, L. (1991). *Healing the addictive mind: Freeing yourself from addictive patterns and relationships.* Berkeley, CA: Celestial Arts.

Jordan, J. V., Kaplan, A. G., Miller, J. B., Stiver, I. P., & Surrey, J. L. (1991). *Women's growth in connection: Writings from the Stone Center.* New York: The Guildford Press.

Jordan, J. (1999). Toward connection and competence. *Work in Progress, No. 83.* Wellseley, MA: Stone Center Working Papers Series.

Jordan, J. (2001). A relational-cultural model: Healing through mutual empathy. *Bulletin of the Menninger Clinic, 65*(1), 92-103.

Kammerman, J. (1993). Latent functions of enfranchising the disenfranchised griever. *Death Studies,* 17, 281-287.

Kellas, J. K., & Manusov, V. (2003). What's in a story? The relationship between narrative completeness and adjustment to relationship dissolution. *Journal of Social and Personal Relationships, 20*(3), 285-307.

Lagrand, L. E. (1988). *Changing patterns of human existence: Assumptions, beliefs, and coping with the stress of change.* Springfield, IL: Charles C. Thomas Publisher.

Lepore, S. J. (1997). Expressive writing moderates the relation between intrusive thoughts and depressive symptoms. *Journal of Personality and Social Psychology, 73*(5), 1030-1037.

Lepore, S. J., & Greenberg, M. A. (2002). Mending broken hearts: Effects of expressive writing on mood, cognitive processing, social adjustment and health following a relationship breakup. *Psychology and Health, 17*(5), 547-560.

Mearns, J. (1991). Coping with a break up: Negative mood regulation expectancies and depression following the end of a romantic relationship. *Journal of Personality and Social Psychology, 60,* 327-334.

Menaghan, E. G., & Lieberman, M. A. (1986). Changes in depression following divorce: A panel study. *Journal of Marriage and the Family, 48,* 319-328.

Miller, J. (1976). *Toward a new psychology of women.* Boston: Beacon Press.

Miller, J., & Stiver, I. (1993). A relational approach to understanding women's lives and Problems. *Psychiatric Annals, 23*(8), 424-431.

Miller, J. V. & Stiver, I. P. (1997). The healing connection: *How women form relationships in therapy and in life.* Boston: Beacon Press.

Nakken, C. (1996). *The Addictive personality: Understanding the addictive process and compulsive behavior.* Center City, MN: Hazelden Publishing.

Peabody, S. (2005). *Addiction to love: Overcoming obsession and dependency* (3rd ed.). PA: Ten Speed Press.

Pennebaker, J. W. (1997). Writing about emotional experiences as a therapeutic process. *Psychological Science, 8,* 162-166.

Pennebaker, J. W., & Beall, S. K. (1986). Confronting a traumatic event: Toward an understanding of inhibition and disease. *Journal of Abnormal Psychology, 95,* 274-281.

Smyth, J. M. (1998). Written emotional expression: Effect sizes, outcome types, and moderating variables. *Journal of Consulting and Clinical Psychology, 66,* 174-184.

Sorenson, K. A., Russell, S. M., Harkness, D. J., & Harvey, J. H. (1993). Account-making, confiding, and coping with the ending of a close relationship. *Journal of Social Behavior and Personality, 8,* 73-86.

Springsteen, B. (1987). One step up. On *Tunnel of Love* [CD]. New York: Columbia Records.

Stack, S. (1990). New micro-level data on the impact of divorce on suicide, 1959-1980: A test of two theories. *Journal of Marriage and the Family, 52,* 119-127.

Sternberg, R. J. (1986). A triangular theory of love. *Psychological Review, 93,* 119-135.

Sternberg, R. J. (1988). Triangulating love. In R. J. Sternberg & M. L. Barnes (Eds.), *The psychology of love* (pp. 119-138). New Haven, CT: Yale University Press.

Sternberg, R. J. (1997). Construct validation of a triangular love scale. *European Journal of Social Psychology, 27,* 313-335.

Stiver, I. (1990). Dysfunctional families and wounded relationships. *Work in Progress, No. 41.* Wellesley, MA: Stone Center Working Paper Series.

Timmerman, G. P. M. (1991). A concept analysis of intimacy. *Issues in Mental Health Nursing, 12,* 19-30.

Watt, B. (1996). Before today. [Recorded by Everything But The Girl]. On *Walking Wounded* [CD]. New York: Atlantic Recording Corporation.

Weber, A. L., Harvey, J. H., & Stanley, M. A. (1987). The nature and motivations of accounts for failed relationships. In R. Burnett, P. McGhee, & D. D. Clarke (Eds.), *Accounting for personal relationships: Explanation, representation and knowledge* (pp. 114-133). London: Methuen.

Wegschieder-Cruse, S. (1987). *Choicemaking.* Pampano Beach, FL: Health Communications, Inc.

Weiss, R. S. (1975). *Marital separation.* New York: Basic Books.

doi:10.1300/J456v01n03_09

Chapter 10

Miscarriage:
A Dream Interrupted

Heather C. Trepal
Suzanne Gibson Semivan
Mary Caley-Bruce

SUMMARY. Pregnancy is a developmental task that requires women to become accustomed to inherent and sometimes profound biological, somatic, and psychological changes. When pregnancy is interrupted by miscarriage, it may become a pivotal crisis point in the development of a woman's maternal identity as well as an issue in family development. This manuscript will discuss the growing body of literature that addresses the emotional and psychological impact of miscarriage, as well as concomitant attachment issues and present therapeutic and treatment implications for counselors working with women and their partners. doi:10.1300/J456v01n03_10 *[Article copies available for a fee from The Haworth Document Delivery Service: 1-800-HAWORTH. E-mail address: <docdelivery@haworthpress.*

Heather C. Trepal, is Assistant Professor at the University of Texas at San Antonio, 501 West Durango Boulevard, San Antonio, TX.
Suzanne Gibson Semivan is affiliated with the University of Akron.
Mary Caley-Bruce is affiliated with the University of Texas at San Antonio.
Address correspondence to: Heather C. Trepal, PhD, University of Texas at San Antonio, 501 West Durango Boulevard, San Antonio, TX 78207-4415 (E-mail heather.trepal@utsa.edu).

[Haworth co-indexing entry note]: "Miscarriage: A Dream Interrupted." Trepal, Heather C., Suzanne Gibson Semivan, and Mary Caley-Bruce. Co-published simultaneously in *Journal of Creativity in Mental Health* (The Haworth Press, Inc.) Vol. 1, No. 3/4, 2005, pp. 155-171; and: *Creative Interventions in Grief and Loss Therapy: When the Music Stops, a Dream Dies* (ed: Thelma Duffey) The Haworth Press, Inc., 2005, pp. 155-171. Single or multiple copies of this article are available for a fee from The Haworth Document Delivery Service [1-800-HAWORTH, 9:00 a.m. - 5:00 p.m. (EST). E-mail address: docdelivery@haworthpress. com].

KEYWORDS. Creativity, miscarriage, maternal identity, attachment issues, family development, counseling

I knew I loved you before I met you.
I think I dreamed you in to life.
I knew I loved you before I met you.
I have been waiting all my life

(Savage Garden, 1999)

INTRODUCTION

My sister called the other day and was in a panic: "I need to share something with you but I'm afraid to tell you." I held in my breath. I knew that she and her husband had been trying for some time and figured that she was going to announce that she was pregnant. "I'm pregnant but the doctor couldn't find a heartbeat. I should be far enough along by now for them to find it. My hormone levels are still rising, so they are going to do another ultrasound on Monday." As my breath returned, my heart sank and memories flooded over me, taking me back 15 years to my miscarriage. Since that time, I have gotten married and carried two successful pregnancies but sometimes when I least expect it, the memory of that unexpected loss jumps back into my mind.

I miscarried my first child at 16 weeks gestation. The baby was a girl. I was a child myself, just seventeen years old at the time. The pregnancy was unacknowledged in a number of ways; school, friends, family, and even my then-boyfriend and his parents pretended that I wasn't pregnant and the whole thing just wasn't happening. In fact, after the miscarriage, most people told me how lucky I was that I would not be "stuck" with a baby; that now I would be able to go to college. Or, they were silent on the issue altogether. It took me many years to sort through the emotional baggage from that chaotic time and I find that the issue forces its way back into my life at certain intervals, including both of my pregnancies as well as during pregnancies of others in my intimate circle. That first pregnancy and subsequent miscarriage changed a lot of things for me, including how I view relationships, my never-ending fears about pregnancy and birth, and how I feel about my own body.

Counselors work with women and their partners who have the misfortune of experiencing a miscarriage. Some view the event as minor; an obstacle on the road to a healthy pregnancy and baby; as fate; or as a relief. For others, a miscarriage signals a time of mourning, yearning, and pain. A need for an empowering view of healing exists for women and their partners following miscarriage. Part of the healing process involves honoring their unique story relative to the loss. This article examines the experience of miscarriage through developmental and attachment lenses and investigates the diverse contexts of reactions held by women and their partners. It also provides recommendations for exploring the healing process following miscarriage.

MISCARRIAGE: DEFINED AND CONCEPTUALIZED

A miscarriage or spontaneous abortion is the unintended end of a pregnancy before a fetus can survive outside of the prenatal environment, at approximately the twentieth week of gestation (Borg & Lasker, 1982). Miscarriage, more repeatedly than not, occurs within the first trimester. Inadequate development of the placenta or umbilical cord, unsuccessful implantation of the embryo due to toxic substances, or the mother's age, health or nutrition can be risk factors that lead to a prenatal loss (Stewart, 1993). Spontaneous abortion is common; between 14-20% of all clinically recognized pregnancies end in this manner (Nybo, Wohlfahrt, Christens, Olsen, & Melbye, 2000). Furthermore, miscarriage is cited as the leading complication during pregnancy and the most prevalent gynecologic condition requiring hospitalization (Hammerslough, 1992; Nybo et al., 2000).

Pregnancy is a task that requires women to become accustomed to profound biological, somatic and psychological changes and involves achieving a maternal identity. When pregnancy is interrupted by miscarriage, a number of issues occur. These issues sometimes lead to existential confusion and a person's coping abilities and resources are tested, while salient attachment issues are exposed.

CONCEPTUALIZING PREGNANCY

Attachment Perspectives

John Bowlby (1969) first developed attachment theory to explain the physical and psychological distress children experience when separated from their primary caregivers. The theory has been expanded, and attachment has been defined as "an enduring affective bond characterized by the tendency to seek and maintain proximity to a preferred caregiver, particularly when under stress" (Ainsworth, 1978, p. 10). Biologically based, these bonds serve to enhance survival of the species (Bowlby, 1969). Additional components of attachment theory include the role of emotions and the impact of early life experiences on the creation of internal working models of attachment during one's life (Bowlby, 1982).

Attachment orientations, affect regulation, and support are the key elements in attachment processes (Bowlby, 1977). These elements are prescriptive and have a rudimentary function in a mother's ability to attach to her child. Simply stated, early bonds with our parents determine our ability to attach to others (Bowlby, 1988). In addition, healthy attachment patterns are analogous to a parent's ability to attach to their child. Studies indicate that the extent of attachment a mother has for the unborn child is highly correlated with the degree of emotional intensity and the length of pregnancy (Moulder, 1994). Further, attachment theory explains varied types of affective disregulation or dysfunction (Bowlby, 1977) subsequent to a maternal loss.

Recognizing the existence of fetal attachment during pregnancy, nurse researchers and child development specialists in the late 1970s called for an extension of Bowlby's theory (Muller, 1992). Prenatal attachment emerged from attachment theory and has been defined by Gaffney (1988) as "the component of the interactional process of attachment that develops within a mother prior to childbirth" (p. 106). This process not only involves tangible behaviors (i.e., feeling movement) but also more abstract things like fantasies about the baby and images of the self as a mother (Robinson, Baker, & Nackerud, 1999). To this end, Cranley (1981) expanded on maternal-fetal attachment and conceptualized it as "the extent to which women engage in behaviors that represent an affiliation and interaction with their unborn child" (p. 282).

The dynamics of prenatal attachment must be understood in contextual, multidimensional terms (Doan & Zimerman, 2003; Zimerman & Doan, 2003). Earlier research suggested a movement from the medical model explanation to a model that promotes understanding of attachment (Moulder, 1994). A universal discourse in the literature emphasizes that variables of attachment stem from situational, demographic and intrapersonal realms (Zimerman & Doan, 2003) and are subjectively controlled by age, culture (Stewart, 1993), and peripheral conditions, such as relationships and resources.

Bowlby's seminal work outlined his theoretical framework of attachment theory, providing a basis to conceptualize how preferences in attachments or affectional bonds to others are made (Bowlby, 1977). Attachment processes feature the development of an internal working model, initiated in infancy, which progresses throughout adulthood. This is matched by a person's cognitive development and can be primarily changed during times of trial and adversity (Bowlby, 1980; Simpson-Rhones, Campbell, & Wilson, 2001). Changes act as motivating forces that require individuals, when confronted with incongruencies, to modify, adapt, and integrate them into their model (Bowlby, 1980). Working models accommodate information about a person's worthiness of being loved; about significant others and whether they will provide security and safety during stressful times; and directives or rules that dictate attention toward or away from others. These directives are based on attachment specific interactions and the meaning assigned to them (Collins & Allard, 2001).

Further, the predisposition a person has in establishing affectional bonds with one individual over another is linked to attachment style and the rules that predispose attachments. These predispositions are based on prior attachment specific experiences with others. In summary, prenatal attachment sprung forth as an extension of Bowlby's attachment theory and attempts to give context to the unique predisposed bond that women may begin to have with their unborn child during pregnancy. Attachment theory may also help explain some of the reactions both women and men have following a miscarriage, based on their existing internal working models of attachment.

Developmental Perspectives

In addition to prenatal attachment, pregnancy can be viewed from other lenses. From a developmental perspective, pregnancy can be conceptualized as one of many potential life tasks that a woman may have, involving separation from her own mother, identification with her own adult body (Pines, 1996), and the construction of a separate maternal identity. This identity involves the reorganization of a woman's sense of self as a mother (Rubin, 1984). This experience is subjective and changes with each experience and child. Pregnancy serves as the preparatory period for this experience. Rubin (1984) writes: "the formation of a maternal identity that binds a woman to this child and to becoming the mother of this child is gradual, systemic, and extensive" (p. 39). Maternal identity development includes dreams and fantasies that a woman has while pregnant; dreams and fantasies that continue even after the child is born (Rubin, 1984).

Miscarriages generally occur during the first trimester. However, in spite of their brief time together, a significant bond may already have been established between the mother and her unborn child (Pines, 1996). This illuminates the attachment process of recognizing life (Speckhard, 2003), even prior to feeling fetal movement. Research examining the psychological antecedents and consequences of miscarriage, including abortion (Speckhard, 2003), show that a woman consciously experiences the emergent fetus as an integral part of herself (Pines, 1996). Thus, both attachment and maternal identity development may play a role in women's reactions to miscarriage.

DIVERSE RESPONSES AND REACTIONS

Women and men frequently have comparable reactions to miscarriage; and in the case of first pregnancies, loss can be exponentially greater as the couple is left with the poignancy of being childless. This fact may also be exacerbated in circumstances of later life pregnancies, which are presently observable in contemporary trends in childbearing. Identifiable themes arising from the aftermath of coping with a miscarriage include grief reactions, depression, anxiety, worries, relational difficulties, sexual dysfunction, attachment considerations, as well as practical concerns relative to provisions for the lost child (Hazen, 2003; Therbert-Wright, 2003). However, grief and depression subsequent to a miscarriage are routinely not acknowledged by professionals or family members (Friedman, 1989; Stirtzinger & Robinson, 1989). Interestingly, it is estimated that between 22-48% of patients suffer from psychological sequelae subsequent to reproductive loss that may extend over a period of six months (Friedman, 1989; Neugebauer et al., 1992).

Emotionally, parents may experience losing a part of themselves, losing a dream, in addition to losing the potential the child may have grown into (Herkes, 2002b). Researchers have found that a key element of mourning is yearning (Bowlby, 1982; Ritscher, 2002) and many parents, isolated in their grief, often attempt to cope with the emotional aftermath with unrecognized and prolonged affects (Anderson & Foley, 1997). Moreover, socially, the potential disenfranchisement, silence and secrecy surrounding unacknowledged grief may interrupt the healing process (Hazen, 2003). Explanations for these reactions are varied and encompass the intrapersonal, interpersonal, social, emotional, and psychological domains. They are, therefore, reflective of the breadth of impact the experience has on individuals and allude to the complexities that clinical treatment protocols will demand.

Herkes (2002a) felt the mourning process could be impacted by the fact that death has become institutionalized and the family no longer cares for their dying. Miscarriages are routinely handled by medical personnel as a medical procedure and sometimes parents are neither given information nor options. Moreover, parents may be forced to reevaluate their religious belief system and make religious connections in order to arrange a religious ceremony (i.e., funeral) to mark their babies' existence. As with any unanticipated death, in the first few days after a miscarriage, there may be a sense of shock and numbness. However, attending a funeral or memorial service may be important because it makes the event feel real. Further, an expression of acceptance may mark the beginning of the process of detachment from the pregnancy (Herkes, 2002a).

Ellen is a 35-year-old woman who suffered her second miscarriage. Distraught and grief-stricken, she sought ways to give place to her unborn children. With the help of her support system, she created rituals for honoring the life of her unborn children. Although she felt isolated by the sheer nature of the loss, Ellen recognized the support of family and close friends. They were there if she needed them.

One of her strongest sources of support is a woman named Sarah. Sarah is ten years older than Ellen and recalls the miscarriages she experienced almost twenty years earlier. Sarah recalls the stark silence in the room as she underwent surgery and the isolation and guilt she experienced following her loss. She asked herself, "Did I do something to cause this? Perhaps I am not fit to be a mother and God knows this." These fears remained unnamed as discussions about miscarriage were seldom held.

Decades later Sarah acknowledged her pain. Since then, enjoying authenticity and mutuality have become very important relational experiences for her. Her unacknowledged pain over her miscarriages triggered feelings of inadequacy and shame she could no longer bear. Now, she feels compassion for herself as the young woman who lost her children years ago and felt ashamed to say so.

There have been a number of psychological conditions linked to miscarriage including depression and anxiety disorders. There is a growing body of literature that discusses the emotional impact of miscarriage. Craig, Tata and Regan (2002) found that 33% of participants suffered from depression, with 9.9% of participants moderately depressed and

7.4% categorized as having severe depression. Twenty-one percent of the participants suffered form clinically significant anxiety. However, the degree of psychiatric morbidity was not affected by age, smoking cigarettes, alcohol intake, previous births, number of miscarriages, and lateness of miscarriage, nor length of time since last miscarriage (Craig et al., 2002).

The research suggested that the subsequent birth of a live child may decrease the psychiatric morbidity of women. However, when women have long term untreated clinically significant depression, it can affect the cognitive and emotional development of children who follow. Medical personnel are encouraged to be proactive and offer counseling to all patients following recurrent miscarriages to prevent later psychiatric problems (Craig et al., 2002).

IMPLICATIONS FOR COUNSELING

Counselors working with people who have suffered miscarriage can help by listening to their clients' stories, acknowledging their feelings, and supporting their right to have those feelings. The grief experience may be layered and the stories complex. For example, a woman might carry several stories about her pregnancy journey. These include her dreams and fantasies about motherhood (possibly stemming from cultural and familial ideas introduced at an early age); stories about conception (i.e., the process including highlights and struggles); the actual pregnancy (how, if relevant, it was confirmed, and the changes she might have noticed in her body); stories about herself as a mother; and stories about the actual child (dreams about them). In addition, there always exists the profound story of the actual miscarriage.

IMPLICATIONS FOR WOMEN

Women may have complex needs with respect to their miscarriage that can be processed in counseling. Initially, there may be issues related to the physical end of a pregnancy (i.e., bodily tissues, hormone levels). Other physical issues may be more complex and may include self- and other-blame (i.e., why can't my body carry a pregnancy to term?), issues associated with multiple miscarriages, body image concerns and even deeper thoughts (perhaps related to feminine archetypes) that may be connected to historical and cultural ideas about the inherent worth of women and the nature of females as nurturers and child-bearers.

Psychologically, there may be issues related to a woman's maternal identity development. For example, in the woman's mind, there are mothers and children all around her. She may well ask: Why not me? Self-doubts arise and questions become pressing. The woman may have had a dream, or story, about this particular pregnancy and child, as well as a vision of herself as a mother. The loss of the pregnancy may represent a challenge to a woman's status as a mother, even if only in her own mind (Layne, 2003).

Finally, there may be developmental needs that arise after the initial crisis has passed. For example, the woman may have been so consumed in the crisis of the moment that her reflections on treatment by medical professionals during the miscarriage catch up with her later (Moohan, Ashe, & Cecil, 1994). Positive contact with health care professionals has been linked with coping abilities after loss (Abboud & Liamputtong, 2005). Finally, there are socially sanctioned forms of grieving and healing and the particular case may or may not have called for a funeral or ritual service.

Further, the research on miscarriage has primarily focused on the grief response of parents and its psychological morbidity. A miscarriage can be devastating to not only the mother but also the entire family. Today's society has removed many of the traditional symbols of mourning (i.e., caring for the dead, wearing black, etc.) which has left family with few means for outward expressions of their grief. Without a socially acceptable means of mourning, parents may turn this grief inward onto themselves, which can result in clinical levels of depression and anxiety. In addition, a *code of silence* exists regarding pregnancy loss in the American culture that communicates remaining silent rather than attempting to understand this type of grief (Layne, 2003).

GRIEF AND LOSS

Given the frequency of miscarriage, counselors will likely encounter a client or family struggling with this issue. Several recommendations from the literature for counselors include: (a) the need for and importance of the counselor to appropriately recognize and address the signs and stages of normal and complex grief, (b) the meaning the pregnancy had for the woman and her family, and (c) the awareness of common reactions to miscarriage by women, their partners and families (De Frain, 1991; Elkin, 1990).

Counselors can listen to the stories parents tell to determine what type and/or stage of grief they may be experiencing. Grief responses may vary by gender and by culture, and people deal with these experiences within their unique social contexts (Abboud & Liamputtong, 2005). Marker and Ogden (2003) discovered that the stories grieving parents tell described their experiences as on-going rather than static because they changed and developed over time.

These researchers noted three stages of grieving seen in parent's stories. These stages include turmoil, adjustment and resolution. During the first stage of grieving, the researchers found that many of the participants felt unprepared, not only for the physical process of having a miscarriage, but also for the intense emotions that followed. As parents begin to transition into the adjustment stage, they search for meaning, share their story, and compare themselves socially to other parents. Many parents report that making social comparisons to others who have had reproductive problems made them feel better. Through sharing their stories, parents obtain support and improve relationships. However, for those that did not get the support they needed–it can be a lonely and isolated experience (Marker and Ogden, 2003).

Many parents try to find meaning respective to the cause of miscarriage. Some blame themselves for not taking better care of themselves, cite medical reasons, or stress at work. However, other parents are more philosophical and think of the miscarriage in terms of fate or destiny (Marker & Ogden, 2003).

Van (2001) found the grief response of African American women to be consistent with those reported by European American women. However, four distinct grief responses were identified in African American women. These included: (a) putting it aside, (b) there was a purpose, (c) heal yourself, (d) and he's in a good place. Some women felt the loss prepared them for a later role as a mother. Others were driven to focus on healing themselves. Life after death was a common theme described by women, with a belief that the baby was in a good place (i.e., heaven, with God, etc.). These healing techniques represent inner and instinctive processes, resources and remedies. It is important to remember that religion and spirituality are extremely valuable to many populations (Van, 2001).

Counselors should also educate couples on the different gendered ways of grieving to reduce miscommunications. Toedter, Lasker, and Alhadeff (1988) found that mothers react to loss through active grieving, sadness, and depression. Conversely, fathers are more likely to deny their grief and internalize feelings of loss. Many subsequently express their loss through higher levels of loneliness and anger. Moreover, the father's response to loss is consistent with the social expectation that men will show minimal affect, which leaves them with fewer social supports and outlets for expression (Stinson, Lasker, Lohman, & Toedter, 1992).

Differences in parental grief patterns can greatly impact a relationship. Couples frequently misunderstand each other or they may not want to burden their partner so they withhold feelings. Some men who are unable to express their grief and are encouraged to stay strong for their partners. Due to the fact that grieving is emotionally, physically, and mentally exhausting, there may not be much energy left to devote to the marriage (Herkes, 2002a).

THE ROLE OF SUPPORT

Given the stressors involved in grief work, support networks are vital to grieving parents. Supportive relationships may impact a family's ability to cope with their loss (Abboud & Liamputtong, 2005). Alternatively, when family and friends make comments that trivialize the loss, the loss becomes disenfranchised and parents may not feel the right to grieve for their baby. Even though this loss may be the first death they experience, many of the couple's friends, relatives and even professionals may find it inappropriate for the parent to grieve (Herkes, 2002b).

Without realizing, family and friends can doing more harm than good when they try to help by using clichés (i.e., you will have more children, you were lucky it was early in your pregnancy, the baby would have been deformed, etc.). Counselors should encourage couples to let their family and friends know how important the baby was to them and to ask them to help by simply listening. It is also important to recognize that young siblings are not too young to experience the loss. Counselors can encourage siblings, as well as other immediate family members, such as grandparents, to share their stories and express their feelings concerning the loss (De Frain, 1991).

COUNSELING CONSIDERATIONS

Initially, when working with clients that have experienced a miscarriage, it is important to listen to their story and to gain an understanding of the meaning the pregnancy may have held for them. There are several themes to be noted including: (a) personal history, (b) if the pregnancy was unacknowledged. If so, the experience may carry additional shame and/or secrecy. Sometimes, the telling and re-telling of a story in a safe place is enough to promote and facilitate healing. However, this process often takes time.

If the client's stories of the miscarriage lack closure–and the child they lost is unacknowledged by others in their lives, they may consider employing a ritual as an intervention. Rituals that provide symbolic acknowledgement help parents to give meaning to the experienced loss (Brin, 2004). In some cases, clients take family portraits and place a teddy bear in an empty seat to acknowledge their deceased child. Others purchase a cemetery marker, usually in a children's section, and participate in a symbolic remembrance ceremony. In second pregnancies where unresolved grief exists, a counselor may utilize interventions that focus on future parenting relationships.

When working with a woman and/or her family who has experienced a miscarriage, it is important for counselors to be aware of common reactions expressed by the bereaved, the unique meaning, including attachment and maternal identity variables attributed to the pregnancy, and common grief responses. This process will be illustrated in the example below.

LUCY'S STORY

Lucy was a 29-year-old woman, a successful graduate student and part-time waitress. She had maintained a long-term relationship with her partner, Colin. Lucy had anticipated delaying marriage and childbearing until her early thirties in order to graduate from school and launch her career. However, she unexpectedly discovered that she was pregnant, and experienced a miscarriage in the beginning of the second trimester.

Lucy was seen in counseling a year after the miscarriage occurred. She reported intermittent sadness and overwhelming feelings related to tasks in family life. When discussing her story of motherhood, Lucy explained that in her family, there was a social imperative, an unwritten rule, that one *must*, above all else, be a mother. During her early dating and college life, she described announcing that she was entering a university program. Instead of expressing joy and congratulations, her mother asked if there would be a financial penalty for withdrawal should she get married and become pregnant.

When she discovered that she was expecting a baby, Lucy delayed telling her family. She did tell Colin, and he was upset, telling her that this baby would chain them together and weigh them down from being able to achieve their individual and collective dreams. He urged her to consider an abortion. Lucy became distraught and spent a few weeks mulling over her options before deciding to have the baby. Lucy's familial and cultural values reflected an image of herself as a mother but she wasn't sure how this unexpected pregnancy would fit into her vision of herself as a married, career women.

Shortly after making her decision, Colin broke up with her. He said that he wanted nothing to do with her or her baby; and, to add insult, he said he wasn't even sure if the baby was his. Lucy was broken-hearted but in her grief, clung to the mental image of the baby growing inside her. She vividly remembered taking a shower and washing and patting her stomach, telling the baby that they, the two of them as a *family*, would be ok. She spent many hours talking to the baby, making mental plans for them, and processing how to tell her family.

One day, Lucy went to the bathroom and noticed a spot of bright, red blood. Terrified, she drove herself to the emergency room and checked in, telling them that she was pregnant. The nurse performing the ultrasound was unable to look her in the face or answer her questions about her child. Soon, two doctors came in and revealed that the baby did not have a heartbeat and that Lucy was in the process of miscarrying. She was quickly checked into the hospital, told that there needed to be something called a D & C, and was given forms to sign. Lucy had a hard time remembering what happened next, but she did remember calling her mother and asking her to come to the hospital where she told her the entire story.

In counseling, Lucy and her therapist worked to examine the dominant narrative stories that she had about herself; particularly her stories about her pregnancy and motherhood. While sad for her own loss, Lucy realized that her concept of motherhood was tied to her concept of being a good daughter; and that she had developed a dominant story about success being tied to parenthood. While she grieved for the baby she lost, Lucy also grieved for the loss of familial identity that a child may have brought her. She did, indeed, feel an attachment or connection to her unborn child. In addition, she had images of herself as a mother. Her inability to share her pregnancy with her family, especially her mother, was also related to the deep level of her grief. Because she had been unable to share the news of the pregnancy, her mother was so shocked when she called her that she was also unable to understand the miscarriage.

ACKNOWLEDGEMENT THROUGH RITUAL

Lucy and her counselor spent some time processing her stories. The counselor saw that Lucy's loss, and especially the connection with her loss of a child, was unacknowledged by her family. After the hospital procedures, Lucy never heard another thing about what happened to the remains of the child. The counselor suggested a ritual to remember the baby and asked Lucy to create a story about an aspect of the pregnancy that was meaningful for her. Lucy shared that when she first learned that she was pregnant, she went out and bought a pair of baby shoes. She still had the little pink shoes and they reminded her of her unborn baby.

The counselor suggested that they design a ritual to commemorate Lucy's unborn child. Lucy named her child and invited her mother and a few other members of her family and close friends to the ceremony. She created an altar in her garden to honor her baby, Macey. She placed the little pink shoes along with some pink roses on the altar. Lucy asked family and friends to contribute to a small stone on which she had her daughter's name, a pair of tiny shoes, and her birthday engraved. While she did not have Macey's physical remains, Lucy was able to create a special place where she could go and remember her child.

CONCLUSION

Miscarriage may be seen by some women and their partners as an expected loss; a minor obstacle on the road to family development. On the other hand, it can also be seen as a pivotal event for some women and their partners. The implications of an interrupted pregnancy can reach down deep into a woman's self-concept, her psyche, the very core of her being. When a client or couple who are struggling with a miscarriage come into counseling, it is important that they tell their story. Stories help us come to terms with our losses and give meaning to life. These stories can be given a place through ritual. In this respect, we have an opportunity to give voice to our experience and to bring dignity to our losses and unrequited hopes and dreams.

REFERENCES

Abboud, L., & Liamputtong, P. (2005). When pregnancy fails: Coping strategies, support networks, and experiences with health care of ethnic women and their partners. *Journal of Reproductive and Infant Psychology, 23,* 3-18.

Ainsworth, M. D. (1978). *Patterns of attachment: A psychological study of the strange situation.* Hillsdale, NJ: Erlbaum.

Anderson, H., & Foley, E. (1997). Experiences in need of ritual. *Christian Century, 114,* 1002-1008.

Borg, S., & Lasker, J. (1982). *When pregnancy fails: Coping with miscarriage, still-birth and infant death.* London: Routledge and Kegan Paul Ltd.

Bowlby, J. (1969). *Attachment and Loss: Vol. 1. Attachment.* New York: Basic Books.

Bowlby, J. (1977). The making and breaking of affectional bonds. *British Journal of Psychiatry, 130,* 201-210.

Bowlby, J. (1980). *Attachment and Loss: Vol. 3: Loss: Sadness and depression.* New York: Basic Books.

Bowlby, J. (1982). *Attachment, separation and loss (Vol. 2-3).* New York: Basic Books.

Bowlby, J. (1988). *Secure-base: Parent-child attachment and healthy human development.* New York: Basic Books.

Brin, D. J. (2004). The use of rituals in grieving for a miscarriage or stillbirth. *Women & Therapy, 27,* 123-132.

Collins, N. L., & Allard, L. M. (2001). Cognitive representations of attachment: The content and function of working models. In G. J. O. Fletcher & M. S. Clark (Eds.), *Blackwell handbook of social psychology: Interpersonal processes* (pp. 60-85). New York: Basic Books.

Craig, M., Tata, P., & Regan, L. (2002). Psychiatric morbidity among patients with recurrent miscarriage. *Journal of Psychosomatic Obstetrics and Gynaecology, 23,* 157-164.

Cranley, M. S. (1981). Development of a tool for the measurement of maternal attachment during pregnancy. *Nursing Residency, 30,* 281-284.

De Frain, J. (1991). Learning about grief from normal families: SIDS, stillbirth, and miscarriage. *Journal of Marital and Family Therapy, 17,* 215-232.

Doan, H., & Zimerman, A. (2003). Conceptualizing prenatal attachment: Toward a multidimensional view. *Journal of Prenatal Psychology and Health, 18,* 109-129.

Elkin, E. F. (1990). When a patient miscarries: Implications for treatment. *Psychotherapy, 27,* 600-606.

Friedman, T. (1989). Women's experience of general practitioner management of miscarriage. *J R Coll General Practice, 39,* 456-458.

Friedman, T. (1989). The psychiatric consequences of spontanious abortion. *British Journal of Psychiatry, 155,* 810-812.

Gaffney, K. F. (1988). Prenatal maternal attachment. *Image: Journal of Nursing Scholarship, 20,* 106-109.

Hammerslough, C. (1992). Estimating the probability of spontaneous abortion in the presence of induced abortion and vice versa. *Public Health Rep, 107,* 269-277.

Hazen, M. A. (2003). Societal and workplace responses to perinatal loss: Disenfranchised grief or healing connection. *Human Relations, 56,* 147-166.

Herkes, B. (2002a). A bereavement counseling service for parents: Part 1. *British Journal of Midwifery, 10,* 79-82.

Herkes, B. (2002b). A bereavement counseling service for parents: Part 2. *British Journal of Midwifery, 10,* 135-139.

Layne, L. (2003). *Motherhood lost: A feminist account of pregnancy loss in America.* New York: Routledge.

Marker, C., & Ogden, J. (2003). The miscarriage experience: More than just a trigger to psychological morbidity? *Psychology and Health, 18,* 403-415.

Moohan, J., Ashe, R. G., Cecil, R. (1994). The management of miscarriage: Results from a survey at one hospital. *Journal of Reproductive and Infant Psychology, 12,* 17-19.

Moulder, C. (1994). Towards a preliminary framework for understanding pregnancy loss. *Journal of Reproductive and Infant Psychology, 12,* 65-67.

Muller, M. E. (1992). A critical review of prenatal attachment research. *Scholarly Inquiry for Nursing Practice, 6,* 5-22.

Nybo, A., Wohlfahrt, J., Christens, P., Olsen, J., & Melbye, M. (2000). Maternal age and fetal loss: Population based register linkage study. *BMJ, 320,* 1708-1712.

Neugebauer, R., Kline, J., O'Connor, P., Shrout, P., Johnson, J., & Skodol, A. et al. (1992). Depressive symptoms in women in the six months after miscarriage. *American Journal of Obstetric Gynecology, 166,* 104-109.

Pines, D. (1996). Pregnancy, miscarriage, and abortion: A psychoanalytic perspective. *Journal of Obstetrics & Gynecology, 16,* 22-27.

Ritscher, J. B. (2002). Perinatal bereavement grief scale: Distinguishing grief from depression following miscarriage. *Assessment, 9,* 31-40.

Robinson, M., Baker, L., & Nackerud, L. (1999). The relationship of attachment theory and perinatal loss. *Death Studies, 23,* 257-270.

Rubin, R. (1984). *Maternal identity and the maternal experience.* New York: Springer.

Savage Garden. (1999). I knew I loved you. On *Affirmation* [CD]. NY: Sony.

Simpson-Rholes, J. A., Campbell, L., & Wilson, L. (2001). Changes in attachment orientations across the transition to parenthood. *Journal of Experimental Social Psychology, 39,* 317-331.

Speckhard, A. (2003). Universal responses to abortion? Attachment, trauma, and grief responses in women following abortion. *Journal of Prenatal and Perinatal Psychology and Health, 18,* 3-37.

Stewart, D. (1993). *Psychological aspects of women's health care.* Washington, DC: American Psychiatric Press.

Stinson, K., Lasker, J., Lohman, J., & Toedter, L. (1992). Parents' grief following pregnancy loss: A comparison of mothers and fathers. *Family Relations, 41,* 218-233.

Stirtzinger, R., & Robinson, G. (1989). The psychological effects of spontaneous abortion. *CMAJ, 140,* 799-806.

Therbert-Wright, C. (2003). Women's experiences with coping after late pregnancy loss: A qualitative study. *Dissertation Abstracts, 64,* 1-B, 433.

Toedter, L., Lasker, N., & Alhadeff, J. (1988). The perinatal grief scale: Development and initial validation. *American Journal of Orthopsychiatry, 58,* 435-449.

Van, P. (2001). Breaking the silence of African American women: Healing after pregnancy loss. *Health Care for Women International, 22,* 229-243.

Zimerman, A., & Doan, H. (2003). Prenatal attachment and other feelings and thoughts during pregnancy in three groups of pregnant women. *Journal of Prenatal and Perinatal Psychology and Health, 18,* 131-148.

doi:10.1300/J456v01n03_10

Chapter 11

Good Grief:
The Part of Arts
in Healing Loss and Grief

Trevor J. Buser
Juleen K. Buser
Samuel T. Gladding

SUMMARY. This manuscript considers the way that several creative media–including music, videography, visual arts, literature, drama, play, and altar-making–can be utilized in assisting the multifaceted grief process of clients. In particular, attention is given to the ability of creative media to enable clients to maintain a connection to the deceased, to access and express complicated emotions, and to gain confidence in authoring a new life story in the midst of loss. doi:10.1300/J456v01n03_11 *[Article copies available for a fee from The Haworth Document Delivery Service: 1-800-HAWORTH. E-mail address: <docdelivery@haworthpress.com> Website: <http://www.HaworthPress.com> © 2005 by The Haworth Press, Inc. All rights reserved.]*

KEYWORDS. Creative media, grief, loss, counseling, mental health

---

Trevor J. Buser and Juleen K. Buser are both graduate students at Wake Forest University.

Samuel T. Gladding is Professor and Chair, Department of Counseling, Wake Forest University, Winston-Salem, NC.

Address correspondence to: Samuel T. Gladding, PhD, Department of Counseling, Wake Forest University, P.O. Box 7406, Winston-Salem, NC 27109.

[Haworth co-indexing entry note]: "Good Grief: The Part of Arts in Healing Loss and Grief." Buser, Trevor J., Juleen K. Buser, and Samuel T. Gladding. Co-published simultaneously in *Journal of Creativity in Mental Health* (The Haworth Press, Inc.) Vol. 1, No. 3/4, 2005, pp. 173-183; and: *Creative Interventions in Grief and Loss Therapy: When the Music Stops, a Dream Dies* (ed: Thelma Duffey) The Haworth Press, Inc., 2005, pp. 173-183. Single or multiple copies of this article are available for a fee from The Haworth Document Delivery Service [1-800-HAWORTH, 9:00 a.m. - 5:00 p.m. (EST). E-mail address: docdelivery@haworthpress.com].

Available online at http://jcmh.haworthpress.com
doi:10.1300/J456v01n03_11

"Good grief!" is a common saying used by Charlie Brown in the popular *Peanuts* cartoons. It is a curious phrase to employ in the midst of unfortunate circumstances–a seeming contradiction in terms. Grief, of course, is rarely viewed in American culture as a positive, growth-promoting, or "good" part of the human story. Although individualized to persons and situations, human grief is a universal response to the losses and absences which indelibly alter life. The first associations for a person facing such loss are typically ones of negative thoughts, emotions, and behaviors, such as depression, isolation, and abandonment (LoCicero, 2006). Counselors, as well, may tend to speak of grief work with negative connotations.

Considering the many ways that grief emerges and is manifested, counseling for the bereaved is rarely simple or singular in form. The literature on grief has underscored a variety of major losses: those associated with the death of loved ones (Bermudez & Bermudez, 2002; Bowman, 1999; Hilliard, 2001a; Le Count, 2000; Mazza, 2001), the sorrow that comes from a mass trauma (Carmichael, 2000; Testa & McCarthy, 2004), the pain correlated with the anticipation of one's own impending death (Hilliard, 2001b; Rigazio-DiGilio, 2001); and the despair connected with the loss of physical movement, quality of life, ability, identity, and social community (Bright, 1999; Reynolds & Prior, 2003; Turetsky & Hays, 2003; Williams, 2000). Additional complexity is introduced by research indicating that responses to loss may vary significantly by gender (Schimmel & Kornreich, 1993; Servaty-Seib, 2004), age (Graham & Sontag, 2001; Kirk & McManus, 2002), and cultural background (Bermudez & Bermudez, 2002; Dalzell, 2005). It is, therefore, not surprising that counselors and clients alike are often quick to locate the negative sides of grief and aim toward "getting through" the stages of its process as expediently as possible.

On the other hand, perhaps Charlie Brown's cries of desperation for "good grief " can best be understood as yearnings and supplications, illustrative of the side of the griever that longs for something hopeful and healing in the very midst of incomprehensible loss. One way counselors may attend to these yearnings and, in some cases, actually make the process of grief "good" and health-promoting, is through use of the creative arts in therapy. By employing creative approaches, counselors access a range of interventions to meet the multifaceted nature of loss. Creative modalities, such as music, writing, video, art, and drama, can also unlock aspects and tasks of the grief process that clients find exceedingly beneficial and enriching. This article explores specifically the use of creativity to enable clients to maintain a connection to the deceased, to access and express emotions in the grieving process, and to gain confidence in authoring a new life story in the midst of loss. Each of these tasks serves as a marker to clients and counselors that grief is a normal part of human experience and may be embraced for its contributions to development throughout the lifespan.

STAYING CONNECTED WITH THE DECEASED

Gradual movement beyond loss and the ability to disconnect from the deceased are themes which are found in many traditional grief theories (Bermudez & Bermudez, 2002; Mystakidou, Tsilika, Parpa, Katsouda, & Vlahos, 2005). Such processes, however, are not always applicable to the individual mourner who values and expects to find a way to maintain a bond with one who has died. Indeed, for many grieving individuals, remaining close to the memory of a deceased loved one is essential to the mourning process. Moreover, several cultures–including Taiwanese culture (Hsu, Kahn, Yee, & Lee, 2003), Greek culture (Mystakidou et al., 2005) and Hispanic culture (Bermudez & Bermudez, 2002)–uphold connection with the dead as a source of strength. Taiwanese families, for instance, may create a symbolic image of the deceased, carry on conversations with the deceased, and strive for a connection with the deceased in the afterlife (Hsu et al.). Similarly, some members of the Hispanic culture maintain connection with the dead through their spiritual faith (Bermudez & Bermudez, 2002). In a related way, technological advances have become an avenue for many of us to maintain expression of lasting bonds with the deceased. The Internet has allowed many individuals to create a virtual record of their lives; Web sites such as *MySpace, Facebook*, and *LiveJournal* assist with such chronicling and allow additional forms of remembrance of those who have died (Shebar, 2006).

Creative therapies are a promising channel of connection between clients and deceased loved ones regardless of tradition. Bermudez and Bermudez (2002) discussed an eight-step therapy model built around an altar-making ritual with Latino/Hispanic families. Altars, or homemade shrines, may be viewed as ways to communicate with spirits, saints, and deceased relatives. The authors noted the memorializing value in this creative endeavor, during which time the client brings in valued objects, mementos, and pictures to attach to the altar:

> Making an altar helps them to reconnect and obtain a greater sense of peace and closeness . . . Clients are able to bring the person into the room and talk about the significance the person has in their life. This process can be healing and comforting and the outcome can serve as a constant reminder of the person they lost. (p. 340)

Music can also facilitate reconnection to the deceased. In an intervention with hospice patients, music therapy was revealed to be a powerful remembrance tool, allowing clients to recall joyous memories of loved ones in tandem with the experience of sorrowful loss (Hilliard, 2001b). Hearing the song *In the Good Old Summertime*, for instance, prompted one individual's warm memories of his deceased wife. The song became for this client a way to "keep her alive in his heart" (p. 163). In a uniquely powerful manner, music allowed this man to paradoxically voice his joy and sorrow in the same moment.

Videography is another creative technique which serves the remembrance purpose in grief counseling. Through the viewing of a video story, a family may re-experience treasured memories of the one who has died (Rigazio-DiGilio, 2001). One family's therapy was structured around the creation of a video with Christina, their adolescent daughter, during the last months of her life. The client family drew upon these videos in therapy "to remember, relive, and reinterpret what occurred, who Christina was, and the role each person played in her life and her caretaking" (p. 340). A motion picture enables this kind of dynamic interaction between individuals and their sense of loss, as clients attend to unsettling memories, unfinished business, or feelings of guilt in regard to the deceased. Rigazio-DiGilio recounted the experience of Christina's brother, who drew a new perspective from the video years after his sister's death. As this man observed his own son viewing the videotape made in therapy long ago, he found himself releasing a lingering sense of guilt over not being a good enough brother to Christina:

> When I watched my son laugh at my video of the woods, I knew I must have had an impact on Christina. A memory from so long ago leaves me with a precious thought of how hard I tried to be there, using the resources I had. Obviously, I did a good job. (p. 340)

An additional creative approach to grief therapy enacts the principles of object-relations theory through the intervention of artwork. Bereaved children who created artwork in this mode of counseling drew much strength from the memories of the deceased, recalling places and times of connection and certain characteristics of the deceased (Graham & Sontag, 2001). In this form of art therapy, several children began to take on specific remembered traits of the deceased, stating their identical likes, dislikes, and talents. The authors postulated that "the memories are the child's internalization of the self object of the deceased," an internalized object which can give the children a source of support, power, and self-esteem (p. 41). In a remarkable way, artwork maintained the bond between these children and their deceased loved ones, thereby endowing a sense of safety and accessibility in the midst of foreign terrain.

EXPRESSING EMOTIONS IN THE MOURNING PROCESS

The ability to express the delicate and potent emotions that arise out of a significant loss has been termed fundamental to the mourning process (Krout, 2005). Giving voice to grief, however, can be profoundly difficult; words seem to fail to capture the intensity of the sorrow and the abyss of distress (Bowman, 1999). The creative arts can enable an expression of emotion that transcends the usual verbal exchanges of therapy. Moreover, creative media may be a less threatening and more natural way for clients to acknowledge feelings of grief. Creative techniques, by virtue of their symbolic and metaphorical nature, afford the client a certain distance from and externalization of emotions. At other times, creative interventions may tap into a "primary process" of communication, in which a client is able to utilize diverse channels of expression that are more immediate and instinctive than the cognitive task of verbalizing emotion (Dokter, 1995, p. 19).

Some clients, such as children, have restricted verbal skills and clearly benefit from the symbolic communication of creative work. In this way, they are able to uncover grief that they have failed to recognize or feared to express (Carbone, 2003; Hilliard, 2001a; Kirk & McManus, 2002). Children may also be drawn to creative therapies because of their similarity to the play which is integral to childhood. The lightheartedness and enjoyment of creative approaches make them particularly well suited for children who have lost touch with the untroubled, blithe nature of childhood play (Johnson & Kreimer, 2005). Various creative media have been used to facilitate grief expression in children. Drama therapy is a technique cited as "a natural way for children to express their feelings and concerns" (Curtis, 1999, p. 184). In one drama therapy group format, children enacted a puppet dialogue, with various animals representing different responses to grief. They then acted out emotions such as denial, anger, and contentment (Curtis, 1999). Sunderland's "Museum of Loss" is another creative technique wherein a child visually places his or her losses on various museum stands, some of which are unlabeled and some of which are titled as "most recent loss," "most painful loss," and "earliest loss" (Le Count, 2000, p. 21). Clay can also be a creative medium which assists children in the expression of grief. In one group setting, children were given clay and were instructed to think of the person who had died; with peaceful music playing, the children were encouraged to make any clay creation that they desired (Carbone, 2003).

In addition, older populations have benefited from the healing properties of creative arts interventions. Reynolds and Prior (2003) reported on a group of women who were able to express their sorrow and loss through artwork: "almost every participant who poured her feelings of anger or sadness into her artwork did so without much awareness of the process at the time" (p. 788). Without intention or conscious thought, grievers were able to let loose their emotions into a creative medium. Furthermore, the words of other people–in music, prose, or poetry–often facilitate emotional expression for those who are developmentally capable of grasping meaning in these forms of communication. The ability of a musical lyric, for instance, to capture the depth of human feeling lends itself well to work with grieving individuals. As Bright (1999) noted, "in many instances, it is only through music that the affective content of the patient's story emerges" (p. 488). Likewise, therapist-composed songs have been used to assist clients in naming and conveying emotions of loss; carefully crafted lyrics can speak to the personal struggles of the grieving client and address a range of losses (Krout, 2005). In one music therapy model, the therapist first listened to the client's story and then played familiar music for the client, linked in some way to their grief experience (Bright, 1999). With this introduction of music, powerful emotions emerged which were not revealed in the client's earlier telling of his or her story. In later parts of the session, the therapist improvised music to document the themes of counseling and left a clear invitation for the client to give personal meaning to this music.

Story metaphors share this quality of enabling the acknowledgement of emotions. Carmichael (2000) chronicled the progress of a group for survivors of a tornado, which used the story *The Wizard of Oz* to provide metaphors for the grief of group members. This creative intervention was particularly useful in normalizing feelings and allowing a safe expression of emotions:

> The group members realize that their emotional responses to the disaster are common or acceptable reactions to situations, without the need for direct personal disclosure. The indirectness is especially powerful with persons who may be expected to be stoic and embarrassed by personal emotional disclosures. (p. 8)

Bowman (1999) further noted that "skilled writers have an ability to find words and phrases which capture the human condition and spirit" (p. 40). When immersed in the confusion, despair, and uncharted territory of grief, the words of poets and writers can voice what a mourning individual is not yet able to express. The tradition of lament can be particularly helpful for expressing a depth of anguish that is not yet hopeful or expectant (Bowman, 1999; Hiltunen, 2003; Wolterstorff, 1987).

CREATING MEANING AND A NEW LIFE STORY

A loss can shake the very foundation of life. It can throw one's sense of personal meaning and identity into a state of chaos (Neimeyer, Prigerson, & Davies, 2002). Therapy in the midst of such upheaval, therefore, may involve the tasks of re-authoring life stories and assigning new meaning to personal experiences. Indeed, Neimeyer (2001) conceptualized "grieving as a process of meaning reconstruction in the wake of loss," terming this the essential task of grief therapy (p. 261). Creative therapies offer grievers a new opportunity for constructing meaning out of their experience. With the aid of these interventions, clients have found the ability and confidence to generate new life stories, to craft enduring legacies, and to begin plans for the future.

Schimmel and Kornreich (1993) documented an art therapy group for widowed individuals, many of whom were struggling with a loss of identity after the end of a fundamental relationship. Through the creation of artwork, many members encountered feelings of empowerment, acceptance, and freedom, which were profoundly divergent from the experiences of frailty and vulnerability surrounding the death of a spouse. Women with chronic illness and disabling conditions may experience a similar undermining of identity; the activities, roles, and goals they once had can be suddenly thwarted. In one creative approach using textile arts, these women were able to gain self-esteem, a sense of capability, and a vision for the future (Reynolds & Prior, 2003). Group members cited many reasons for these outcomes of increased self-confidence and new perspectives on life, including the individual fulfillment of working with art, the encouraging responses of others, the ongoing nature of the art project, and the new social relationships centered on ties other than illness and disability.

The metaphorical group intervention mentioned above, which incorporated the story of *The Wizard of Oz* into therapy, also enabled participants to gain confidence and strength. Dorothy's magical shoes were discussed as symbolic of Dorothy's inner strength, a power that eluded her attention until later in the story. Through this metaphor, the group members were able to turn to their own "emotional strength" during the grief process and see signs of vitality instead of only weakness (Carmichael, 2000, p. 13).

Poetry and narrative writing may also be helpful for clients in fashioning a new life story and locating pockets of meaning. A new narrative can be crafted through creative writing exercises such as sentence stems, family poetry, and letters (Mazza, 2001). Such creation of a story may allow a client to leave a legacy which counter-balances the finality and sorrow of grief. Rigazio-DiGilio (2001), as noted above, chronicled the journey of one adolescent cancer patient, whose stories were recorded on videotape in order to leave an account of her life. "Ultimately, sessions end, but stories live on. The tapes, and how they were made, shared, and discussed become the living legacy. This legacy can be shared with future generations to create a sense of continuity of family" (p. 340). In such processes, the feelings of powerlessness of a terminally ill client may be considered alongside the generative effects of creative interventions.

Loss associated with large scale trauma can be positively impacted by creative techniques, as well. The painting of a mural to commemorate the tragedy of September 11th assisted one group of psychiatric inpatients in creating a legacy for others to see (Testa & McCarthy, 2004). Through the means of this creative approach, the group members would not allow death and destruction the last word: "they were able to communicate a powerful message of hope and remembrance for themselves and for viewers while rebuilding shattered trust in their future and in the world" (p. 41). As is demonstrated by these creative interventions, the grief associated with various losses in life can be influenced powerfully with the creation of artwork. The creative arts seed new meaning in the midst of the most despairing and vulnerable moments of life (Turetsky & Hays,

2003). With these approaches, counselors furnish opportunities for clients to re-vision life stories and establish enduring legacies.

CONCLUSION

The experience of grief is not easily understood or shared. Theorists have noted commonalities in the grief experiences of many individuals, yet the distinctive voice of each person in grief remains the guiding theme in the literature (Servaty-Seib, 2004). Creative techniques–and the sense of connection, reassurance, and possibility that they encourage–offer numerous opportunities for good expression of the multifaceted experience of mourning. These interventions facilitate recognition and utilization of the positive, enriching aspects of grief work.

As pointed out in this article, creativity may assist clients with three grief-related tasks: maintaining a bond to a deceased loved one, accessing and expressing complicated emotions surrounding loss, and shaping meaning in the face of distress and chaos. By way of these experiences, individuals may come to appreciate the process of grief as a very constructive part of the life journey. Clients, with the support of a creative counselor, may even uncover their own resolution to the cries for good grief, which leads them further along the path of development as persons. Through using creativity and the creative arts, rebirth and redirection may occur with all involved in the process.

REFERENCES

Bermudez, J. M., & Bermudez, S. (2002). Altar-making with Latino families: A narrative therapy perspective. *Journal of Family Psychotherapy, 13*(4), 329-347.

Bowman, T. (1999). Literary resources for bereavement. *The Hospice Journal, 14*(1), 39-54.

Bright, R. (1999). Music therapy in grief resolution. *Bulletin of the Menninger Clinic, 63*(4), 481-498.

Carbone, L. M. (2003). Using the arts in a bereavement group for children. In D. Capuzzi (Ed.), *Approaches to group work: A handbook for practitioners* (pp. 2-11). Upper Saddle River, NJ: Merrill Prentice Hall.

Carmichael, K. D. (2000). Using a metaphor in working with disaster survivors. *Journal for Specialists in Group Work, 25*(1), 7-15.

Curtis, A. M. (1999). Communicating with bereaved children: A drama therapy approach. *Illness, Crisis & Loss, 7*(2), 183-190.

Dalzell, R. (2005). Making sense of grieving. *Healthcare Counselling and Psychotherapy Journal, 5*(3), 20-22.

Dokter, D. (1995). Fragile board: Arts therapies and clients with eating disorders. In D. Dokter (Ed.), *Arts therapies and clients with eating disorders* (pp. 7-22). Philadelphia: Jessica Kingsley Publishers.

Graham, M., & Sontag, M. (2001). Art as an evaluative tool: A pilot study. *Art Therapy: Journal of the American Art Therapy Association, 18*(1), 37-43.

Hilliard, R. E. (2001a). The effects of music therapy-based bereavement groups on mood and behavior of grieving children: A pilot study. *Journal of Music Therapy, 38*(4), 291-306.

Hilliard, R. E. (2001b). The use of music therapy in meeting the multidimensional needs of hospice patients and families. *Journal of Palliative Care, 17*(3), 161-166.

Hiltunen, S. M. S. (2003). Bereavement, lamenting, and the prism of consciousness: Some practical considerations. *The Arts in Psychotherapy, 30,* 217-228.

Hsu, M., Kahn, D. L., Yee, D., & Lee, W. (2003). Recovery through reconnection: A cultural design for family bereavement in Taiwan. *Death Studies, 28,* 761-786.

Johnson, M., & Kreimer, J. (2005). Guided fantasy play for chronically ill children: A critical review. In L. A. Reddy, T. M. Files-Hall, & C. E. Schaefer (Eds.), *Empirically based play interventions for children* (pp. 105-122). Washington, DC: American Psychological Association.

Kirk, K., & McManus, M. (2002). Containing families' grief: Therapeutic group work in a hospice setting. *International Journal of Palliative Nursing, 8*(10), 470-480.

Krout, R. E. (2005). Applications of music therapist-composed songs in creating participant connections and facilitating goals and rituals during one-time bereavement support groups and programs. *Music Therapy Perspectives, 23*(2), 118-128.

Le Count, D. (2000). Working with 'difficult' children from the inside out: Loss and bereavement and how the creative arts can help. *Pastoral Care, 1,* 17-27.

Lo Cicero, J. P. (2006). *Complicated mourning: Assessment and intervention.* Paper presented at Wake Forest University, Winston-Salem, NC.

Mazza, N. (2001). The place of the poetic in dealing with death and loss. *Journal of Poetry Therapy, 15*(1), 29-35.

Mystakidou, K., Tsilika, E., Parpa, E., Katsouda, E., & Vlahos, L. (2005). Death and grief in the Greek culture. *Omega, 50*(1), 23-34.

Neimeyer, R. A. (2001). The language of loss: Grief therapy as a process of meaning reconstruction. In R. A. Neimeyer (Ed.), *Meaning reconstruction and the experience of loss* (pp. 261-292). Washington, DC: American Psychological Association.

Neimeyer, R. A., Prigerson, H. G., & Davies, B. (2002). Mourning and meaning. *American Behavioral Scientist, 46*(2), 235-251.

Reynolds, F., & Prior, S. (2003). "A lifestyle coat-hanger": A phenomenological study of the meanings of artwork for women coping with chronic illness and disability. *Disability and Rehabilitation, 25*(14), 785-794.

Rigazio-DiGilio, S. A. (2001). Videography: Re-storying the lives of clients facing terminal illness. In R. A. Neimeyer (Ed.), *Meaning reconstruction and the experience of loss* (pp. 331-343). Washington, DC: American Psychological Association.

Schimmel, B. F., & Kornreich, T. Z. (1993). The use of art and verbal process with recently widowed individuals. *American Journal of Art Therapy, 31*(3), 91-97.

Servaty-Seib, H. L. (2004) Connections between counseling theories and current theories of grief and mourning. *Journal of Mental Health Counseling, 26*(2), 125-145.

Shebar, A. (2006). *Logged off: Increased use of Internet in life leads to digital memories with death.* Retrieved March 12, 2006, from The Chronicle of Higher Education Web Site: http://wiredcampus.chronicle.com/

Testa, N., & McCarthy, J. B. (2004). The use of murals in preadolescent inpatient groups: An art therapy approach to cumulative trauma. *Art Therapy: Journal of the American Art Therapy Association, 21*(1), 38-41.

Turetsky, C. J., & Hays, R. E. (2003). Development of an art psychotherapy model for the prevention and treatment of unresolved grief during midlife. *Art Therapy: Journal of the American Art Therapy Association, 20*(3), 148-156.

Williams, R. M. (2000). Art, poetry, loss, and life: A case study of Ann. *Journal of Poetry Therapy, 14*(2), 65-78.

Wolterstorff, N. (1987). *Lament for a son.* Grand Rapids, MI: Wm. B. Eerdmans Publishing Company.

doi:10.1300/J456v01n03_11

Chapter 12

Keeping the Music Alive:
Using the "Grief and Hope Box"
with Adult Offenders
with Co-Occurring Mental Health
and Substance Use Issues

Robert Gee
Paul Springer
George Bitar
Faith Drew
Chad Graff

SUMMARY. Individuals with co-occurring mental health and substance use disorder (COD) present unique challenges for counselors.

Robert Gee is Assistant Professor, Department of Neuropsychiatry and Behavioral Science, Texas Tech University Health Sciences Center.

Paul Springer, George Bitar, and Faith Drew are PhD Candidates in the Marriage and Family Therapy Program, Department of Applied Studies, College of Human Sciences, Texas Tech University.

Chad Graff is Research Assistant, Department of Neuropsychiatry and Behavioral Science, Texas Tech University Health Science Center.

Address correspondence to: Robert Gee, Department of Neuropsychiatry and Behavioral Science, Texas Tech University Health Sciences Center, 3601 4th Street, Lubbock, TX 79430 (E-mail: robert.gee@ttuhsc.edu).

[Haworth co-indexing entry note]: "Keeping the Music Alive: Using the "Grief and Hope Box" with Adult Offenders with Co-Occurring Mental Health and Substance Use Issues." Gee, Robert et al. Co-published simultaneously in *Journal of Creativity in Mental Health* (The Haworth Press, Inc.) Vol. 1, No. 3/4, 2005, pp. 185-204; and: *Creative Interventions in Grief and Loss Therapy: When the Music Stops, a Dream Dies* (ed: Thelma Duffey) The Haworth Press, Inc., 2005, pp. 185-204. Single or multiple copies of this article are available for a fee from The Haworth Document Delivery Service [1-800-HAWORTH, 9:00 a.m. - 5:00 p.m. (EST). E-mail address: docdelivery@haworthpress.com].

Available online at http://jcmh.haworthpress.com
doi:10.1300/J456v01n03_12

When individuals are incarcerated, they suffer unique forms of losses, including the loss and grief of their family members. In addition, they often struggle with stigma and cultural stereotypes that are oppressive and devastating. The purpose of this manuscript is to help counselors and clients access creativity in a manner that facilitates client self-disclosure about grief and loss related issues, leading to a more coherent personal narrative, increased social integration, and enhanced psychological and physiological health. doi:10.1300/J456v01n03_12 *[Article copies available for a fee from The Haworth Document Delivery Service: 1-800-HAWORTH. E-mail address: <docdelivery@haworthpress.com> Website: <http://www.HaworthPress. com> © 2005 by The Haworth Press, Inc. All rights reserved.]*

KEYWORDS. Creativity, mental health, substance abuse, criminal justice, group counseling

> She never mentions the word addiction
> In certain company
> Yes, she'll tell you she's an orphan
> After you meet her family
> She talks to angels
> Says they call her out by her name
>
> (Robinson & Robinson, 1990)

INTRODUCTION

Individuals with co-occurring mental health and substance use disorder (COD) present special challenges for counselors. Many community members, including family members, health care providers, and counselors often convey that they feel inadequate and unprepared to help confront the multitude of losses they encounter. The problem of treating individuals with COD is especially challenging when psychosocial losses interact with loss associated with incarceration. It is important to recognize that individuals in this population often struggle with stigma and may be subjected to cultural stereotypes. It is equally important that counselors recognize that labeling them "alcoholics," "offenders," or "addicts" can be devastating.

Additionally, in not acknowledging the interaction between dynamics of power, oppression, privilege, gender, race, and social class we further perpetuate what is often viewed as individual pathology. While challenging, treating individuals with COD in the criminal justice system can be a positive experience when clinicians are able to access the innate creativity in themselves and their clients. The purpose of "The Grief & Hope Box" presented in this article is to access creativity in a manner that facilitates client self-disclosure about grief and loss related issues, leading to a more coherent personal narrative, increased social integration, and enhanced psychological and physiological health.

DEFINING THE PROBLEM

Substance Use

The Diagnostic and Statistical Manual of Mental Disorders (DSM-IV-TR) (American Psychiatric Association [APA], 2000) divides substance-related disorders into substance use disorders (which include both substance abuse and dependence disorders) and substance-induced disorders. According to the DSM-IV-TR (2000), substance abuse is a "maladaptive pattern of substance use manifested by recurrent and significant adverse consequences related to the repeated use of substances" (APA, 2000, p. 198). In contrast, substance dependence involves "a cluster of cognitive, behavioral, and physiological symptoms indicating that the individual continues use of the substance despite significant substance-related problems" (APA, 2000, p. 192). Substance-induced disorders include substance intoxication, substance withdrawal, and groups of symptoms that are in excess of those related to intoxication or withdrawal. In such cases, clinical attention is warranted.

Mental Health

Mental health terms and diagnoses are also derived from the DSM-IV-TR (2000). Due to the extent and variety of mental disorders, a full discussion of each one in this article is prohibitive. However, major disorders relevant for adults with COD are mood disorders (e.g., major depressive disorder, anxiety disorders) and personality disorders (e.g., narcissistic, histrionic, antisocial, etc.). It is important to note that these examples are not exhaustive and are meant only as illustrations of possible relevant mental health issues that co-occur with substance use issues.

Co-Occurring Disorders

The mental health and substance abuse fields have made considerable progress in defining a common language and providing a conceptual framework for addressing the needs of adults with COD (Center for Substance Abuse Treatment [CSAT], 2005a). Adults with COD have at least one diagnosable mental disorder, as well as, at least one diagnosable substance-related disorder (CSAT, 2005b). The range and combination variability of COD is extensive (Dixon et al., 2001). Counselors should be aware that each one of these disorders may interact differently within any one person (Drake & Wallach, 2000; Mueser et al., 2000). Indisputably, compared to adults with only one psychiatric concern, adults with COD are more severely impaired and more likely to experience negative social consequences (Minkoff, 2001).

The Substance Abuse Mental Health Services Administration's (SAMHSA) new Co-Occurring Center for Excellence (COCE) encourages the use of language and strategies that reflect the realities of clinical practice. Indeed, for many counselors, COD are inexplicably intertwined and have become the expectation, rather than the exception (Minkoff, 2001). In the United States, existing incidence rate studies estimate that 6 million to 10 million people have COD (Mueser, Essock, Drake, Wolfe, & Frisman, 2001; U. S. Department of Human and Health Services [USDHHS], 1999) and is expected to double to 15 million in the next 30 years (Substance Abuse Mental Health Services Administration [SAMHSA], 2002). If counselors fail to treat one disorder, both disorders usually become more severe (New Freedom Commission on Mental Health [NFCMH], 2003). Clearly, COD among the adult population warrants attention.

COD Among the Criminal Justice Population

Tragically, approximately 3% or 6.5 million adult men and women in the U.S. are under some form of correctional supervision (Bureau of Justice Statistics, 2001). Unfortunately, the likelihood that a person will be incarcerated increases dramatically if the person has COD (Beck & Harrison, 2001). Individuals in this population are incarcerated not because they have committed a violent or other serious crime, but because the service delivery system is ill-equipped to manage them (Drake, Wallach, Alverson, & Mueser, 2001). The magnitude of this problem can be seen in the landmark prevalence study, the National Comorbidity Study (NCS). (Kessler et al., 2005) and his colleagues estimate that 10 million Americans of all ages and in both institutional and non institutional settings have COD in any given year. The rate of special needs among this population is simply astonishing.

GRIEF AND LOSS ISSUES
AMONG ADULT OFFENDERS WITH COD

Grief and loss issues frequently occur for adult offenders with COD, including the loss of physical health (Ridgely, Lambert, Goodman, & Chichester, 1998), loss of significant relationships (Drake, Mercer-McFadden, Mueser, McHugo, & Bond, 1998), loss of shelter (Rahav et al., 1995), loss of freedom (Ditton, 1999), and loss of employment/ career (Drake, Wallach, Alverson, & Mueser, 2002). Above all, it could be argued that they experience a tremendous loss of future dreams.

In many ways, the loss and grief these individuals feel are unique. For example, when a father or mother is incarcerated, they may lose years of being able to interact with their child, missing important and irreversible events such as the child's first steps, first day of school, loss of first teeth, first dates, holidays, important cultural events (e.g., Quinceaneras, Bar Mitzvahs, etc.), weddings, and funerals. Often, other family members, friends, or state agencies step in to raise the children with little input from the incarcerated parent. The issues of grief and loss are compounded when incarcerated parents live with their children's grief and loss issues through letters, telephone conversations, and visitations. Furthermore, their family members and children suffer tremendous loss and grief as a result of the abandonment and incarceration of their loved one. Although the above example is limited to parental issues, it may be expanded to loss of career, health and freedom.

In her book, *Life Beyond Loss: A Workbook for Incarcerated Men*, Welo (1999) addresses the different types of grief and loss issues found in this population, including the loss of material goods, loss of job, loss of freedom, loss of dreams, loss of self control, loss of relationships, and loss through death. Further, many incarcerated men and women experience "disenfranchised" grief (Doka, 1989). Disenfranchised grief is defined as the situation where a person is not given the opportunity to "publicly grieve or acknowledge the loss" (Doka, 1989, p. 5).

Other researchers have investigated helping this population address grief and loss issues, as well. Schetky (1998) found that many offenders experience unresolved issues with grief and loss. With the help of a peer facilitator, she formed a prison-based support group to provide others an opportunity to cope with their grief. Olson and McEwen (2004) facilitated grief counseling groups with male offenders that explored disenfranchised grief and gender and cultural issues related to grieving. Woolfenden (1997) also characterized the benefits of a bereavement and loss group conducted in a closed women's prison. In summary, strong scientific evidence supports the reality that adult offenders with COD represent a major concern for counselors working with grief and loss issues.

CREATIVELY WORKING WITH ADULT OFFENDERS WITH COD

Multiple definitions of creativity exist depending on discipline, time, and culture however Dowd (1989) provides a simple, yet concise definition of the concept, "True creativity is invention or the process of making something new" (p. 233). In working with clients who may find therapy difficult, it is beneficial to provide novelty and ingenuity to enhance the therapeutic process. In addition to enhancing the therapeutic process for the client, creativity is also a way to decrease the likelihood of counselor burnout (Carson & Becker, 2003) when working with challenging populations (i.e., mandated clients with COD). The following section delineates the benefits of creativity for both client and therapist and, in so doing, describes the benefits of "The Grief & Hope Box" activity.

Creativity is essential in therapy (Carson & Becker, 2004; Deacon & Thomas, 2000; Hecker & Kottler, 2002), lending itself to the therapeutic process in multiple ways. For example, creativity assists clients in problem solving (Nickerson, 1999), viewing problems differently while enhancing divergent thinking (Dowd, 1989), and facilitating the development of coping skills while producing variety and amusement (Carson & Becker, 2003). More generally, creativity works to improve the quality of life, for both client and counselor, while enhancing knowledge related to making individual lives more interesting and productive (Csikszentmihalyi, 1996). Finally, in the therapeutic context, creativity works to decrease the problem of "stuckness" for both counselor and client (Hecker & Kottler, 2002). Clearly, creativity plays a vital role in therapy in general and, perhaps, plays an even more crucial role in the treatment of mandated clients with COD, a population that can be particularly challenging in treatment (Carlson & Garrett, 1999).

"The Grief & Hope Box" activity is intended to infuse treatment with creativity and the associated benefits. Particularly when clients struggle in the process of disclosing information, using creativity creates space for change and introspection, in addition to leaving an imprint on the minds and souls of all participants (Schofield, 2002). Creativity is a valuable aspect of the therapeutic process and should be integrated into treatment to enhance the overall experience of therapy for both counselor and client. "The Grief & Hope Box" activity provides one way of making creativity possible.

Self-Disclosure in Adults with COD

In addition to the benefits described, creativity creates space for change and introspection (Schofield, 2002) and facilitates the discussion of stressful and traumatic experiences related to grief and loss. Healing takes place, in part, through allowing clients to express their experiences around the stressful and traumatic events associated with imprisonment (i.e., separation from children and other significant family members). The following section establishes the empirical support for the benefits of self-disclosure.

The physiological and psychological benefits of self-disclosure are strongly supported in the literature. Expressing emotional thoughts, feelings, and/or memories (relative to writing about superficial control topics) has been associated with significant declines in healthcare visits (Pennebaker & Beall, 1986), long-term immune system benefits (Pennebaker, Kiecolt-Glaser, & Glaser, 1988), more rapid re-employment following job loss (Spera, Buhrfiend, & Pennebaker, 1994), decreased absenteeism from work (Francis & Pennebaker, 1992), an improved college adjustment process, and higher grade point averages in undergraduate college students (Cameron & Nichols, 1998). Additionally, several other studies have examined the positive biological effects of disclosure, highlighting the dynamic relationship between the mind and body (Christenson et al., 1996; Dominguez et al., 1995; Francis & Pennebaker, 1992; Pennebaker, Hughes, & O'Heeron, 1987; Petrie & Booth, 1995).

Three Hypotheses: Inhibition, Cognition, and Social Integration

In hypothesizing *why* research consistently supports the benefits of disclosure, Pennebaker proposes three inter-related theories for an explanation: (a) inhibition theory, (b) cognitive organization, and (c) social integration (Pennebaker, 1997). Pennebaker (2001) describes inhibition theory as follows:

> To actively inhibit ongoing thoughts, emotions, or behaviors, requires work–physiological work. We can see the work of inhibition in autonomic nervous system activity as well as brain and even hormonal activity. Over time, inhibition serves as a long-term, cumulative, low-level stressor that affects the body. This inhibitory stress, then, can cause or exacerbate a number of psychosomatic illnesses. The reverse side to this theory is that if we can get people to stop inhibiting, their health should improve. (Pennebaker, 2001, p. 34)

Pennebaker supports the rationale for the theory by citing the numerous studies that have found an association between disclosure, higher immune-functioning, and decreased physician visits.

Pennebaker (2001) explains that the limits of inhibition theory were realized during follow-up research when participants were asked to describe what was helpful about the expressive activity. The researcher explains that the participants "kept using words like 'understandable,' 'realize,' 'come to terms,' 'getting past,' at high rates," leading to the belief that there was "something very cognitive going on besides just a reduction in inhibition" (Pennebaker, 2001, p. 39). Pennebaker uses the metaphor of a "story" or "narrative" and hypothesizes that there is a relationship between an individual's ability to construct a personal narrative and a cessation of negative affect. Pennebaker states that the process of constructing a story "allows one to organize and remember events in a coherent fashion, while integrating thoughts and feelings . . . Once an experience has structure and meaning, it would follow that the emotional effects of that experience are more manageable" (Pennebaker, 2001, p. 39).

Finally, the third hypothesis that Pennebaker (2001) proposes involves the process of greater disclosure leading to increased social integration. Pennebaker explains that keeping a secret or feelings or thoughts related to a stressful or traumatic experience has an isolating effect,

> If I have a traumatic experience and can't tell anyone about it, no one in my social world will know what I'm thinking and feeling. I will be preoccupied with the emotional event. The longer I live with this secret, the more detached I will be from others in my social world. Almost by definition, I will become more and more iso-

lated. I'll be a poor listener, and will be guarded in my discussions with others. (Pennebaker, 2001, p. 42)

Pennebaker, therefore, hypothesizes that one of the effects of writing and talking about traumatic experiences may be a greater level of social integration, as isolating emotions are expressed and their effects are reduced in intensity. In integrating all three hypotheses, Pennebaker (2001) states the following, "When we write about upsetting experiences, we no longer need to inhibit, we find cognitive coherence and closure, and we are able to return to our normal, healthy social lives" (p. 43).

The research on self-disclosure has direct application to this activity. As clients write down issues related to grief and loss and then discuss their experiences in the context of this activity, they are more likely to create a coherent narrative, they are less likely to inhibit emotion, and they are more likely to experience an increase in social integration, both within the group therapy and outside of group therapy. This activity, therefore, has the potential to move clients one step closer to improved psychological, physiological, and social health.

THE GRIEF AND HOPE BOX

The purpose of this activity is to provide a safe structure where individual group members may begin to externalize the pain surrounding the grief and loss they have experienced in their life. In addition, this activity may also help the group members develop insight into their own healing process and ways they can fully mourn the loss.

Volkan and Zintl (1993) speak to the importance of understanding grief and loss in the following passage:

> Three things are fundamental to an understanding of mourning. First, each loss launches us on an inescapable course through grief. Second, each loss revives all past losses. Third, each loss, if fully mourned, can be a vehicle for growth and regeneration. (p. 22)

Consequently, the meanings attributed to personal loss may provide a rich window into intra-psychic and interpersonal realms of how group members are processing and dealing with their grief and loss. "The Grief & Hope Box" activity is a process and should be conducted in such a manner that allows group members the necessary time and space needed to explore the meanings behind their loss. As group members begin to externalize their grief, and explore the meanings behind it, therapy can be used as a catalyst to enhance insight and growth in their lives.

Instructions

When working with adult offenders with COD, it is important to understand that grief and loss are a part of their everyday life. From the moment of incarceration, they are faced with the loss of their freedom, loss of employment, loss of choice, loss of their children, and loss of their spouse, family members and friends. However, these individuals rarely talk openly about this loss, in fear of being portrayed as vulnerable or weak. As a result, this activity is most effective when used with an established group after cohesion and safety issues have been established. It is our experience that in a safe environment, group members are more likely to be open and sincere about their loss, and that group members readily demonstrate support to one another throughout this process.

Items Needed for Exercise

1. Scissors (enough for each group member);
2. Markers, crayons and colored pencils;
3. Tape or glue; and
4. Box outlines (enough copies for each group member).

Ground Rules

At the beginning of the group session, the facilitator introduces the idea of the "The Grief & Hope Box" activity, explaining how each member of the group has experienced loss that often holds them back into becoming the person they want to become. Examples of this grief or loss might be the shame or guilt emotions that the group member experiences in the separation from their children or family members. Another possible example may be the emptiness felt in a spouse not waiting for them, or the pain of having a love one die while the group member was incarcerated in prison. The facilitator explains that just like a box, grief builds a wall that may prevent us from growing into the person we want to become. As a result, group members may fail to reach out to others, or express their emotions in a positive way. The facilitator then asks the group to reflect on their own lives and think of what issues of grief and loss are keeping them captive and from truly finding and living their dreams.

Process

1. Each group member goes to different parts of the room, where they can be alone.
2. Group members are instructed to cut out their own "Grief & Hope Box."
3. They are then asked to draw and or write what issues of grief and loss are keeping them captive; on each of the four sides of the box. Group members are encouraged to be as creative as possible.
4. Next, group members are instructed to assemble their "Grief & Hope Box."
5. Once the boxes are assembled, the group facilitator asks the group member to look within themselves and think of the positive attributes that are locked inside of their box. These attributes may be the vulnerable aspects of their lives that they would like to express, but do not because of the "walls" surrounding them. Again, group members are encouraged to be as creative and reflective as possible and to write these attributes on the inside of their box.
6. Once they have completed this task, the groups members are asked to return to their seats with their "Grief & Hope Box" in hand.

At this point, the facilitator may choose to self-disclose and model the exercise, explaining his/her issues of grief or loss in his/her life to begin the exercise. Having the facilitator begin "The Grief & Hope Box" activity has the advantage of illuminating the significance of one's grief and loss. This can be an important first step, since many people do not generally realize the impact and meaning of grief and loss in their lives. Additionally, as the facilitator displays vulnerability by beginning the activity, group members may be more likely to also respond in a more vulnerable manner. As with any disclosure, the facilitator must be sure that his/her own vulnerability adds to the therapeutic context and does not distract from the therapeutic process. If the facilitator feels uncomfortable participating, he/she may choose to take the one down position and ask the group members to help him/her understand the impact of their experiences with grief and loss issues. During this process, the group facilitator may choose to ask clarifying questions and use reflective comments during the group members' disclosure.

THE GRIEF & HOPE BOX: CASE EXAMPLE

The following are a few examples of how this activity was applied to a "Working Group" of adult offenders with COD facing community reintegration issues. In this case example, the first group session is spent on exploring issues of grief and loss. The next or second group session focused on the group member's positive attributes that are held hostage within their box. Please note that fictional names are used in the following two illustrations.

Tom's Loss

Tom was an active participant in our group, having been recently released from prison after serving seven years on a drug-related offense. While Tom reported that he was glad to be out of prison, he stated that he was struggling with family and employment reintegration issues. Specifically, Tom stated that he was not able to forgive himself for "not being there" for his children. Accordingly, Tom was able to use this activity to express his grief and loss in a supportive and understanding environment. In addition, Tom met the DSM-IV-TR criteria for a depressive and substance use disorder.

Tom began the activity in describing his box of "loss" as "un-scalable walls of guilt and shame." On each wall, Tom drew bricks enclosing around himself with the words: "BAD PARENT," "SELFISH," and "LOST MOMENTS" in large black letters. He described each of these words as "suffocating" and "immobilizing." In fact, Tom reported that these words often flashed in his mind when he was at home, and kept him from taking present action in being the father his children needed. Whenever he tried to take a more active role in parenting, he reported that he would often feel shame as his children frequently lashed out in anger because he "was not there" for them. Tom reported that this experience would further reinforce his behavior to withdraw and remained uninvolved with his family, perpetuating a vicious cycle.

As group facilitators, we felt that Tom's experience was not isolated and probed other group members if they experienced some of the same or similar emotions. The response was almost universal. Several group members were able to describe feeling identification with Tom, and provided insight into how they overcame their own shame and guilt surrounding parenting issues, incarceration, and COD. Another group member described her parenting struggle, as a process of learning how to "accept the time she lost" with her kids, while at the same time, recognizing that she could not allow herself to lose what little precious time she had left with them. As Tom listened to her story, it became clear that he felt supported and heard. He seemed to have felt empowered by the group members' altruism and their empathic stance. By overtly identifying the problem, Tom was able to verbalize what the tasks he needed to accomplish in order to overcome the problem, even at the risk of being rejected by his children. This therapeutic process also allowed Tom and other group members an opportunity to self-disclose their emotions surrounding grief and loss issues, facilitating the development of more coherent personal narratives and increasing feelings of connection that would, hopefully, carry over to their relationships outside the group process. Figure 1 illustrates an example of the completed outside walls of the "Grief & Hope Box."

FIGURE 1. The Grief and Hope Box–Tom's Outside Walls

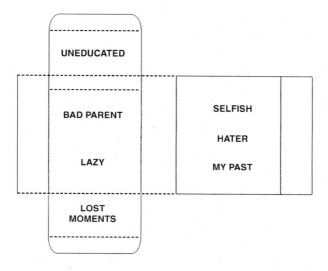

Chris' Shame

Chris was the youngest member of the group, age 23, and had served over two years in prison for drug-related offense. Unlike Tom, Chris had no children, and was struggling with entirely different issues of grief and loss that were preventing him from accepting the responsibility of his life. Likewise, at the intake assessment, Chris met the DSM-IV-TR criteria for an anxiety-related and substance use disorder.

Chris' box was less detailed than other group members. However, the meaning Chris associated with the "Grief & Hope Box" activity was just as emotionally laden. On each wall of his box, Chris had written in large letters: "LOSS of FAMILY" and "SCHOOL." He described losing contact with his family, and his uncertainty of enrolling in school and pursuing an education. Chris described himself as someone who was "never really in trouble," but was "involved with the wrong crowd" when he attended college. As a result, he reported that began using drugs, eventually selling substances "to earn extra cash." Unfortunately, Chris stated, this led to his arrest and subsequent conviction.

Chris described the loss of his family as "devastating." He stated that he has had little contact with them since his incarceration. In fact, Chris reported that his father had not spoken or communicated with him in over two years. Chris stated that he was extremely "hurt and depressed" by this experience, and that he longed to have a relationship with his father. Nevertheless, Chris reported that he "felt too much shame and guilt to even attempt to contact them." Much like a ship without a rudder, Chris felt directionless in his life, and stated that he did not know how to reach out to his family. Chris then turned to the group for help.

One group member quickly shared his own experience of his family's initial reaction to his legal troubles. However, the group member shared that after time, his family slowly began reaching out to him. The group member shared that he believed his family was struggling with grief and loss, as well, and that they were unsure of what or how to support him. His fellow peer indicated that his family was afraid that he had not changed and may again become involved with drugs. Other group members encouraged Chris to take the responsibility of reaching out to his family. Still other group members supported Chris by providing positive feedback of his current behavior (e.g., employment, compassionate, genuineness, etc.). Another group member indicated that Chris was responsible for his actions and not for his family's actions. Chris seemed to appreciate the feedback, and began to formulate concrete tasks he could accomplish in order to begin rebuilding his family relationships. At the end of the group session, Chris told his group peers that he intended to send his family a card letting them know how he was doing.

SECOND GROUP SESSION

During the second group session of "The Grief & Hope Box" activity, group members shared their positive attributes that may often be "held hostage" by their feelings of grief and loss. In addition, group members discussed possible avenues and strategies for empowering these positive attributes.

Tom's Strengths

When it was Tom's turn to discuss what he had written inside his "Grief & Hope Box," he disclosed the difficulty of identifying his positive attributes. He reported that it wasn't until the previous group session that he realized the incredible impact that his grief and loss issues had taken on his perception of self, especially in relation to his children. Tom then opened his box and stated that his greatest strength was often his greatest liability, his CHILDREN. Tom self-disclosed how he finds strength in wanting to be a good father, and that he recognizes the COMPASSION and LOVE he has for them. Even after his children lash out at him, Tom stated that he hangs on to the HOPE that things can be better. Tom declared that HOPE keeps him "from quitting."

As group facilitators, we praised Tom for identifying the compassion and love he feels for his children and challenged him on ways he can make his HOPE a reality. As Tom explored possibilities, several group members assured him that in redefining parental boundaries, things may become worse before stabilizing and enjoying a healthier, productive life with his children. His fellow group peers encouraged him to demonstrate stability and consistency with his children "showing that he is home to stay." Interestingly, at the end of sharing his positive attributes, Tom smashed his "Grief & Hope Box" symbolizing the freedom of his positive attributes. Figure 2 illustrates an example of the completed inside walls of the "Grief & Hope Box."

FIGURE 2. The Grief and Hope Box–Tom's Inside Walls

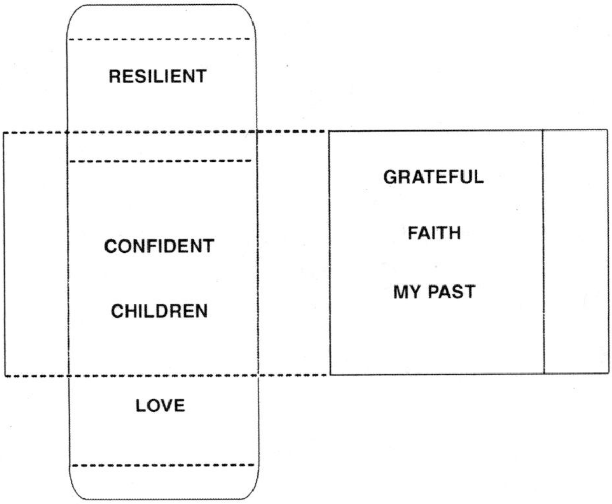

Chris' Strengths

Chris identified his strengths as his FAITH in God and DESIRE TO BE DIFFERENT. Chris stated that he believes that God has a life purpose for him, and that he believes that his life experiences happen purposefully. Chris shared that this faith has helped him find meaning in his struggles and perseverance in his life.

He identified with a strong desire to "make something" of himself, and to "prove to himself and his family" that he can "be someone." He reported that he realizes being extremely fortunate that he was not sentenced to a longer period of incarceration, and that he still has an opportunity to go to school. Group members encouraged Chris to take advantage of his opportunity to go to school and better his life. At the end of his sharing, Chris emphatically smashed his box several times.

DISCUSSION

As demonstrated in the above case illustration, "The Grief & Hope Box" activity is a way to access client creativity in a manner that facilitates self-disclosure surrounding issues of grief and loss among adult offenders with COD. This activity also provides a creative way for clients to identify strengths that may be constrained by issues of grief and shame, thus facilitating discussions related to growth and healing. While treating individuals with COD in the criminal justice system can be challenging, creative activities such as "The Grief & Hope Box" activity provide a method of accessing and exploring previously unidentified and suffocating feelings and beliefs related to grief and loss. The activity may also help to build group cohesion, decrease feelings of isolation outside of the group experience, and improve psychological functioning. Moreover, creative activities, such as "The Grief & Hope Box" provides opportunities for incarcerated parents to grieve their losses and build a new dream.

REFERENCES

American Psychiatric Association. (2000). *Diagnostic and statistical manual of mental disorders* (4th ed.). Washington, DC: American Psychiatric Association.

Beck, A. J., & Harrison, P. M. (2001). *Prisoners in 2000* (NCJ 188207). Washington, DC: U.S. Department of Justice, Office of Justice Programs, Bureau of Justice Statistics.

Bureau of Justice Statistics. (2001). *National corrections population reaches new high grows by 117,400 during 2000 to total 6.5 million adults.* Washington, DC: U.S. Department of Justice, Office of Justice Programs, Bureau of Justice Statistics.

Cameron, L., & Nichols, G. (1998). Expressions of stressful experiences through writing: Effects of self-regulation manipulation for pessimists and optimists. *Health Psychology, 17*(1), 84-92.

Carlson, P. M., & Garrett, J. S. (1999). *Prison and jail administration: Practice and theory.* Gaithersburg, MD: Aspen Publishers.

Carson, D. K., & Becker, K. W. (2003). *Creativity in psychotherapy: Reaching new heights with individuals, couples, and families.* New York, NY: Haworth Clinical Practice Press.

Carson, D. K., & Becker, K. W. (2004). When lightning strikes: Re-examining creativity in psychotherapy. *Journal of Counseling & Development, 82*(1), 111-115.

Center for Substance Abuse Treatment. (2005a). Definitions and terms relating to co-occurring disorders (COCE Overview Paper No. 1). Rockville, MD: Substance Abuse and Mental Health Services Administration, and Center for Mental Health Services.

Center for Substance Abuse Treatment. (2005b). Substance abuse treatment for persons with co-occurring disorders, treatment improvement protocol tip series 42 (DHHS Publication No. SMA 05-3922). Rockville, MD: Substance Abuse and Mental Health Services Administration.

Christensen, A. J., Edwards, D. L., Wiebe, J. S., Benotsch, E. G., McKelvey, L., & Andrews, M. et al. (1996). Effect of verbal self-disclosure on natural killer cell activity: Moderating influence of cynical hostility. *Psychosomatic Medicine, 58,* 150-155.

Csikszentmihalyi, M. (1996). *Creativity: Flow and the psychology of discovery and invention.* New York, NY: HarperCollins Publishers.

Deacon, S. A., & Thomas, V. (2000). Discovering creativity in family therapy: A theoretical analysis. *Journal of Systemic Therapies, 19*(3), 4-17.

Ditton, P. M. (1999). *Mental health and treatment of inmates and probationers.* Washington, DC: Bureau of Justice Statistics.

Dixon, L., McFarlane, W. R., Lefley, H., Lucksted, A., Cohen, M., & Falloon, I. et al. (2001). Evidence-based practices for services to families of people with psychiatric disabilities. *Psychiatic Services, 52,* 903-910.

Doka, K. J. (1989). Disenfranchised grief. In K. J. Doka (Ed.), *Disenfranchised grief: Recognizing hidden sorrow* (pp. 3-11). Lexington, MA: Lexington Books.

Dominguez, B., Valderrama, P., Maria de los Angeles, M., Perez, S., Silva, A., & Martinez, G. et al. (1995). The roles of disclosure and emotional reversal in clinical practice. In J. Pennebaker (Ed.), *Emotion, disclosure, and health* (pp. 255-270). Washington, DC: American Psychological Association.

Dowd, E. T. (1989). The self and creativity: Several constructs in search of a theory. In J. A. Glover, R. R. Ronning, & C. R. Reynolds (Eds.), *Handbook of creativity: Perspectives on individual differences* (pp. 233-242). New York, NY: Plenum Press.

Drake, R. E., Mercer-McFadden, C., Mueser, K. T., McHugo, G. J., & Bond, G. R. (1998). Review of integrated mental health and substance abuse treatment for patients with dual disorders. *Schizophrenia Bulletin, 24,* 589-608.

Drake, R. E., & Wallach, M. A. (2000). Dual diagnosis: Fifteen years of progress. *Psychiatric Services, 51,* 1126-1129.

Drake, R. E., Wallach, M. A., Alverson, H. S., & Mueser, K. T. (2002). Psychosocial aspects of substance abuse by clients with severe mental illness. *The Journal of Nervous and Mental Disease, 190,* 100-106.

Francis, M. E., & Pennebaker, J. W. (1992). Putting stress into words: The impact of writing on physiological, absentee, and self-reported emotional well-being measures. *American Journal of Health Promotion, 6*(4), 280-287.

Hecker, L. L., & Kottler, J. A. (2002). Growing creative therapists: Introduction to the special issue. *Journal of Clinical Activities, Assignments & Handouts in Psychotherapy Practice, 2*(2), 1-3.

Kessler, R. C., Birnibaum, H., Demler, O., Falloon, I. R. H., Gagnon, E., & Guyer, M. et al. (2005). The prevalence and correlates of nonaffective psychosis in the national comorbidity survey replication (NCS-R). *Biological Psychiatry, 58*(8), 668-676.

Minkoff, K. (2001). Developing standards of care for individuals with co-occurring psychiatric and substance use disorders. *Psychiatric Services, 52,* 597-599.

Mueser, K. T., Essock, S. M., Drake, R. E., Wolfe, R. S., & Frisman, L. (2001). Rural and urban differences in patients with a dual diagnosis. *Schizophrenia Research, 48,* 93-107.

Mueser, K. T., Yarnold, P. R., Rosenberg, S. D., Swett, C., Miles, K. M., & Hill, D. (2000). Substance use disorder in hospitalized severely mentally ill psychiatric patients: Prevalence, correlates, and subgroups. *Schizophrenia Bulletin, 26,* 179-192.

New Freedom Commission on Mental Health (NFCMH). (2003). Achieving the promise: Transforming mental health care in America–Final Report (DHHS Pub. No. SMA-03-3832). Rockville, MD: Author.

Nickerson, R. S. (1999). Enhancing creativity. In R. J. Sternberg (Ed.), *Handbook of creativity* (pp. 392-430). New York, NY: Cambridge University Press.

Olson, M. J., & McEwen, M. A. (2004). Grief counseling groups in a medium-security prison. *Journal for Specialists in Group Work, 29*(2), 225-236.

Pennebaker, J. (1997). Writing about emotional experiences as a therapeutic process. *Psychological Science, 8,* 162-166.

Pennebaker, J. (2001). Explorations into the health benefits of disclosure: Inhibitory, cognitive, and social processes. In L. L'Abate (Ed.), *Distance writing and computer assisted interventions in psychiatry and mental health* (pp. 25-55). London: Westport.

Pennebaker, J. W., & Beall, S. K. (1986). Confronting a traumatic event: Toward an understanding of inhibition and disease. *Journal of Abnormal Psychology, 95*(3), 274-281.

Pennebaker, J. W., Hughes, C. F., & O'Heeron, R. C. (1987). The psychophysiology of confession: Linking inhibitory and psychosomatic processes. *Journal of Personality and Social Psychology, 52,* 781-793.

Pennebaker, J. W., Kiecolt-Glaser, J. K., & Glaser, R. (1988). Disclosure of traumas and immune function: Health implications for psychotherapy. *Journal of Consultation and Clinical Psychology, 56,* 239-245.

Petrie, K., & Booth, R. (1995). Disclosure of trauma and immune response to a Hepatitis B vaccination program. *Journal of Consulting and Clinical Psychology, 63*(5), 787-793.

Rahav, M., Rivera, J. J., Nuttbrock, L., Ng-Mak, D., Sturz, E. L., Link, & B. G. et al. (1995). Characteristics and treatment of homeless, mentally ill, chemical-abusing men. *Journal of Psychoactive Drugs, 27,* 93-103.

Ridgely, M. S., Lambert, D., Goodman, A., & Chichester, C. S. (1998). Interagency collaboration in services for people with co-occurring mental illness and substance use disorder. *Psychiatric Services, 49,* 236-238.

Robinson, C., & Robinson, R. (1990). She talks to angels (Recorded by The Black Crowes). On *Shake Your Money Maker* (CD). Burbank, CA: Def American. (1990).

Schetky, D. H. (1998). Mourning in prison: Mission impossible? *The Journal of The American Academy of Psychiatry and the Law, 26*(3), 383-391.

Schofield, M. J. (2002). Creative mediation to enhance positive feeling states and inner resources. *Journal of Clinical Activities, Assignments, & Handouts in Psychotherapy Practice, 2,* 59-75.

Spera, S., Buhrfeind, E., & Pennebaker, J. (1994). Expressive writing and coping with job loss. *Academy of Management Journal, 37,* 722-733.

Substance Abuse Mental Health Services Administration's (SAMHSA) (2002). Report to Congress on the Prevention and Treatment of Co-Occuring Substance Abuse Disorders and Mental Disorders. Rockville, MD: Author.

U.S. Department of Health and Human Services. (1999). Mental health: A report of the Surgeon General. Rockville, MD: Author.

Volkan, V. D., & Zintl, E. (1993). *Life after loss: The lessons of grief.* New York, NY: Scribner Paper.

Welo, B. K. (1999). *Life beyond loss: A workbook for incarcerated men* (2nd ed). Lanham, MD: American Correctional Association.
Woolfenden, J. (1997). A bereavement and loss group in a closed women's prison. *Psychodynamic Counseling, 3*(1), 77-82.

doi:10.1300/J456v01n03_12

Chapter 13

Shattered Dreams
of Professional Competence:
The Impact of Client Suicides
on Mental Health Practitioners
and How to Prepare for It

Gerald A. Juhnke
Paul F. Granello

SUMMARY. This article reviews the frequency of suicide, compares and contrasts suicide prediction to suicide assessment and provides a succinct overview of suicide high risk factors that mental health practitioners should be aware. Finally, the article describes common symptoms experienced by mental health practitioners who survive their clients' suicides, and presents a Pre-suicide Preparation Plan that mental health practitioners can implement prior to a crisis to hopefully enable them for a less demanding post-suicide experience. doi:10.1300/J456v01n03_13 *[Article copies available for a fee from The Haworth Document Delivery Service: 1-800-HAWORTH. E-mail address: <docdelivery@haworthpress.com> Website:*

Gerald A. Juhnke is Professor and doctoral program Director, Department of Counseling, Educational Psychology, and Adult & Higher Education, The University of Texas at San Antonio.

Paul F. Granello is Associate Professor of Counselor Education, School of Physical Activity and Educational Services, The Ohio State University.

Address correspondence to: Gerald A. Juhnke, CEPAHE/DB, UTSA Campus, 501, West Durango Boulevard, San Antonio, TX 78207 (E-mail: Gerald.juhnke@utsa.edu).

[Haworth co-indexing entry note]: "Shattered Dreams of Professional Competence: The Impact of Client Suicides on Mental Health Practitioners and How to Prepare for It." Juhnke, Gerald A., and Paul F. Granello. Co-published simultaneously in *Journal of Creativity in Mental Health* (The Haworth Press, Inc.) Vol. 1, No. 3/4, 2005, pp. 205-223; and: *Creative Interventions in Grief and Loss Therapy: When the Music Stops, a Dream Dies* (ed: Thelma Duffey) The Haworth Press, Inc., 2005, pp. 205-223. Single or multiple copies of this article are available for a fee from The Haworth Document Delivery Service [1-800-HAWORTH, 9:00 a.m. - 5:00 p.m. (EST). E-mail address: docdelivery@haworthpress.com].

doi:10.1300/J456v01n03_13

KEYWORDS. Suicide, mental health practitioners, creativity, pre-suicide preparation plan, post suicide

INTRODUCTION

Melinda was new to the profession and eager to practice psychology; she joined a group practice soon after receiving her license. Melinda's professional future looked bright and her practice seemed to thrive quickly. Unfortunately, within the first year of her work, one of her clients committed suicide. The client was new to therapy and did not show evidence of being in danger. Melinda was, of course, shocked by the suicide and suffered feelings consistent with the literature: sorrow, shame, fears that she was not competent, and fear of retribution.

Melinda was fortunate in many respects. Her colleagues were supportive, and she did not experience any problems with her licensing board. Still, she was shaken by the experience, and in time, shifted her therapeutic focus to the practice of assessment. Melinda was a talented psychologist, by all accounts, and had the support and trust of her colleagues. Still, the experience was difficult and had long-lasting implications for the direction of her professional focus.

Suicide is the 13th leading cause of worldwide deaths and the 11th overall leading cause of deaths in the U.S. (Centers for Disease Control and Prevention [CDC], 2004). Among Americans ages 25-34, suicide is the second leading cause of death (CDC, 2003). For Americans ages 10 to 24, suicide is the third leading cause of death (CDC, 2004). Nearly 12% of all deaths among this last population result from suicide.

The most recent statistics published by National Center for Health Statistics (National Center for Health Statistics [NCHS], 2004) HS, 2004) indicate that 31,655 Americans died as a result of suicide in 2002. This equates to approximately 87 suicides a day, nearly one every 17 minutes. In 1993 the Youth & Alcohol, Selected Reports to the Surgeon General (U. S. Department of Education, 1993) reported, "Suicide among American teenagers is increasing at an alarming though underestimated rate" (p. 3). It became apparent in the 1980s that younger persons were killing themselves in increasing numbers (U.S. Department of Health and Human Services (USDHHS), 1989) and by the 1990s weekly deaths among American children ages 5-14 attributed to suicide reached nearly one per day (M. Bradley, personal communication, February 10, 1994). Mental health practitioners are especially concerned with this rise in suicidality among young people. Persons with diagnosable mental disorders (especially affective disorders), and those abusing alcohol or other drugs (Maris, 1991; Nekanda-Trepka, Bishop, & Blackburn, 1983; Rich, Young, & Fowler, 1986; Stillion, McDowell, & May, 1989) are also at higher risk of suicide and by the nature of their mental health problems are often in treatment at the time of their suicide (Granello & Granello, 2006).

DEVASTATION OF SUICIDE

The above data clearly denote suicide's frequency in the US. However, it fails to adequately describe the emotional pain experienced by family suicide survivors. Many family members are adversely affected by the suicide of a loved one and frequently face one of the most challenging and difficult forms of bereavement (Farberow, Gallagher, Dorothy, Gilewski, & Thompson, 1992; McIntosh & Kelly, 1992; Osterweis, Solomon, & Green, 1984; Van Dongen, 1991). Bereavement reactions to a family member's suicide often induce feelings of significant shame, guilt and anger (Danto & Kutsher, 1977), as well as suicidal thoughts, suicidal attempts, and successful suicides (Gyulay, 1989). Most surviving family members experience profound disruptions in their lives including changes in cognitive, emotional, physical and social functioning as a direct result of their family members' suicide (Van Dongen, 1990). Furthermore, Posttraumatic Stress Disorder (PTSD) is experienced by many surviving friends and family members (Brende & Goldsmith, 1991; Brent, Perper, Moritz, Allman, & Liotus, 1993; Cleiren, Diekstra, Kerkhof, & Van der Wall, 1994; Pynoos & Nader, 1990).

Given the frequency of comorbid negative consequences of suicide, the first intent of this article is to provide a succinct overview of risk factors commonly associated with suicide. All mental health practitioners should become familiar with these risk factors so as to be able to properly assess clients' suicidality. Additionally, despite using commonly accepted clinical practices, many practitioners will experience a client's suicide. This article will address the experiences of practitioners' post-client suicide. Finally, we will outline a pre-suicide plan that can be implemented for mental health professionals should they experience a client's suicide.

SUICIDE RISK FACTORS

As one can imagine, there is not one single risk factor that adequately predicts inevitable suicide among all people. Motto (1991) eloquently stated, "Uncomfortable as it is, we have no realistic choice but to deal in levels of risk, which can vary from day to day or hour to hour, subject to the influence of numerous uncontrollable and unpredictable events." (p. 884). For mental health practitioners the truth is simple–we can not predict with 100% certainty that a client will or will not commit suicide. Instead, we must seek to provide the most thorough suicide risk assessment possible and evaluate interventions based upon immediate suicide risk levels. Thus, effective practitioners assess for risk factor clusters that are highly correlated with suicide. Below is a list of suicide risk-factors that we have found critically important to the suicide assessment process. Minimally, each of these factors must be assessed with potentially suicidal clients and their significant others.

Demographics: Sex, Ethnicity, and Age

Although the research indicates that women attempt suicide more often then men, men complete suicide more often than women. When reviewing sex and ethnicity, Caucasian males are by far the most likely group to suicide. Caucasian females are second, followed by African American males, and African American females (Granello & Granello, 2006).

In general, males are at increased suicide risk as they age. Female suicide risk, however, typically peaks around middle age. While it is beyond the scope of this article to provide an extensive review of the multicultural, age, and sex related information concerning suicide risk, it is important for competent practitioners to learn about the differences in suicide risk that are relevant to their clients' specific demographics and respond accordingly. However, one simply cannot lump all clients into risk categories based upon their sex, ethnicity or age.

The key factor is assessing clients for clusters of suicide risk factors. No mental health practitioner should haphazardly "identify" clients as being at risk simply due to their sex, ethnicity, sexual orientation, or age. Likewise, mental health practitioners should not discount clients' self-reported suicidal intent, simply because they fail to fall into high risk categories. The intent of this manuscript is to provide a thorough assessment and respond to the specific client's statements and needs.

Intervention Through Assessment: Depression/Hopelessness

Depression has long been associated with suicide (Brown & Blanton, 2002; Brown, Beck, Steer, & Grisham, 2000; Keller, 1994; Zweig & Hinrichsen, 1993). Specifically, depression or depressive symptoms have been historically noted in approximately 54% to 85% of those who suicide (Robins, 1986). Of course, not all depressed person's suicide. One potential explanation for this fact may be that not all depressed persons have lost the hope that their condition or situation will improve. Beck, Steer, Kovacs, and Garrison (1985) noted in their 10 year study that hopelessness was a strong suicide predictor. Thus, the intersection where depression and hope intersect may be a more important risk factor to assess than either alone. In our professional experiences, we have found it vitally important to assess both the levels of depression and hopelessness with clients presenting with suicidal ideation. When both are noted as present, we believe significant care should be taken to insure the client does not act upon the present suicidal ideation.

One way we assess hope is to ask a question such as, "When do you believe things will get better for you?" This is an important question. The client's response suggests whether or not hope for improvement actually exists. Should a client respond, "Things will never get better for me. I want to die so I won't have to continually suffer," such a response may suggest no future hope and no perception of pending improvement.

Another method for determining clients' immediate perceptions of hope is to utilize scaling questions (Cade & O'Hanlon, 1993). Again, in our professional experience, we have found scaling questions central to our work with depressed and potentially suicidal clients. Scaling questions allow clients to assign numerical values to their perceived levels of hope. The numerical values we seek reflect clients' perceptions in two distinct but overlapping areas. The first of these areas is related to immediate and pressing stressors that engender feelings of hopelessness. The second hopeless numerical value we seek relates to reasons for continued living. For example, mental health practitioners could ask two important hopelessness assessment scaling questions. The first is, "We have found it helpful to use a scale when asking about the situations or concerns that you may be experiencing. The scale is comprised of numbers from zero to 10. The number zero indicates the situations or concerns that are most overwhelming for you right now will *never* get better. The number 10 indicates that over time as you continue to choose to live, that the most overwhelming things you are facing today will *slowly improve* and get better. What number between zero and 10 best reflects how you see your current concerns over time?"

Should clients select a low number such as zero or four, this may well suggest a greater perception that their chief presenting problems will never fade or improve over time. Thus, their self-report suggests they perceive the situation as "hopeless." Clients endorsing low scores (e.g., zero to four) could be considered at greater risk for suicide, because they don't perceive an end to their immediate problems or stressors. Suicide, in such cases, could then mean an escape to end their suffering.

Higher numbers such as five and above may suggest that clients perceive some hope for improvement. Therefore, those indicating a higher number may have less immediate risk, because they self-report the hope that their immediate overwhelming concerns will likely diminish over time. In other words, someone who would respond "10" is indicating that although she is experiencing emotional pain or turmoil currently, the discomfort is temporary. Thus, they have hope that things are improving or could ultimately improve.

The second hopeless numerical value we seek relates to reasons for continued living. Utilizing a similar scaling question, we attempt to determine whether or not clients see positive life experiences on their horizon. In other words we are assessing reasons to live. This question is slightly different. Here a mental health professional might say, "Often people will be able to peer into the future and see some upcoming events or positive reasons for continuing to live. Similar to the question I previously asked, if zero suggests that in the future you will continue to encounter no positive life experiences or happiness and 10 suggests that you will certainly experience reasons to live and enjoy life, what score do you believe best indicates how you will experience your life in the next six months to 12 months?"

Again, low scores between zero and four could suggest that clients' view few if any upcoming rewarding experiences. In other words, they are self-reporting that there exists very little hope for a favorable future. Contrarily, high scores of five or more might suggest potential reasons to continue living are on the horizon. In such cases, practitioners could work with clients to help them increase their reasons for living by both helping to identify new reasons and reinforcing those reasons that the client is currently aware.

Robert is a 17-year-old who experienced the death of his last surviving parent and the amputation of his arm. As a result of his amputation, he lost a scholarship to a prestigious university and took it upon himself to help his aging grandparents raise his younger siblings. This meant

Robert stayed at home and attended a local junior college. Robert was heartbroken and depressed. When asked the first scaling question about his immediate situation, he reported a score of " . . . Zero. My arm's gone, and it's never growing back. My mother's dead, and I'll never see her again." However, for the second question he indicated a " . . . Six. I'm going to graduate in June, and I'm going to see my sister get married." Here we can see the benefit of asking two different questions regarding hopelessness. This young man felt no hope related to either having his arm repaired or his mother returned. However, he did view positive things on the horizon. Despite his depression and grief, he was able to identify hope for the future and reasons to live.

Diagnosable Axis I and/or Axis II Disorders

The literature suggests that a significant number of clients who complete suicide had one or more diagnosed Axis I or Axis II disorders (Glowinski et al., 2001, Fernquist, 2000; Harris & Barraclough, 1994, Hiroeh, Appleby, Mortensen, & Dunn, 2001; Maris, 2002). This seems especially true when clients have either an Axis I substance-related disorder (e.g., Alcohol Dependence) (Foster, 2001) or affective disorder (e.g., Major Depression) (Glowinski et al., 2001; Maris, 2002). Axis II personality disorders also have high suicide comorbidity (Brent et al., 1994; Maris, 2002). This also appears to be true for persons presenting with personality disorders with existing issues of impulsivity.

Frequently, one of the most challenging aspects for counselors involves the clients' lack of coping skills and significant other support. There are times when clients will use suicidal behaviors as a means to resolve conflicts with significant others. For example, clients may indicate suicidal ideation as a means to either seek reconnection with persons they feel are abandoning them or to bring conflict to a close. When they repeatedly use suicidal behaviors as a means to cope, therapists will often find their significant others beginning to question the validity of the threats. When suicidal threats and behaviors become suspect, clients can enter into an increasingly lethal matrix that challenges them to "prove" their dangerousness to self via more life-threatening behaviors that have fewer survival opportunities.

To illustrate, Henry slashed his wrist which created a superficial wound. In talking to Henry, the counselor saw this to be his attempt to re-connect with his partner, whom he perceives is abandoning him. Henry's partner responded to his actions by saying "This is the third time this month you cut your wrists and claimed to be suicidal. If you really intended to kill yourself, you would not have failed." The counselor could conceptualize that, from Henry's perspective, the lethal matrix now required him to "prove" that he actually intended to kill himself and to utilize a more lethal suicidal behavior. As some mental health professionals conclude, chances for survival can diminish with each attempt. Based on this conclusion, the person's behaviors must become more lethal and frequent in an effort to prove dangerousness to self. Additionally, with each attempt there is an increased risk of something going wrong with the parasuicide plan and the person accidentally completing the suicide.

Substance Use

Substance abuse and dependence are diagnosable mental disorders that deserve special attention related to suicide. Contrary to the misunderstanding of some practitioners, clients do not have to be physically or psychologically substance dependent to be at greater suicide risk. Many clients who abuse substances or who binge are at increased suicide risk. When under the influence of certain substances such as alcohol or cocaine, clients often present as more impulsive, daring, and reckless in behavior. In such cases, they often lack caution and internal monitoring that tend to inhibit life-threatening behaviors. This combination increases the probability that substance abusing clients will act upon their suicidal impulses without thinking of the dangerousness of their behaviors. We have encountered a number of clients who were not suicidal when sober and substance free. However, once they were under the influence of drugs and other drugs, they would become highly impulsive and act upon their desires to die. From foolishly running back and forth across a multilane highway to playing Russian roulette with a loaded revolver, these clients did things while under the influence that put them in danger. Thus, when you have clients who are abusing substances, suicide risk should be assessed.

Recent Previous Suicide Attempts

Unfortunately, one of the better predictors for suicide risk is the recent attempt of suicide by a client. This is especially true when the attempt was highly lethal (e.g., hanging). Suicidal clients often are in such emotional pain that they don't want to live. When they attempt suicide and survive, many will become less fearful of their own death. Some even become angry at themselves for failing to complete their suicides. For example, a client who attempts suicide by hanging herself may find that upon struggling to breathe, she was able to regain footing on an object and ultimately break free from the noose. Learning from her failed suicide, she might then identify a new location where she will be unable to regain her footing when she hangs himself or she may select a more lethal means to end her life (e.g., gunshot to the head).

The implication to mental health practitioners is striking. Should a client have a recent suicide attempt, the initial issues that brought about that suicide attempt likely have gone unresolved. More importantly, the client likely learned more lethal means to end his life and is at greater chance of using his enhanced suicide knowledge to ultimately bring about his death.

Suicidal Ideation

Although, most all adolescents and adults have at one time or another thought about suicide, the vast majority never act upon those thoughts. Persons presenting with frequent and obsessive thoughts about suicide and death are at a more significant risk for suicide, because they increasingly think about ending their lives. As they begin to ruminate about suicide, many aspects of their lives are overshadowed by their thoughts of death. Such suicidal ideation becomes central to their daily lives. Little by little they become myopic to things other than suicide. Ultimately, everything revolves around their suicide.

Therefore, whenever we have clients who note suicidal ideation, it is important that we intervene. Whatever methods they are contemplating as a means to bring about their deaths should be removed. Some may argue that clients will merely turn from one suicide plan to another. This likely is true with the intensely suicidal. However, we have also found that when the major suicide instruments (e.g., gun, car, etc.) are removed from the clients' immediate access, that clients are less apt to impulsively kill themselves. The more difficult it is to carry out the suicide plan, the greater the chance that the client will have the energy or determination to access the instrument of death.

Georgia, a client, who, at one time was intent upon killing herself, reported in session, "Once you talked my father into removing the garage door so I couldn't asphyxiate myself, I couldn't figure out how to kill myself. Shooting myself in the head or jumping off a bridge sounded too painful. The only thing I wanted to do was die, but I didn't want to die in pain."

Relational Challenges to Clear Thinking

Any time clients experience some factor that impedes their ability to problem solve or accurately interpret perceptual information, they are at increased suicide risk. Although the relationship of mental disorders was previously discussed and certainly relates here, this section is included, because it is also important to note that clients may experience emotions such as anger or betrayal apart from a diagnosed mental disorder that can impair their judgment and lead to impulsive behavior and suicide.

Additionally, there are cases where persons are clearly out of touch with reality and will experience significant auditory or visual hallucinations. We have experienced cases where suicidal persons believed God or the devil told them to kill themselves. Clearly, when persons are experiencing bizarre thinking or active hallucinations that are interpreted as an indication by a higher power prescribing suicide, there exists imminent danger that requires antipsychotic medications and a restricted environment.

Family Dysfunction, Abuse, and Family Suicidal Modeling

There exists a number of suicide risk factors related to clients' family of origin experiences that warrant discussion. Clients who have experienced physical, emotional, or sexual abuse within their family systems are believed to be at increased suicide risk. Additionally, clients reared in families where familial dysfunction compromised typical supportive functions are also a risk factor. Further, another known suicide risk factor is previous suicidal modeling within the family system.

Such was the case when the senior author assessed a teenage girl for suicide risk. Taylor was a teenage girl who presented with her family for therapy at a community mental health and substance abuse agency because she appeared suicidal. When entering the family counseling room, the senior author commented about the mother's hand. Each finger of her hand was attached to a separate spring. The individual springs were attached to a large metal loop that outlined the mother's hand. During the opening conversation, we discovered that both mother and father had extensive suicide histories. In fact, the mother's hand was in traction because she had damaged her tendon via multiple self-inflicted parasuicides. According to the mother, the lacerations were her attempts to end her life. The mother than pointed to the father's missing ear and commented that he had attempted suicide via a self-inflicted gunshot blast. The injury damaged his skull and blew off his ear. The pain in this family could be seen across generations.

Access to Lethal Means

Client suicide risk is directly related to the lethality of the methods. Firearms are a highly lethal means for suicide. Males complete suicides more than females, because more males use guns in their suicide attempts. Men typically use guns, hanging, and self-asphyxiation (car exhaust or other gas), while females typically attempt suicide via overdose, hanging, and then guns. Clients reporting suicidal ideation and having ready access to guns are in grave danger. When clients have direct access to guns, the guns need be removed from immediate access.

This requires more than placing the gun into a locked location at a client's home. Most people who reside in homes know either where keys to locked guns are or can gain access to guns by breaking into locked gun cabinets. Thus, in our professional endeavors, we have made it a rule that if someone within the home is suicidal all guns, weapons, and ammunition must be removed from the home and placed in a locked location away from their primary residence where the client cannot gain access. We have made this a rule without exception, and trust that you will too.

Recent and Chronic Stressors

Clients' coping ability is related to many factors. It is important to understand both the clients' chronic stressors, such as a relational support, chronic disease, poverty, or cultural adjustment. Other potential stressors include marital discord, job loss, or life transition. Once these stressors are understood, appropriate supports can be implemented to help.

One example of such chronic stressors was experienced by Mabel, an, 83-year-old female, with chronic breathing difficulties. Upon the senior author's arrival, the client indicated she no longer wanted to live. She reported chronic sores in her throat and nose, and expressed feelings of loneliness, and anger. After speaking with the client's family, we were able to create a "family schedule" where each of her adult children and their families identified one weekend per month to visit. The psychiatrist who interviewed the client at our urging prescribed antidepressants. The client's primary physician was unaware that the prescribed oxygen was causing sores and quickly changed the manner in which the oxygen was administered.

Within a month this client reported significant positive change and a desire to live. She no longer experienced sores in her nose or throat.

And, she began participating in two group experiences per week. Addressing her relational needs and these chronic stressors enhanced Mabel's life to a degree that she reported a balance between positive experiences and negative stressors. Her desires to suicide faded.

RESPONDING TO MENTAL HEALTH PRACTITIONERS WHOSE CLIENTS SUICIDE

Regretfully, even though the vast majority of suicides are preventable, there will be times when a client suicide is not foreseeable. Since 1987, we have conducted suicide assessment and intervention workshops to mental health practitioners. It is not uncommon to have three or more mental health practitioners remain after these workshops to describe their clients' suicides. The stories are poignant. Displayed emotions are often raw. Many report these experiences as a first time admitting to other mental health practitioners the loss of their clients to suicide. Nearly all who speak report feelings of loss and abandonment by their fellow professional colleagues. Some have reported that as a direct result of the suicide, they were voted out of group independent practices; others report that they were terminated from mental health or substance abuse agencies. One professional reported that the day after she informed another practitioner within her joint practice that her client had committed suicide, she was called at home and informed her books and belongings would be boxed up and available for removal the next day.

Apparently her experience is not atypical. Concomitantly, the literature reports that mental health practitioners who experience client suicide frequently encounter a number of post-event cognitive and emotional aftershocks that are significant on both a professional and personal level. These include:

- Loss: The loss of a life.
- Guilt: The practitioner may think that if only he or she had done "x" or said "y," then the client suicide could have somehow been averted.
- Doubts about professional competence: Practitioners may question their ability to provide care to others. These doubts may even be accompanied by feelings of shame, even if they did everything possible to ensure their clients' safety.
- Feelings of fear about being blamed for their clients' suicide by the clients' families or by other mental health practitioners.

- Irrational feelings of anger, betrayal, and disappointment directed at client for having completed the suicide.
- Existential grief (Hendin, Lipschitz, Maltsberger, Haas, & Wynecoop, 2000).

A PRE-SUICIDE PREPARATION PLAN

The emotional needs of practitioners who suffer the loss of a client can be substantial. These needs are best tended in connection with supportive others. Certainly, the death of a client can be extraordinarily painful for counselors who have had the privilege of walking through aspects of their lives with them. The death of a human being one has come to know creates suffering that few could fathom. Given that, it is important that counselors develop mutually supportive peer relationships and trusting supervisory relationships where processing tragedies such as a client suicide is possible. In addition, counselors must also consider practical issues that can arise during these tragic times. With this need in mind, we have created a Pre-Suicide Plan for counselors who encounter the heartrending experience of client suicide.

Although we can never anticipate anyone's every need during such stressful situations, it is important that counselors have a plan in mind should such a tragedy occur. Having a plan enables us to better understand the immediate steps necessary for taking care of ourselves and protecting our professional practice should a client suicide. Because many mental health practitioners are contacted at home regarding a client's suicide, we suggest creating two, three ring, Pre-Suicide Preparation Plan binders. Each should contain an index page, and color-tabbed, clear vinyl sheet protection pages. One Plan should be kept at home. The other should be kept at the practice.

Tab One: The Insurance Carrier Policy

Create a Tab One cover sheet that indicates the insurance policy number and the company's 24-hour, emergency contact telephone number. The following pages should include copies of the actual insurance policy. Many insurance carriers offer free risk management seminars and educational materials, as well as free legal telephone consultation privileges to their customers. It is important to determine whether their suggested procedures match the needs of our professional practice. For example, should the carrier not have risk management representatives or should the risk management representative report the insurance carrier does not have suggested standardized procedures to help insulate us from potential liability blunders, this might be a good time to seek a different insurance carrier. Once we have identified an insurance carrier that provides a logical risk management strategy, we can create an easy to follow flow-chart of that strategy. This flow chart should be posted on the second page of Tab One.

Tab Two: Clinical Supervision

The second tab of the Pre-Suicide Preparation Plan indicates the clinical supervisor's name and emergency contact numbers. This should include her home, cell, office, and common contact telephone numbers where she can be reached (e.g., cottage, boat, etc.). Furthermore, a list of secondary or "back up" supervisors and resources identified as acceptable and appropriate to the clinical supervisor should be listed along with corresponding telephone numbers.

It is critical to determine whether the supervisor of record is a clinical supervisor or simply an administrative manager. A supervisor who is an administrative manger is a representative of the agency and has little or no commitment to us. If the supervisor is an agent of the agency and provided by the agency, we need to learn how she and the agency interpret her supervision charge. Specifically, is her charge solely to protect the agency from liability and to insure that we comply with the agency's rules and procedures, or is her charge to train and mentor us? Next, we document the supervisor's response in the Pre-Suicide Preparation Plan and determine if we need to hire an external clinical supervisor. Once we have a supervisor who is dedicated to our development and tutelage, we can begin addressing the additional concerns listed below.

Finally, when creating a supervision relationship, it is vitally important to understand how the supervisee and the supervisor will interface should a client suicide occur. For example, we can ask how the clinical supervisor helped other supervisees successfully navigate their clients' suicides. It would be important to know what our supervisor's experience is with client suicide and to learn how she was able to help the supervisee and what the limits of her support would be. It is also important that as we consider forming this relationship, that we brainstorm and agree on ways of making the supervision mutually effective.

Given the power differentials between supervisor and supervisee, naming express needs is also important. What is it that we need our supervisors to do should we experience such a crisis? What is it that we expect from our supervisor should a client ever suicide? How do these supervisors wish to be informed should we perceive a client to be at significant suicide risk? Secondarily, we need to understand how supervisors wish us to address any perceived anger or frustration they may express towards us or toward the client. Similar to the way we create a counseling contract with our clients, it is helpful to create a supervision contract that specifies goals and objectives for negotiating the trials of a suicidal client.

Tab Three: Professional Mentors and Peers

It is also important that we identify a list of professional mentors and peers, including their telephone and emergency contact numbers. As we establish these relationships, it is important that we discuss with them whether they would be willing to help us process a client suicide should one ever occur (Bosco, 2000). If so, it would be important to know how they would like to be contacted should such a crisis occur and what we can expect with respect to support. In other words, would they be willing for us to come immediately to their offices? Would they be willing to listen to what happened and provide support and suggestions? Their responses can be written in Tab Three. If they seem disinterested or reluctant, it is not likely that a mutual growth-fostering relationship would occur. In that case, it would be important to find other mentors or peers with whom we could find this support.

Tab Four: Personal Counseling

Counselors in training are often encouraged to seek personal counseling services. Established counseling professionals also benefit from this practice. Within that setting, we can identify how we typically respond to stressful situations and identify new, more helpful ways to respond when faced with tragedies such as a client suicide. In this forum, we can discuss any unrealistic professional goals we carry (e.g., to cure every client who comes to counseling) and potential underlying reasons for these unrealistic goals. It is important that we gain insight related to our needs, and to then secure healthy, appropriate means to meet our professional and personal needs.

Tab Five: Speak with Your Nonprofessional Significant Others

Friends and family love us. When we are suffering, often they suffer too. It is important that we speak to our significant others regarding the possibility of a client suicide occurring sometime in our professional career. Let them know how the issues of confidentially will need to prevail to protect clients and their families. However, as we discuss potential ways that they can help us through a client suicide, we invite them to enter a part of our professional world and create a forum for mutual support and safety. In the case of a client suicide, we must let our friends and family know what they can do to help us. Further, we can develop a schedule that will insure that we speak with one friend or family member each morning, afternoon, and night for the first 30 days following the suicide.

Tab Six: Create a Realistic Statement for Yourself Related to Client Suicide

Create a maximum five sentence statement regarding client suicide. One example might be, "Because I work with people who suffer unique forms of distress, and because some of my clients will be at-risk to suicide, the odds are that someday one of my clients will complete this tragic act. This will occur despite my very best efforts and intentions."

CONCLUSION

The impact of a client's suicide on well-meaning, conscientious counselors cannot be minimized. As we learn more about the risks and consequences of suicide on the person and professional of the counselor, we become better equipped to offer each other empathic support and create a culture where shame and isolation following this very tragic experience are no longer prevalent. We enter this field to support and assist people in their healing. What, then, do we do when despite our best efforts, we fail to save our clients from harm? How do we come to terms with the limitations of our power? And finally, how do we accept that we have done all we know to do, and that sometimes what we do will not be enough? Coming to terms with our limitations for affecting change outside our control leads us one step closer toward healing the shattered dream that comes with client loss by suicide.

REFERENCES

Beck, A. T., Steer, R. A., Kovacs, M., & Garrison, B. (1985). Hopelessness and eventual suicide: A 10-year prospective study of patients hospitalized with suicidal ideation. *American Journal of Psychiatry, 142,* 559-563.

Bosco, A. F. (2000). Caring for the care-giver: The benefit of peer supervision group. *Journal of Genetic Counseling, 9,* 425-430.

Brende, J. O., & Goldsmith, R. (1991). Post-traumatic stress disorder in families. *Journal of Contemporary Psychotherapy, 21,* 115-124.

Brent, D. A., Johnson, B. A., Perper, J., Connolly, J., Bridge, J., & Bartle, S. et al. (1994). Personality disorder, personality traits, impulsive violence, and completed suicide in adolescents. *Journal of the American Academy of Child and Adolescent Psychiatry, 33,* 1080-1087.

Brent, D. A., Perper, J. A., Moritz, G., Allman, C., & Liotus, L. (1993). Psychiatric sequel to the loss of an adolescent peer to suicide. *Journal of the American Academy of Child and Adolescent Psychiatry, 32,* 509-517.

Brock, G. W., & Barnard, C. P. (1988). *Procedures in family therapy.* Boston, MA: Allyn and Bacon.

Brown, D. R., & Blanton, C. J. (2002). Physical activity, sports participation, and suicidal behavior among college students. *Medicine and Science in Sports and Exercise, 34,* 1087-1096.

Brown, G. K., Beck, A. T., Steer, R. A., & Grisham, J. R. (2000). Risk factors for suicide in psychiatric outpatients: A 20-year prospective study. *Journal of Consulting and Clinical Psychology, 68,* 371-377.

Cade, B., & O'Hanlon, W. H. (1993). *A brief guide to brief therapy.* New York: Brunner/Mazel.

Center for Disease Control and Prevention. (2003). 10 Leading causes of death, United States, *http://webappa.cdc.gov/cgi bin/broker.exe*

Center for Disease Control and Prevention. (2004). Suicide and Attempted Suicide, MMWR Weekly June 11, 2004, 53(22); 47. *http://www.cdc.gov/mmwr/preview/mmwrhtml/mm5322al.htm*

Cleiren, M. P., Diekstra, R. F., Kerkhof, J. F., & Van der Wall. (1994). Mode of death and kinship in bereavement: Focusing on "who" rather than "how." *Crisis, 15,* 52-58.

Cohn, B., & Osborne, W. L. (1992). *Group counseling: A practical self-concept approach for the helping professional.* Chappaqua, NY: L. S. Communications.

Danto, B. L., & Kutsher, A. H. (Eds). (1977). *Suicide and bereavement.* New York: MSS Information Corporation.

Farberow, N. L., Gallagher, T., Dorothy, E., Gilewski, M. J., & Thompson, L. W. (1992). Changes in grief and mental health of bereaved spouses of older suicides. *Journal of Gerontology, 47,* 357-366.

Fernquist, R. M. (2000). Problem drinking in the family and youth suicide. *Adolescence, 35,* 551-558.

Foster, T. (2001). Dying for a drink: Global suicide prevention should focus more on alcohol use disorders. *British Medical Journal, 323,* 817-818.

Glowinski, A. L., Bucholz, K. K., Neslon, E. C., Qiang Fu, P., Madden, A. F., & Reich, W. et al. (2001). Suicide attempts in an adolescent female twin sample. *Journal of the American Academy of Child and Adolescent Psychiatry, 40,* 1300-1308.

Granello, D. H., & Granello, P. F. (2006). *Suicide: Essential guide for helping professionals and educators.* Boston, MA: Allyn & Bacon.

Gyulay, J. E. (1989). What suicides leave behind (Special issue: The death of a child). *Issues in Comprehensive Pediatric Nursing, 12,* 103-118.

Harris, E. C., & Barraclough, B. M. (1994). Suicide as an outcome for medical disorders. *Medicine, 73,* 281-297.

Hendin, H., Lipschitz, A., Maltsberger, J. T., Haas, A. P., & Wynecoop, S. (2000). Therapists' reactions to patient's suicides. *American Journal of Psychiatry, 157,* 2022-2027.

Hiroeh, U., Appleby, L., Mortensen, P., & Dunn, G. (2001). Death by homicide, suicide and other unnatural causes in people with mental illness: A population-based study. *The Lancet, 358,* 2110-2112.

Jenkins, S. R. (1996). Social support and debriefing efficacy among emergency medical workers after a mass shooting incident. *Journal of Social Behavior & Personality, 11,* 477-492.

Keller, M. (1994). Depression: A long-term illness. *British Journal of Psychiatry. 165,* 9-15.

Kirchner, J. T. (1997). Health status and risk of suicide in elderly patients. *American Family Physician, 56,* 1188-1189.

Kleespies, P. M., Smith, M. R., & Becker, B. R. (1990). Psychology interns as patient suicide survivors: Incidence, impact, and recovery. *Professional Psychology: Research & Practice, 21,* 257-263.

Maris, R. W. (2002). Suicide. *The Lancet, 360,* 319-326.

Maris, R.W. (1991). Introduction. *Suicide and Life-Threatening Behaviors, 21*(1), 1-17.

Matthew, L. R. (1998). Effect of staff debriefing on posttraumatic stress symptoms after assaults by community housing residents. *Psychiatric Services, 49,* 207-212.

McIntosh, J. L. (1991. January 12). U.S. suicide: 1988 official final data. *Michigan Association of Suicidology,* 10-11.

McIntosh, J. L., & Kelly, L. D. (1992). Survivors' reactions: Suicide vs. other causes. *Crisis, 13,* 82-93.

Motto, J. A. (1991). An integrated approach to estimating suicide risk. *Suicide and Life-Threatening Behaviors, 7*(4), 883-886.

National Center for Health Statistics (May 28, 1998). *FASTATS A to Z,* http://www.cdc.gov/nchswww/fastats/suicide.htm

National Center for Health Statistics. (2004). Deaths: Final data for 2002, National vital statistics reports 53(5) October 12, 2004.

Nekanda-Trepka, C. J., Bishop, S., & Blackburn, I. M. (1983). Hopelessness and depression. *British Journal of Clinical Psychology, 22*(1), 49-60.

O'Hara, D. M., Taylor, R., & Simpson, K. (1994). Critical incident stress debriefing: Bereavement support in schools developing a role for an LEA educational psychology service. *Educational Psychology in Practice, 10,* 27-34.

Osterweis, M., Solomon, F., & Green, M. (Eds.). (1984). *Bereavement: Reactions, consequences, and care.* Washington, DC: National Academy Press.

Pilkinton, P. (2003). Encountering suicide: The experience of psychiatric residents. *Academic Psychiatry, 27,* 93-99.

Pynoos, R. S., & Nader, K. (1990). Children's exposure to violence and traumatic death, *Psychiatric Annals, 20,* 334-344.

Rich, C. L., Young, D., & Fowler, R. C. (1986). San Diego suicide study. *Achieves of General Psychiatry, 43,* 577-582.

Robins, E. (1986). Completed suicide. In A. Roy (Ed.), *Suicide* (pp. 123-133). Baltimore, MD: Williams & Wilkins.

Schneidman, E. S. (1985). *Definition of suicide.* New York, NY: John Wiley & Sons.

Sewell, J. D. (1993). Traumatic stress of multiple murder investigations. *Journal of Traumatic Stress, 6,* 103-118.

Smith, K., & Crawford, S. (1986). Suicidal behavior among normal high school students. *Suicide & Life Threatening Behavior, 16,* 313-325.

Spitzer, W. J., & Neely, K. (1992). Critical incident stress: The role of hospital-based social work in developing a statewide intervention system for first-responders delivering emergency services. *Social Work in Health Care, 18,* 39-58.

Stillion, J. J., McDowell, E. E., & May, J. H. (1989). *Suicide across the span: Premature exits.* Washington, DC: Hemisphere Publishing.

Thompson, R. A. (1993). Posttraumatic stress and posttraumatic loss debriefing: Brief strategic intervention for survivors of sudden loss. *The School Counselor, 41,* 16-22.

U.S. Department of Education (1993). *Youth and alcohol, selected reports to the Surgeon General* (DE Publication No. ED1.2:Y8). Washington, DC: U.S. Government Printing Office.

U.S. Department of Health and Human Services (USDHHS). (1989). *Report of the Secretary's Task Force on Youth Suicide. Volume 3: Prevention & Interventions in Youth Suicide.* (DHHS Publication No. ADM89-1623). Washington, DC: U.S. Government Printing Office.

Van Dongen, C. J. (1990). Agonizing questioning: Experiences of survivors of suicide victims. *Nursing Research, 39,* 224-229.

Van Dongen, C. J. (1991). Experiences of family members after a suicide. *Journal of Family Process, 33,* 375-380.

Weinberg, R. B. (1990). Serving large numbers of adolescent victim-survivors: Group interventions following trauma at school. *Professional Psychology: Research and Practice, 21,* 271-278.

Zweig, R. A., & Hinrichsen, G. A. (1993). Factors associated with suicide attempts by depressed older adults: A prospective study. *American Journal of Psychiatry, 150,* 1687-1692.

doi:10.1300/J456v01n03_13

Chapter 14

The American Reincarnation of the Superfluous Experience: Finding Meaning in Generation Y

Madelyn Elizabeth Duffey
Thelma Duffey

SUMMARY. The superfluous man became a prominent literary figure in Russia during the 19th century. This article makes a comparison of the superfluous experience to the "celebutante" phenomenon, as reflected in the media. It also includes a discussion on the impact that the celebutante influence may have on the dreams, values and meaning-making experience of members of Generation Y. A values clarification exercise is included. doi:10.1300/J456v01n03_14 *[Article copies available for a fee from The Haworth Document Delivery Service: 1-800-HAWORTH. E-mail address: <docdelivery@haworthpress.com> Website: <http://www.HaworthPress.com>* © 2005 by The Haworth Press, Inc. All rights reserved.]

KEYWORDS. Russian literature, superfluous man, generation Y, "celebutante," creativity, counseling, values clarification

---

Madelyn Elizabeth Duffey is affiliated with University of Colorado at Boulder. Thelma Duffey is the Counseling Program Director at the University of Texas at San Antonio.

Address correspondence to: Madelyn Elizabeth Duffey, 3726 Marymount, San Antonio, TX 78209 (E-mail: Madelyn.duffey@colorado.edu).

[Haworth co-indexing entry note]: "The American Reincarnation of the Superfluous Experience: Finding Meaning in Generation Y." Duffey, Madelyn Elizabeth and Thelma Duffey. Co-published simultaneously in *Journal of Creativity in Mental Health* (The Haworth Press, Inc.) Vol. 1, No. 3/4, 2005, pp. 225-235; and: *Creative Interventions in Grief and Loss Therapy: When the Music Stops, a Dream Dies* (ed: Thelma Duffey) The Haworth Press, Inc., 2005, pp. 225-235. Single or multiple copies of this article are available for a fee from The Haworth Document Delivery Service [1-800-HAWORTH, 9:00 a.m. - 5:00 p.m. (EST). E-mail address: docdelivery@haworthpress.com].

Available online at http://jcmh.haworthpress.com
© 2005 by The Haworth Press, Inc. All rights reserved.
doi:10.1300/J456v01n03_14

We buy our way out of jail, but we can't buy freedom
We'll buy a lot of clothes when we don't really need 'em
Things we buy to cover up what's inside
Cause they make us hate ourself and love their wealth

(West, 2004)

There has not been a generation whose dreams for the future have been more influenced by what can appear to be infinite possibilities than Generation Y. Members of this generation, also known as Echo Boomers and The Millennial Generation (CBS, Inc., 2005; Odle, 2006; Zemke, Raines, & Filipczak, 2000) are the first to have access to technological innovations such as personal computers, cable television, and the Internet since childhood (Chester, 2002). The development of technology during Generation Y has offered exposure to lifestyles and possibilities that many people could not have imagined. Among these possibilities is a "celebutante" lifestyle, currently popularized by the media. Coined from the words, debutante and celebrity, celebutantes, in popular culture, are now depicted in many television shows and magazines. Just by turning on the television, we see these depictions in such shows as "My Super Sweet Sixteen" (Reid, 2005), "Filthy Rich Cattle Drive" (Berfield, 2005), "Laguna Beach" (Brumels, 2004), "Rich Girls" (Ricks, 1993), and "The Fabulous Life Of . . . " (Saavedra, 2005).

Children, adolescents, and young adults throughout the country witness daily the lifestyles of these "rich and famous." Given that our value system becomes integrated into our belief system through the exposure we receive in childhood and adolescence (Chester, 2002), it becomes interesting to consider what the impact of this celebutante exposure will have on the dreams and aspiration of members of Generation Y.

In this manuscript, we will discuss the effects of mass media coverage of the celebutante phenomenon on the dreams, values, and meaning-making experiences of young adults. Using a popular character in Russian literature as a metaphor, this article will conclude with suggestions for a values centered group experience for counselors working with young adults as they evaluate future life goals and choices. Because this manuscript is a thought piece based on observations and as-sumptions, personal positions and generalizations will be made which are yet to be explored or supported in research. However, written from the perspective of a student in English and History studies and a member of Generation Y, this piece presents an opportunity for counselors to consider unique challenges discussed and deliberated by some Generation Y members, and to explore some potential means for creatively addressing these challenges.

For purposes of this article, celebutante will be defined as a person of wealth and unearned fame celebrated and emulated in popular culture. In this manuscript, this phenomenon is compared with a noted literary figure from Russian literature, the "superfluous man." By using experiences illustrated in other cultures; and by focusing on a literary character removed from our contemporary culture, we can consider the impact that our own evolving cultural values may have on our dreams for the future. Through this experience, we can also consider what matters to us; what we find important; and what we ultimately aspire to create in our lives.

THE USE OF RUSSIAN LITERATURE TO DESCRIBE THE SUPERFLUOUS EXPERIENCE

Among the numerous literary contributions of 19th century Russian authors, perhaps one of the most notable is the creation of the "superfluous man" (Lermontov, 1840/2001; Nock, 1994). A staple in 19th century Russian literature, the "superfluous man" is a character that possesses wealth, intelligence, education, and charisma but who is ultimately unable to make any meaningful societal contributions, or commit to any one person or cause. He has become a national literary archetype in Russia, a representation of a polarized economy where the majority of national wealth is concentrated in a minute faction of the population. In the superfluous man, one can see the consequences of unchecked wealth and privilege. While the superfluous man is most often associated with 19th century Russia, it is the position of this manuscript that his character has seen a recent rebirth within American popular culture.

Far from the dismal economic conditions of imperial Russia, it is curious that there appears to be a growing trend among a small but visible group of well-educated, financially secure Americans to reject any form of commitment or obligation. Waiting patiently for the reign of the baby boomers to subside, this group is discarding the dreams and influences of previous generations and forming a new generational set of values, similar to those of the "superfluous man."

The "superfluous man" is the antithesis of the archetypal hero. While the traditional hero will successfully complete a quest, restoring order to the land, the "superfluous man" ventures on numerous quests, never satisfied with any one pursuit, or any one woman (Lermontov, 1840/

2001; Nock, 1994). He yearns to positively impact those around him, but is unable to yield anything substantial, and often negatively affects the women he courts. The "superfluous man" is unable to form consequential connections, and perennially searches for adventure and personal fulfillment (Lermontov, 1840/2001; Nock, 1994).

One of the greatest works detailing the exploits of the "superfluous man" is Mikail Lermontov's *A Hero of Our Time* (1840/2001). The book was initially met with critical trepidation and poor reviews, as many reviewers were shocked by the roguish hero, Pechorin. The book is split into multiple adventures, as Pechorin leaves Russian society to travel throughout the Caucasus, making friends and enemies along the way. Pechorin tries to reject society and to lead a more fulfilled life away from the aristocracy, but is ultimately unable to do so. He pursues numerous women throughout his expedition, enjoying the novelty of their naiveté and un-worldliness, but soon becomes bored and moves on to his next conquest.

The "superfluous man" was representative of the frustration that Russian classes had with an autocratic and authoritarian government. With all his faults, the "superfluous man" helped to display the ineffectuality and futility felt by Russians. If the small wealthy and educated population of 19th century Russia was unable make effective change, then who could? These were the questions Russian author's sought to answer through the proliferation of the "superfluous man."

A notable distinction between the character in Russian literature and the celebutante icon is that the new American "superfluous man" is not restricted to one gender, but can be seen most readily in the rising generation of wealthy Americans who are dominating the media and idealized and emulated for their spending habits, chronic relationship shifts, and sense of entitlement. With excessive wealth and privilege, the new "superfluous people" are not respected for any academic, philanthropic, or professional accomplishments, but rather, for the fact that they do not need any accomplishments to finance their extravagant lifestyle. They are celebrated for their wealth, power, and nonchalant attitudes, all characteristics common to the superfluous man (see Lermontov, 1840/2001; Nock, 1994).

Perhaps the most popular example of the exploits of the new "superfluous person" is the "Simple Life" series (Bunim & Murray, 2003) on the Fox television network, featuring Paris Hilton and Nicole Richie. The show's first season placed two enormously affluent girls with a family in rural Altus, Arkansas for a month. Paris and Nicole were filmed doing chores and common tasks such as milking cows, and working for a day at a Sonic Drive-In restaurant. Unable to complete these tasks, the girls ruined the milk supply, took advantage of their employer's credit card, and were unable to successfully complete everyday responsibilities. The show became a huge success and was renewed for multiple seasons. Audiences reveled in the antics of two indulged women who are now seen in nearly every pop culture magazine publication. Like Pechorin, the characters abandoned high society for a short duration, disrupted the lives of the people they met, and were ultimately glorified on their return to society. They epitomize the new set of "superfluous people" dominating American culture.

In contrast to Pechorin, one could suggest that the modern "superfluous person" has arisen, not to bring attention to the moral isolation brought on by social, political, or economic inequalities, but rather, to glorify these inequalities. We see in the media how common it is to idealize a "superfluous lifestyle" by focusing on purchasing the newest Louis Vuitton clutch rather than creating substantial dreams, independent of the influences of popular culture. While celebutantes ride a wave of publicity, perhaps the lessons learned from the "superfluous man" can come into play. With every advantage in the world, he is ultimately left restless, unfulfilled, and isolated. We are at a turning point in American pop-culture history, straddling the American dream of white picket fences and the emerging phenomenon of "celebutante" worship. Perhaps Pechorin, in the form of the superfluous man, can shed light on this inner experience. Then, we, too, can reconsider our opinions about the meaning and value we give to wealth, power, and privilege, and in so doing, broaden our perspectives and possibilities for creating authenticity and meaning in our lives and relationships.

VALUES IN THE AGE OF THE SUPERFLUOUS PERSON

Taking a look at the cultural environment in which members of a generation experience life provides counselors with a contextual understanding of clients who seek their services. Indeed, the values we carry are influenced by what we have known, by what we have come to appreciate, and by what we believe to be possible. The basic values experienced by every generation are characterized by their life experiences and by the historical events that shaped them (Chester, 2002). By drawing context from the historical backdrop experienced by members of a generation, counselors are better able to help people clarify what is important to them, while understanding some of the unique issues they may face. Members of the Generation Y are no exception.

Ultimately, members of this generation share a challenge faced by others: finding meaning in their experiences and living purposeful lives. Indeed, how we make meaning of our experiences is directly related to the connections we share with others and the values we carry. According to Chester (2002), "Psychologists remind us that our core values are programmed into us during our first fifteen to sixteen years of life, through a combination of five major life shaping influences; Parent/ Family; Schools/Education; Religion/Morality; Friends/Peers; and Media/Culture" (p. 12). This article addresses the influence of media/ culture, specifically the focus on celebutantes, on the development of values and the aspiration of dreams for members of Generation Y.

Corinne

In one example, Corinne, a 32-year-old single mother and counselor-in-training describes her experience. Corinne acknowledges that her value system is characterized by investment in family through self sacrifice. She explains, "I took in my 16-year-old younger brother. After he came to live with me, we experienced significant conflicts and our time together was short-lived." With regret, she adds, "Although we both grew up in the same ethnic background, and within the same lower socio-economic strata, and although we were raised within the same family, our values are completely different." Corinne reports, "My brother would become very angry and sad if he could not have some of the things that he saw his more affluent friends and classmates have; things he saw others have on television. He felt entitled to have a car, which we could not afford. He felt entitled to have the latest cell phone, which we could not afford."

Corinne notes how sometimes, people who do not have the financial foundation to live the lifestyle portrayed by celebutante figures aspire to live similarly and can be keenly disappointed when it remains out of their reach. She states, "They see people who have not done anything to earn their lifestyle. As a result, they don't feel they should have to do anything to earn the means by which to live a luxurious life either." She adds, "In some cases, older Generation Y members, those of working age, feel that the sole purpose of work is to provide for material goods." Corrine speaks about a relative from an otherwise financially stable middle class family:

My cousin, Lauren, is 25 years old. She lives at home with her parents but drives a very expensive luxury car. She shops at expensive specialty stores, such as Gucci and Prada. Her family is not a wealthy family. It is a working class family. Her mother is a principal at an elementary school and her father sells insurance. Still, Lauren glorifies an affluent lifestyle and the people who live it. She measures her worth by what she has and lives her life in pursuit for more. (Corinne, personal communication, April 24, 2006)

Corinne is not alone in her concerns about the focus on materialism and the glorification of celebutante living among young adults. Regardless of race, class, or gender, the perpetuation of messages by the media influence and infiltrate our thinking (Kilbourne, 1999). These messages directly impact our dreams for the future, what we value, and how we relate to others as a result of our value system.

VALUES CLARIFICATION

According to Edwards (2005), unproductive behavior may be related to an unfocused and vaguely defined value system. He purports that by participating in a clarification process, we can better decide which values to maintain and which to discard. Three phases of this process include: (1) discovery/awareness, (2) claiming/reclaiming, and (3) acceptance (Edwards, 2005).

In the first phase, clients are asked to identify some of their values. They assess whether these values are personally suitable, and whether they are consistent with family and community life. Clients then assess whether the value contributes to the larger order (Edwards, 2005). The second phase of this process is one of claiming and reclaiming (Edwards, 2005). Here we see how values relate to a person's emotional experience: "How does this value feel to me? Does it add to my quality of life?" In this phase, we also consider how others have behaved towards us and how we behave towards them. In the final phase, we accept or reject the examined values. Accepted values are assimilated into our daily lives and can be seen in our interactions and relationships with others (Edwards, 2005).

Values can be clarified through group process. For example, a counselor working with a group of eight to ten 18-24 year olds could use readings from literature to discuss the impact of popular culture on their values and desires. The group format offers participants opportunities to develop connections with others, to "explore behaviors practiced within relationships that impede or promote growth and resilience" (Hartling, 2005, p. 348), and to reflect upon their value system in a relationally supportive environment. Groups can be organized to meet once a week for a two hour block over an academic term. Counselors can introduce the concept of pop culture and elicit discussion from the group members on their experiences relative to cultural mores, while the group members engage in discussions and read books or stories that carry related themes. The following are questions that counselors can use to facilitate these discussions.

GUIDING QUESTIONS

1. What do we know about the protagonist that we would want to emulate? How do these values and behaviors manifest in current times?
2. What do we see as the benefits of living life as depicted in this literary example? What examples can we find in popular culture that speak to these benefits?
3. Imagine what it could feel like to be the protagonist. What would our relationships look like? How would we express affection? How would we experience love? How do we express love now? How would we want to express love?
4. Imagine what it would feel like to live as the protagonist. How does this life compare to the lives we perceive celebutantes to live? In what ways can we imagine this life to be satisfying? In what ways can we imagine satisfaction to be elusive?
5. What do you perceive the protagonist's values to be and how have they affected his or her lifestyle? How do these values seem to compare with the values promoted in pop culture? In what ways can these values add or detract from the overall quality of life you hope to have?
6. What do you hope life will bring to you and what do you see yourself doing to create that life?

When we have an opportunity to discuss important concerns within a safe and thought-provoking context, we may find that some of our concerns are also shared by others. For some, this discussion creates a feeling of connection, and in some cases, feelings of relief. Thematic group discussions also provide a forum for people to collaboratively problem solve solutions to their concerns and to create alternative possibilities. In the forum described above, we can reconsider what we value at the same time that we learn more about the literary and cultural experience of people and literary figures from another culture or country. Group experiences of this nature not only serve to give us context for exploring our own values and beliefs, they offer opportunities for promoting greater understanding of the complex and intricate influences that context and culture have on the development of values among its members.

CONCLUSION

Members of any generation face the challenge of defining their life choices, aspirations, and dreams. This challenge is not only influenced by our hopes, investment, drive, and potential, but is also influenced by the possibilities and alternatives available to us. Members of a generation for whom unearned wealth and power is normalized, at a time when pride in work, accomplishment, relationships, and contribution are publicly minimized, face additional challenges. It is the position of this manuscript that mass consumerism, as it stands, has the potential to create financial consequences and feelings of disconnection and disillusionment if we are not able to establish meaningful connections and goals (see Kilbourne, 1999). The intent of this manuscript is to propose a forum, using a literary figure as a context, where individuals can explore their interests, relationships, and personal sets of values. The intended outcome of this exercise is for participants to deepen their understanding of their values; to grow as individuals; and to connect with the larger societal experience.

Russian literature and the archetypal hero, the Superfluous Man, remind us that struggles come to all of us. If we do not find our contributions to be meaningful, can we experience anything more than intermittent satisfaction? If our goal is to acquire rather than to support, will the meaning we make of our experiences be substantive? And if we begin our adult life with expectations of indiscriminate access, can we appreciate the value that effort, success, and genuine connection with others can bring?

History, culture, and literature have much to offer us as we examine what we value and why. In looking at historical and cultural contexts, we can look at diverse belief systems and lifestyles claimed by prominent figures, with the benefit of seeing the eventual outcome of their experiences. Along the same vein, literature, through fictional characters, creates a means for us to "enter the shoes" of another and "try on" an experience. Sometimes the experience can appear appealing, and at times, it is. Few of us would reject monetary, material, or other pleasure-seeking opportunities. However, if our dreams do not go beyond these to include care, investment, mutuality, and vision, would they be ultimately fulfilling? And if our exposure and perspective are limited, would we have the psychological and relational context to identify more fulfilling dreams? Members of Generation Y have the opportunity to use history and literary figures to inspire their dreams and clarify hopes for their futures. Counselors working with this population can use these historical or literary figures to help clients identify what they value and create a context for seeing their dreams and values realized.

REFERENCES

Berfield, J. (Producer). (2005). *Filthy rich cattle drive* (Television series). Culver City: CNET Networks, Inc.

Brumels, C. (Producer). (2004). *Laguna Beach* (Television series). New York: CNET Networks, Inc.

Bunim, M. (Producer) & Murray, J. (Producer). (2003). *The simple life* (Television series). Beverly Hills, CA: Fox.

CBS, Inc. (2005). *The Echo Boomers*. Retrieved on April 27, 2006 from http://www.cbsnews.com/stories/2004/10/01/60minutes/main646890_page2.shtml

Chester, E. (2002). *Employing Generation Why?* Colorado: Tucker House Books.

Edwards, A. W. (2005). Values clarification as a therapeutic process. *North American Association of Christians in Social Work Convention.*

Hartling, L. (2005). Fostering resilience throughout our lives: New relational possibilities. In D. Comstock (Ed.), *Diversity and development–Critical contexts that shape our lives and relationships* (pp.337-354). Belmont, CA: Wadsworth Publishing.

Kilbourne, J. (1999). *Deadly persuasion: Why women and girls must fight the addictive power of advertising.* New York: Free Press, Inc.

Lermontov, M. (2001). *A hero of our time* (P. Foote, Trans.). New York: Penguin Book. (Original work published 1840).

Nock, A. J. (1994). *The memoirs of a superfluous man.* Tampa, FL: Hallberg Publications.

Odle, T. G. (2006). The new generation of leaders. *Unique opportunities: The physician's resource.* Retrieved May 01, 2006 from http://www.uoworks.com/articles/generation.html

Reid, L. A. (Producer). (2005). *My super sweet sixteen* (Television series). New York: CNET Networks, Inc.

Ricks, S. (Director/Producer). (1993). *Rich girls* (Television series). Los Angeles, CA: CNET Networks, Inc.

Saavedra, C. (Producer). (2005). *The fabulous life of . . .* (Television series). Los Angeles, CA: CNET Networks, Inc.
West, K. (2004). All falls down. On *The College Dropout* (CD). New York: Roc-a-Fella Records.
Zemke, R., Raines, C., & Filipczak, B. (2000). *Generations at work: Managing the clash of veterans, boomers, Xers, and Nexters in your workplace.* New York, NY: American Management Publications.

doi:10.1300/J456v01n03_14

Chapter 15

Superheroes and Heroic Journeys: Re-Claiming Loss in Adoption

Lawrence C. Rubin

SUMMARY. This manuscript addresses adoption and the related gifts and challenges faced by adoptees. Challenges such as the search for identity, reconciliation, and identifying how they belong are also discussed. This manuscript also addresses common myths and misconceptions about the adoption experience. A creative intervention, using super heroes and science fiction, is illustrated through case study. doi:10.1300/ J456v01n03_15 *[Article copies available for a fee from The Haworth Document Delivery Service: 1-800-HAWORTH. E-mail address: <docdelivery@haworthpress. com> Website: <http://www.HaworthPress.com> © 2005 by The Haworth Press, Inc. All rights reserved.]*

KEYWORDS. Adoption, identity, reconciliation, counseling, creativity, superheroes, science fiction

Ever since my childhood nights with flashlight and comic book in hand, superheroes have fascinated me. To this day, my life seems to be an unintentional spare closet for items super heroic, such as lunch boxes, action figures, clothing, and movies. As the father of two young

---

Lawrence C. Rubin is affiliated with the St. Thomas University.

Address correspondence to: Lawrence C. Rubin, St. Thomas University, 16401 NW Avenue, Miami, FL 33054 (E-mail: lrubin@stu.edu).

[Haworth co-indexing entry note]: "Superheroes and Heroic Journeys: Re-Claiming Loss in Adoption." Rubin, Lawrence C. Co-published simultaneously in *Journal of Creativity in Mental Health* (The Haworth Press. Inc.) Vol. 1, No. 3/4, 2005, pp. 237-252; and: *Creative Interventions in Grief and Loss Therapy: When the Music Stops, a Dream Dies* (ed: Thelma Duffey) The Haworth Press, Inc., 2005, pp. 237-252. Single or multiple copies of this article are available for a fee from The Haworth Document Delivery Service [1-800-HAWORTH, 9:00 a.m. - 5:00 p.m. (EST). E-mail address: docdelivery@haworthpress.com].

Available online at http://jcmh.haworthpress.com
© 2005 by The Haworth Press, Inc. All rights reserved.
doi:10.1300/J456v01n03_15

children who enjoy the exploits of superheroes, I have enjoyed the opportunity of retaining an important connection to my own superhero fantasies of flight, strength, speed and unswerving morality. As a scholar and an individual who continually strives for enlightenment, power, and a glimpse into eternity, the hero's journey is also a particularly resonant theme in my life. As a clinical psychologist who values superhero fantasy and the hero metaphor, as well as one who works with adoptive families, I work toward deepening my understanding of the adoption experience. I must also mention that my two children are adopted, which firmly anchors me at one corner of the so-called "adoption triangle." Their adoption journey is mine as well. Therefore, a chapter combining superheroes, heroic journeys, and adoption is an inevitable crossroads on my own personal, professional and spiritual journey.

While I was not raised a particularly privileged child, I nevertheless enjoyed many privileges. In retrospect, and through the eyes of my own children, one of those privileges was not having to question whether or not the people I called mom and dad were my "real parents." I never wondered who my biological parents were, whether I had other siblings out there somewhere, why someone would have given me away, or when I would finally meet the people who came before my mother and father. Compared to my own two children, I was freed from the burden of these questions that they continually ask in many ways, on many days, with intense emotion. My wife and I encourage our children to ask any questions about adoption that they see fit, and we attempt to answer them as best we can. Perhaps for reasons related to their own unique worldviews, or because of our attempt to explore their journeys with them, adoption is part of our ongoing family discourse. It is not surprising; therefore, that superheroes find their way into our conversations about adoption. After all, one of the main motifs in the superhero genre is challenging early-life circumstances, including adoption. As a result, I have come to appreciate the power of the superhero adoption narrative in my role as parent, teacher, scholar, and clinician. With that in mind, I turn to an overview of the literature on adoption.

THE REALITY OF ADOPTION

Much has been written about adoption; from the deeply personal stories of adoptees, birth-parents and adoptive parents–the adoption triangle, to the clinical and empirical work of mental health professionals and social scientists respectively. The American adoption narrative has been influenced by the depictions in, and interests of the mass media. Additionally, the issues surrounding adoption have become part of the national discourse on the volatile associated topics of race, culture, genetics and homosexuality. However, and regardless of the scope of adoption-related issues, the most powerful voice in the narrative is that of the adoptee (Ryan & Nalavany, 2003).

It has been estimated that over the last seventeen years, close to 125,000 children are adopted annually, and of these, the percentage of domestic inter-racial and international placements has steadily risen (National Adoption Information Clearinghouse, 2004). Growing up in contemporary American society is challenging, even in the best of circumstances; however, growing up adopted is for many, a special challenge. It is not that adopted children are maladjusted, per se. Interestingly, empirical meta-analytic studies have suggested that they are generally well adjusted (Smith & Brodzinsky, 2002). And certainly, non-adopted children experience a variety of disturbing events including illness, parental divorce and abuse. However, the challenge of mastering each of life's obstacles is compounded along the adopted child's developmental trajectory by the emerging reality and implications of their adoptive status.

With regard to this "developmental" perspective to adoption, Brodzinsky, Smith, and Brodzinsky (1998) discovered through extensive interviews with adoptees, that each phase of their life presents unique challenges, consistent with Erik Erikson's stages. During infancy, the adoptee's task, like that of the child raised by their biological parents, is to adjust to a new home, surroundings, and people, particularly the primary caretaker. This is an even greater challenge to the infant removed from the care of his biological mother during this critical period. During toddler-hood, the adopted child may first become exposed to information about adoption, and begin to notice physical differences between herself and her adoptive parents. However, it is during the school-age years that the child first wrestles with the implications of being adopted and must begin to consider that if someone adopted them, someone must have "given them away." This is the period when emotional reactions to adoption, both positive and negative, begin to emerge. Adolescence brings the additional challenge of integrating adoptive status into their emerging identity, and reconciling the differences between themselves, their families and others who are not adopted.

During young adulthood, adoptees who search for their birth parents begin to do so in earnest as they learn to integrate their adoptive identity into their emerging self-hood. The added challenges of beginning a romantic relationship and having children contribute to the challenge of creating a legacy and choosing whether to adopt or to have biological children. Middle adulthood carries with it the task of further integrating their adoptive identity into their own aging, beginning to construct their history, and making peace with the loss of the inevitable loss of parents, both adoptive and biological. Finally, the elder adoptee must reconcile their status with end-of-life issues, and in so doing, solidify their legacy.

As this developmental perspective suggests, adjustment to adoption is a lifelong process. However, two prominent themes emerge in the adoptive journey: the search for identity and loss. According to Brodzinsky, Schecter, and Henig (1992):

> The struggle to understand who you are, where you fit in and how you feel about yourself is universal; it is a unique part of being human. Adoptees go through the search for self in some unique characteristic ways and many of the differences (between them and non-adoptees) can be explained by the fact that adoption cuts off people from a part of themselves. To understand the psychology of adoption from the perspective of the adoptee is (also) to recognize and appreciate the unique role played by loss in the search for self. (p. 3)

So potentially profound is the loss associated with adoption, it has been referred to as a 'primal wound' (Verrier, 1993). As the adoptee grows better able to cognitively appreciate loss, she comes to realize that regardless of how wonderful it was to be 'wanted' (by the adoptive parents), someone, somewhere, for whatever reason, "gave her away." Loss becomes potentially fused to the adopted child's narrative, and search for identity and self invariably becomes a search, in one form or another, either literal or figurative, for the birth parent. According to Verrier, " . . . the search for self is a mission for many adoptees (and) seems to be intimately connected to the search for the birth-mother (or birth-father) . . . " (1993, p. 33). In addition, the unfolding narrative of loss in the child's life is compounded by the real, felt, or imagined losses experienced by the other members of the adoption triangle: the birth and adoptive parents.

The challenges of loss and the search for self are compounded in the cases of domestic inter-racial and trans-national adoption. In each of these situations, the adopted child can be reminded, typically by virtue of appearance, that she came from another family. According to Pertman (2000), " . . . children who look nothing like their parents (or extended families) are more deeply steeped in reminders that they are adopted" (p. 121). In addition to the dissimilarity in appearance with his adoptive parents, the trans-national adoptee may experiences a "genealogical bewilderment," which is " . . . the feeling of being cut off from your heritage, your religious background, your culture and your race" (Brodzinsky, Schecter, & Henig, 1992, p. 108). Importantly, and as in the case of adoption outcome research in general, there is little empirical evidence supporting the long-term adverse impact of inter-racial or trans-national adoption (Brodzinsky, Smith, & Brodzinsky, 1998). However, these are obstacles, no less, for the adopted child.

Regardless of the nature and circumstances of their adoption, research suggests that adoptees express curiosity about and search for their birth parents. It has been estimated that in countries that provide access to birth records (after the age of majority), 50% of adoptees initiate a search for their birth parents at some point in their lives (Muller & Perry, 2001-A). The search is more often for birth mothers than it is for birth fathers. It initially has a positive outcome and typically follows a period of internal struggle over such issues as identity and genealogy (Muller & Perry, 2001-B). While children in families more open to adoption-related communication freely ask questions about their origins, it is during late adolescence that the questions increase. And, it is in early adulthood that adoptees more actively search for and contact their birth parents.

MYTHS AND MISCONCEPTIONS ABOUT ADOPTION

As the above discussion suggests, adoption is a complex psychological, social and cultural phenomenon; and as such, has potential for misunderstanding. In the public forum, this is called stigma, myth and misconception. In academia and clinical practice, it is seen in unsubstantiated theory and unfounded technique. Regardless of their origin and the name they go by, myths and misconceptions about adoption permeate our culture through all forms of popular and professional media; from daytime television to college and professional texts. With regard to adoption, and particularly in the context of clinical intervention with members of the adoption triangle, erroneous beliefs, myths and presumptions on the part of the clinician can undermine treatment and cause unintended harm.

One of the more prominent of these adoptions myths is that of the 'bad seed phenomenon' (Hartman & Laird, 1990). This refers to the inevitable adverse impact of genetics on the adoptee's emotional, psychological, and behavioral functioning. According to this line of thinking, the genetic legacy of domestic violence, learning disability, substance abuse, and mental illness can not be mitigated by even the best of adoptive placements: nature trumps nurture. Empirical research does not support this 'biology is destiny' hypothesis (Smith & Brodzinsky, 2002). Equally prevalent is the fallacy that adoptees are far more likely than non-adopted peers to manifest psychiatric disturbance, receive psychological services, psychotropic medication and residential treatment. In fact, the results of empirical and meta-analytic studies suggest that, in general, adoptees are well adjusted (Smith & Brodzinsky, 2002).

In a study comparing the information on adoption in college textbooks and readers with empirical research, it was determined that "the coverage provided (of adoption), was predominantly negative, stressing the potential problems of adoption about twice as often as its probable successes and rewards" (Fisher, 2003, p. 154). Some of the more glaring misrepresentations of adoption in this analysis included its inaccessibility to homosexuals, inevitable legal entanglements, inextricable racial and cultural dilemmas, unavoidable stigmatization and the rarity of truly positive outcomes.

Along similar lines, Horner (2000) turned a critical adoptee's-eye view to the adoption literature, advocating that clinicians familiarize themselves with empirical research in order to avoid the adverse impact of mythology on their treatment. Some of the more clinically dangerous myths included the belief that all adoptees feel compelled to search for their birthparents, ethnic differences between adopted children and adoptive parents plague all inter-racial adoptions, open adoptions undermine adoptive family ties and that there is an extensive body of empirical research on psychological treatment in adoption.

A CAVEAT

The previous discussions on the empirical literature and mythology surrounding adoption suggest a growing body of credible scientific research in this area dating back several decades. That the notion "there is an extensive body of empirical psychological treatment in adoption" is more myth than reality, seems counter-intuitive. However, at closer inspection, and from the perspective of psychotherapy, the absence of a body of evidenced based treatment outcome research makes good sense.

In my clinical practice, as well as those of colleagues who work with adoption, it is uncommon for a child or family to be referred to counseling because of adoption, per se. This population of clients is demographically and clinically broad. Clients who are adopted struggle with issues similar to those of people raised by their biological parents. These issues include depression, peer and family problems, and self-esteem. The major difference is that they also wrestle with the additional impact of their adoption on otherwise "normal" developmental challenges, such as attachment, relationships, identity, aging and loss (Brodzinsky, Schecter, & Henig, 1992). There are far more treatment models and techniques available for these issues than there are for adoption, because adoption is not a clinical problem to be solved or a symptom to be eliminated. Therefore, it is at the clinician's discretion to decide whether individual, group or family therapy is warranted; whether to apply cognitive, psychoanalytic or gestalt techniques; and whether to utilize traditional verbal therapies or creative-expressive modalities. In the absence of either a commonly accepted modality of treatment or specific techniques for "adoption," I have chosen to apply the superhero adoption narrative in the context of play therapy in order to help certain clients who struggle with adoption related issues.

FANTASY PLAY AND SUPERHEROES

Fantasy play has long been regarded as a valuable component of clinical work with children. While not a child-therapist, Sigmund Freud was reportedly moved by a young client who was play-acting separation from his mother. He noted "in their play, children repeat everything that has made a great impression on them in real life, and that in doing so, they abstract the strength of the impression and make themselves a master of the situation" (1955, p. 17). Freud's daughter, Anna, who specialized in the treatment of children, was concerned that fantasy play had the potential to undermine a child's healthy psychological development (1965). However, she also considered it to be a powerful means of working through intra-psychic sexual and aggressive conflicts, as well as a therapeutic tool for understanding the child's worldview. Other important voices, both within and beyond the realm of psychoanalysis, have addressed the importance of fantasy and fantasy play in healthy cognitive and emotional development (Bettleheim, 1987; Bruner, 1986; Erikson, 1963; Landreth, 2002; Piaget, 1962; Vygotsky, 1978). The consensus of this interdisciplinary chorus is that fantasy provides the child with a means of both deepening their understanding of, and experimenting with reality, working through feelings related to both positive and negative experiences, and gaining a sense of mastery that is inaccessible to them because of their tender years.

Of the innumerable fantasies available to children, adolescents and adults, the superhero has become a mainstay in our cultural consciousness, as well as a part of our collective unconscious. A mere three years after Superman was introduced to the American public, psychoanalysts Bender and Lourie (1941) advocated for the use of superhero fantasy play in psychotherapy. Since that time, hundreds, if not thousands of superheroes have flown from the pages of comic books into movies, literature, television, video games, music and material culture. The ubiquity of superheroes in our culture begs the question, "what is their appeal,?" and in the context of this discussion, how can this appeal be constructively channeled psychotherapeutically?

According to Lawrence and Jewett (2002):

> The (American) mono mythic superhero is distinguished by disguised origins, pure motivations, a redemptive task and extraordinary powers. He originates outside of the community he is called to save, and in those exceptional instances when he resides therein, the superhero plays the role of the idealistic loner. His identity is secret, either by virtue of his unknown origins or his alter ego: his motivation is a selfless zeal for justice. By elaborate conventions of restraint, his desire for revenge is purified. Patient in the face of provocations, he seeks nothing for himself and withstands all temptations. He renounces sexual fulfillment for the duration for the mission, and the purity of his motivation ensures his moral infallibility in judging persons and situations. When he is threatened by violent adversaries, he finds answers in vigilantism, restoring justice and thus lifting the siege of paradise. In order to accomplish this mission without incurring blame or causing undue injury to others, he requires superhuman powers. The superhero's aim is unerring, his fists irresistible, and his body incapable of suffering fatal injury. (p. 47)

In addition to these core elements of the genre, innumerable superheroes have been challenged by early life circumstances that even the most conservative of clinicians would regard as traumatic: violent parental loss, abandonment and adoption. According to Reynolds, "the (super) hero is marked out from society . . . often reaching maturity without having a relationship with his parents" (1992, p. 16). While plot-lines, such as early life adversity, incredible powers and vulnerabilities and crucial missions of salvation are certainly compelling to fans of comics and movies, they can also be therapeutically useful.

HOW CAN SUPERHEROES HELP?

The answer to the preceding question becomes clear when we consider that each traditional superhero has a powerful origin story, possesses unique powers and vulnerabilities, conceals their true power beneath a benign façade (secret identity), struggles to find a connection to the society he serves, undergoes a life-changing transformational journey, and battles with demonic villains. These rich and varied components of the superhero fantasy provide a child with limitless therapeutic metaphors and vehicles with which to explore and resolve their own personal dilemmas.

In the same way that superheroes begin their journeys from unique starting points and places and undergo transformative changes along the way, clients too, embark on lifelong adventures to reconcile their present with their past, and to make peace with early challenges, including the losses inherent in adoption. Just as superheroes are influenced by adversity and trauma, so, too, are clients altered by painful experiences, such as abuse, divorce, illness, loss and relocation. While clients do not have super powers or fatal flaws, per se, identifying with the strengths and weaknesses of their favorite superhero can help a client come to terms with disabilities and deficiencies, either real or perceived.

Most germane to the current discussion is the superhero adoption narrative. Some of the most historically prominent superheroes are adopted. Superman, was born Kal-El, son of Jor-El and Lara, prominent scientists on the doomed planet of Krypton. Knowing that the end was near, they sent their infant son hurtling to Earth in a space-craft equipped with the entire history of their civilization; a home study that would impress even the most diligent of adoption workers. The rest is history, at least to comic book fans. The super infant was lovingly raised as Clark Kent by adoptive parents Jonathan and Martha, who nurtured both his mortal and super soul as he experimented with his emerging God-like powers. While Clark was devoted to the Kents, he clung to the memories and lessons taken from his biological parents.

Peter Parker was the son of American patriots Richard and Mary, who were violently murdered while serving their country. Peter was subsequently adopted by his paternal uncle and aunt, Ben and May, who taught him among other things "with great power comes great responsibility." This axiom was prophetic for young Parker, who became the Amazing Spiderman after being bitten by a radioactive spider. While Peter never forgot the important and loving lessons of his uncle and aunt, those who follow the adventures of Spiderman are continually reminded of the deep sense of loss he carried within him.

Then there is Bruce Wayne, son of Thomas and Martha, who was orphaned following the brutal murder of his parents. While Bruce was adopted by Alfred, the loyal and loving family butler, it is not difficult to see how Bruce's childhood trauma shaped his future identity as the vigilante dark knight, known as Batman.

All three of these superheroes, Superman, Spiderman, and Batman were adopted. Their lives and heroic journeys were, in large part, shaped by the experiences of their early lives, most prominently adoption. Let us now turn to one other heroic fantasy figure, Luke Skywalker of the Star Wars saga, who, while not a "superhero," he embodies the genre that will form the foundation for the clinical case hero.

THE STAR WARS ADOPTION NARRATIVE

For those familiar with the original Star Wars saga (episodes IV-VI), the names Luke Skywalker, Princess Leah, Darth Vader, Obewan-Kenobi and Yoda conjure tales of great adventure. While not ostensibly a superhero tale, Star Wars contains all of the core elements of the genre as outlined above by Lawrence and Jewett (2002). In addition, and according to Champlin, "Lucas devoured the great themes: epic struggles between god and evil, heroes and villains, magical princesses and ogres, heroines and evil princes, (and) the transmission from father to sons of the powers of both good and evil" (1992, p. 41). True to the superhero genre, Lucas utilized fantasy and science fiction in order to draw our attention to issues affecting societies, planets, star systems, and individual protagonists.

Foremost among these protagonists is Luke Skywalker, whose name is not usually associated with the traditional superhero. His adventures have more in common with Joseph Campbell's classical heroes, Ulysses, Hercules, and Prometheus (1949). However, Luke Skywalker is arguably akin to Superman, Captain America, and Green Lantern. Like many of his super-relatives, Luke's birth and early childhood is cloaked in secrecy and adversity. While he can neither leap tall buildings in a single bound, travel faster than a speeding locomotive, nor lift imponderable weights, Luke has inherited the power of *the force*. With the aid of this legacy, he wields powerful weapons, moves objects telekinetically, and "senses" events happening far away or before they happen. Not least among his super heroic characteristics, Luke fights against evil.

Luke Skywalker's heroic adventures are clearly the predominant narrative underscoring the first Star Wars trilogy. Equally compelling, however, particularly as it relates to the clinical case to be described in this chapter, is the sub-narrative surrounding his adoption. Luke's adventure is rooted in a childhood lost, a traumatic disconnection from his biological parents, and the dramatic subsequent search for his true identity and his father Anakin Skywalker, also known as Darth Vader.

Luke and his sister, Leia Organa, are the children of Padame Amidala and Anakin Skywalker. Their relationship is destroyed by the ongoing battle between the Federation and the Empire. After their mother's death, the twins are separated and Luke is raised by his paternal uncle and aunt. After they are killed by the Empire, Luke embarks on a journey of self-discovery, which includes finding his father. In doing so, he must reconcile the powerful opposing forces within himself, and both confront and accept his legacy before re-claiming a rightful place in his family.

Ironically, Anakin Skywalker, who also shares in the adoption narrative, is not as fortunate as his son. While Luke is guided along his journey by the benevolent Obiwan-Kenobi and Yoda, who lead him to the light, Anakin was corrupted by the Evil Emperor, Palpatine, to join the Dark Side as Darth Vader. Both Luke and his father struggle, each in their own way, to reconcile early losses and subsequent adoption. Let us now turn to a real-life story no less epic in scope or mythic in its significance than the one of Luke and Anakin Skywalker–the story of Alex.

CASE PRESENTATION

Intake

Alex, a previously happy, seemingly self-contented and compliant eleven-year-old, had become a great concern to his parents. More argumentative both at home and at school, Alex had also begun complaining of feeling sad and much to his parent's dismay, curious about his "real parents." According to his parents, Alex had become much more self-conscious about the differences in appearance between himself and his family, both nuclear and extended. During moments of defiance, Alex would say things like "I don't have to listen to you. You're not my real parents!" This hurt them deeply and opened old wounds.

Alex, like his older brother, was adopted at birth; however, unlike his brother who was blond-haired and fair-skinned, he was of Asian descent. While the adoption had initially been uneventful and legally unencumbered, his biological father emerged within several months to assert his paternal rights. This man argued that Alex's biological mother had failed to tell him she was pregnant, and had moved away after their relationship ended. When he discovered that she had given birth to their child, he hired an investigator and an attorney, the result of which was a fierce litigation with Alex's adoptive parents. In response, they agreed to grant him visitation with the child.

By the time the biological father's interest in Alex had waned, along with the visitations, the adoptive parents had been traumatized by the surrounding media attention and their continuous fear that they would somehow lose their son. They made a pact, more unknowingly than consciously, not to discuss the adoption with Alex, unless of course, he asked. Over the next several years, Alex became increasingly aware of the physical differences between himself and family members, both nuclear and extended. During these moments, questions arose, but were only nominally addressed. Otherwise, Alex proceeded on a relatively uneventful development journey and was described by his parents as an intelligent, highly verbal and creative child who loved the History and Discovery channels as well as all things Star Wars.

As the intake session drew to a close, I better understood Alex through his parent's eyes. I also began to appreciate how difficult the journey had been for them. Although they gained a son, Alex's entry into their life was surrounded by loss, and they were continually threatened by losing him during those early contentious years. While it had become easy for them to conceal painful memories between scrapbook covers, Alex's parents were now threatened by the feared loss of his affection as he began questioning his origins. I then realized that in order to help Alex to continue on his journey to self-discovery and healing, I would have to help his parents do the same.

Initial Contact

Alex was immediately engaging, greeting me with warmth and a wide smile. He was attentive as I introduced him to my therapy room–

sand box, miniatures, doll-house, arts and crafts materials, puppets, comic books, board games and action figures. As Alex discussed his growing sense of alienation, both at home and at school, along with a sadness that was taking him over, he rummaged through the various superheroes: Batman, Wonder Woman, Iron Man, Green Lantern and Luke Skywalker. Alex shared his fascination with time travel, wondering what it would be like to travel back and change his life. He reflected upon the magnificent accomplishments of Michelangelo and Leonard Da Vinci, reflecting on what he would do if he were a great inventor. Without prompting, Alex brought up his adoption and the fact that he looked very different than everyone else in his family. He thought that he might have met his biological father, but he wasn't sure. When asked what his parents had discussed with him about the adoption, he offered "not much." Alex then began to discuss Star Wars, musing that if he could change his name, it would become Michelangelo Skywalker, a cross between his favorite inventor and superhero. When I asked Alex to describe the story of Michelangelo, he eagerly rose to a challenge that would set the stage for the remainder of our work.

Heroic Journeys and Mortal Goals

Over the next several sessions, Alex dictated, and together we refined the narrative which he entitled "Star Wars, Episode VII: The Search for Luke." It chronicled the as yet untold story of Luke Skywalker's marriage and entry into parenthood by way of adoption. Still bereft and grieving the loss of his own father, Luke was compelled to place his child Michelangelo into foster care. Michelangelo grew to be a great Jedi warrior, who then set out on an adventure of his own to conquer evil and find his father. At the end of Alex's narrative, father and son were united, and each was rendered whole in the process.

In the course of discussing the narrative, Alex composed a series of questions he hoped that he could someday ask his biological parents, particularly his father, including:

- Why did you give me up for adoption?
- Why haven't I been able to see you all of these years?
- Do I have any other brothers, sisters or cousins?
- Who will I be when I grow up?

In attempting to answer these questions through our discussions, Alex became aware of questions that would form the foundation of his own heroic journey toward understanding and healing which included:

- What are my true powers?
- How do I reconcile the fantasies of my biological parents with the realities of my adoptive life?
- To whom may I reveal my secret (adoptive) identity?
- How do I learn to accept painful feelings related to the losses I experienced?
- How do I find hope for the future so that I may confront life's challenges
- Can I look different from my family and still be a part of it?

Accomplishments

In the course of developing his Star Wars narrative, Alex had begun his healing journey. His story was a first attempt to openly share the pain of losing someone close to him, as well as the loss of a part of himself that he could not get back, other than through fantasy. Through the narrative story-telling, Alex was able to express sadness related to the loss of his biological legacy, as well as the other life he would never have. He seemed quite enthusiastic in the telling, as if a burden had been lifted from him.

Alex also began to construct an identity that included, rather than excluded, loss. While adoption formed a cornerstone of his identity, he could acknowledge that as with any great and complex structure, there are many foundational elements. Thus, he began to see that the love of his adoptive family, and a safe and secure place in the world are additional and equally important essential ingredients of "self." While the journey to wholeness would no doubt take him down perilous paths fraught with new challenges, he had hopefully gained some strength to take the first steps.

For Alex, sadness and anger would no longer be viewed so dramatically as arch enemies, but instead as parts of himself–as allies. His willingness to rise to the challenge of re-writing his narrative signaled a growing inner strength that had likely been there all along, hidden in his creative pursuits. This inner strength was further exemplified in the courageous questions he had prepared for his birth parents, should he someday meet them.

While Alex's parents remained ambivalent about proactively addressing adoption issues with him, they nevertheless signed on for the healing journey by entrusting him to my care. In my last meeting with them, they had shared with me Alex's adoption scrapbook, complete with all of the newspaper headlines that had surrounded the adoption years before. Perhaps they would someday share those images and stories with Alex.

Reflections

When Alex showed an initial interest in superheroes, science fiction and Star Wars, I was optimistic that we would find a common ground for communication around difficult issues. However, I was also concerned that I might push too hard by being overly directive around the issue of adoption. In the past, around the time that I been relatively new to the role of adoptive parent, I treated a young adopted client. My anxiety over having him express feelings about the adoption led me to push him into unwanted conversations about it. After only a few sessions, he complained to his mother, "he makes me talk about stuff I don't want to!" I worried that I might do the same with my next adopted client.

In retrospect, I believe that I learned from that early therapeutic misstep and respected Alex's ability to set his own therapeutic goals and work creatively towards accomplishing them. I was able to do this by trusting my own creative process; my healer's voice. I have come to understand that as an adoptive parent working with adoptive families, I become a necessary, albeit temporary link in their "adoption triangle." I have since learned that this so-called adoption triangle is truly forged in bonds of hope. It is, however, also built upon loss; that of the biological parents' connection to their child, that of the adoptive parents' relationship to a biological child they will never have, and that of the adopted child's biological legacy. The journey towards healing in adoption is truly a heroic and lifelong adventure.

REFERENCES

Bender, L., & Lourie, R. (1941). The effect of comic books on the ideology of children. *American Journal of Orthopsychiatry, 11*(3), 540-550.

Bettelheim, B. (1987). The importance of play. *The Atlantic Monthly, 259,* 35-46.

Brodzinsky, D., Schecter, M., & Henig, R. (1992). *Being adopted: The lifelong search for self.* New York: Doubleday.

Brodzinsky, D., Smith, D., & Brodzinsky, A. (1998). *Children's adjustment to adoption: Developmental and clinical issues.* New York: Sage Publications.

Bruner, J. (1986). Play, thought, and language. *Prospects: Quarterly Review of Education, 16*(1), 77-83.

Campbell, J. (1949). *The hero with a thousand faces.* Princeton, NJ: Princeton University Press.

Champlin, C. (1992). *George Lucas: The creative impulse.* New York: Harry N. Abrams, Inc.

Erikson, E. (1963). *Childhood and society.* New York: W.W. Norton.

Fisher, A. (2003). A critique of the portrayal of adoption in college textbooks and readers on families. *Family Relations, 52*(2), 154-160.

Freud, A. (1965). *Normality and pathology in childhood: Assessments of development.* New York: International Universities Press, Inc.

Freud, S. (1955). Beyond the pleasure principle. In J. Strachey (Ed. & Translator), *The standard edition of the complete psychological works of Sigmund Freud* (1st ed.) (pp.17-29). London: Hogarth.

Hartman, A., & Laird, J. (1990). Family treatment after adoption: Common theories. In D. Brodzinsky & M. Schecter, (Eds.), *The psychology of adoption* (pp. 221-239). New York: Oxford University Press.

Horner, R. D. (2000). A practitioner looks at adoption research. *Family Relations, 49*(4), 473-477.

Landreth, G. (2002). *Play therapy: The art of the relationship.* New York: Brunner Routledge.

Lawrence, J. S., & Jewett, R. (2002). *The myth of the American superhero.* Grand Rapids, MI: William B. Eerdmans Publishing Company.

Muller, U., & Perry, B. (2001a). Adopted persons' search for contact with their birth parents I: Who searches and why? *Adoption Quarterly, 4*(3), 5-37.

Muller, U., & Perry, B. (2001b). Adopted persons' search for and contact with their birthparents II: Adoptee-birth parent contact, *Adoption Quarterly, 4*(3), 39-62.

National Adoption Information Clearinghouse. (2004). How many children were adopted in 2000 and 2001–Highlights. Retrieved December 20, 2005 from http://naic.acf.hhs.gov/pubs/s_adoptedhighlights.cfm

Pertman, A. (2000). *Adoption nation: How the adoption revolution is transforming America.* New York: Basic Books.

Piaget, J. (1962). *Play, dreams and imitation in childhood.* New York: Norton.

Reynolds, R. (1992). *Super heroes: A modern mythology.* Jackson, MS: University of Mississippi Press.

Ryan, S., & Nalavany, B. (2003). Adopted children: Who do they turn to for help and why? *Adoption Quarterly, 7*(2), 29-52.

Smith, D., & Brodzinsky, D. (2002). Coping with birthparent loss in adopted children. *Journal of Child Psychology and Psychiatry and Allied Disciplines, 43*(2), 213-223.

Verrier, N. N. (1993). *The primal wound: Understanding the adopted child.* Baltimore, MD: Gateway Press, Inc.

Vygotsky, L. S. (1978). *Mind in society.* Cambridge, MA: Harvard University Press.

doi:10.1300/J456v01n03_15

Chapter 16

Coping Responses and Emotional Distress in Fathers of Children with Special Needs and "Redreaming" as a Creative Intervention

Andrew P. Daire
Montserrat Casado-Kehoe
Chang-Hui Lin

SUMMARY. Parents dream that their children will have every benefit possible to survive and thrive in the world. When their children have special needs, these dreams are challenged. Parents must adjust to the needs of their child and to the loss of this aspect of their dream. Common challenges and considerations when working with fathers of children with special needs are presented. "Redreaming," an intervention to facilitate positive reappraisal, and creative approaches are also presented. doi:10.1300/J456v01n03_16 *[Article copies available for a fee from The Haworth Document Delivery Service: 1-800-HAWORTH. E-mail address: <docdelivery@haworthpress.com> Website: <http://www.HaworthPress.com> © 2005 by The Haworth Press, Inc. All rights reserved.]*

Andrew P. Daire and Montserrat Casado-Kehoe are affiliated with the University of Central Florida.

Chang-Hui Lin is affiliated with the Brigham Young University, HI.

Address correspondence to: Andrew P. Daire, PhD, Assistant Professor, Counselor Education, University of Central Florida, P.O. 161250, Orlando, FL 32816-1250 (E-mail: adaire@mail.ucf.edu).

[Haworth co-indexing entry note]: "Coping Responses and Emotional Distress in Fathers of Children with Special Needs and 'Redreaming' as a Creative Intervention." Daire, Andrew P., Montserrat Casado-Kehoe, and Chang-Hui Lin. Co-published simultaneously in *Journal of Creativity in Mental Health* (The Haworth Press, Inc.) Vol. 1, No. 3/4. 2005, pp. 253-271; and: *Creative Interventions in Grief and Loss Therapy: When the Music Stops, a Dream Dies* (ed: Thelma Duffey) The Haworth Press, Inc., 2005, pp. 253-271. Single or multiple copies of this article are available for a fee from The Haworth Document Delivery Service [1-800-HAWORTH, 9:00 a.m. - 5:00 p.m. (EST). E-mail address: docdelivery@haworthpress.com].

KEYWORDS. Creative intervention, coping responses, distress, fathers, children, special needs, counseling, mental health

O, I believe
Fate smiled and destiny
Laughed as she came to my cradle
Know this child will be able . . .
With love, with patience, with faith
She'll make her way

(Merchant, 1995)

Parents with young children face many challenges and stressors. For most parents, the role of parent requires commitment and specific obligations and responsibilities to meet the needs of children on a daily basis (Simmerman, Blacher, & Baker, 2001). Ideally, both the mother and the father play a role in providing resources and opportunities that assist in the child's development. Although the topic of fathers' involvement in children's development remains understudied, more recent research has examined how fathering impacts children's growing up in a variety of ways in the last 20 years (Carpenter, 2002; Cummings & O'Reilly, 1997; Navalkar, 2004; Pelchart, Lefebvre, & Perreault, 2003). Fathers play an important role in helping children develop positive identities and children need fathers to make them feel competent and worthy, as well as to learn life skills. Successful fathers see their role as important and worthwhile (Ballantine, 2000). Without a doubt, these factors impact children's well-being and development (Cummings & O'Reilly, 1997).

But, what do we know about the experiences of parents whose children have special needs? When parents have a child with a special need, a dream for what they hoped their child would experience dies. Given that, parent needs time to grieve and to find coping skills for the challenges they will encounter. However, a gap in the research exists on how fathers are affected psychologically, emotionally and relationally by their children's disabilities (Carpenter, 2002; Lamb & Billings, 1997). In this manuscript, the authors will provide an overview of the literature on the specific needs of fathers with children who have special needs. The authors will also provide creative interventions for working with these fathers and present the findings of a study investigating the relationship between the emotional distress experienced by these fathers and the coping responses they utilized.

The U.S. Department for Health and Human Services (USDHHS) defined children with special needs as those who, " . . . have or are at increased risk for a chronic physical, developmental, behavioral, or emotional condition and who also require health and related services of a type or amount beyond that required by children generally" (USDHHS, 2004). According to the 2001 National Survey of Children with Special Health Care Needs, it was estimated that 12.8%, or 9.4 million, children in the United States have special needs (USDHHS, 2004). The survey results also indicated that 20% of U.S. households were raising children with special needs.

However, a challenge exists in specifying the types of special needs because over 40 definitions existed at the federal level based on programs and research (Westbrook, Silver, & Stein, 1998). Additionally, the Americans With Disabilities Act (ADA) defined disabilities as a "physical or mental impairment that substantially limits one or more of the major life activities of such individual" (ADA, 1990). However, types of disabilities included visual (mild visual impairment to blindness), hearing (mild hearing loss to deafness), physical or orthopedic (weakness or loss of motor control), learning (see DSM-IV-TR), psychiatric (see DSM-IV-TR), and medical (medical condition that requires medical intervention or accommodation) (American Psychiatric Association, 1994). Another category, developmental disabilities, was defined by the the Administration for Children and Families (ACF) as " . . . severe, life-long disabilities attributable to mental and/or physical impairment, manifested before age 22" (ACF, n.d.).

How then, does one begin to understand the various types of disabilities and conditions that contribute to a child having a special need? Westbrook et al. (1998) found it beneficial to consider three areas of consequence when a child had a special need: Functional limitations (FL), dependence on compensatory mechanisms or assistance (CD), and service use or need beyond routine care (SU/N) when defining disabilities and special needs in children. They conceptualized functional limitation "as limitation of the function, activities, or social role compared with healthy age peers in the general areas of physical, cognitive, emotional, and social growth and development" (p. 1026). Dependence on compensatory mechanisms or assistance was "conceptualized as dependency on an accommodating mechanism to compensate for or minimize limitation of function, activities, or social role" (p. 1024). And, service use or need beyond routine care was "conceptualized as the use of or need for medical care or related services, psychological services, or educational services beyond the norm for the child's age, or use of or need for special ongoing treatments, interventions, or accommodations at home or in school" (p. 1024).

It is beyond the scope of this manuscript to provide a detailed description of the many different conditions that contribute to a child having a special need. However, what may be relevant for counselors to consider when working with fathers of a child with special needs are the functional limitations, dependence on compensatory mechanisms or assistance, and service use or need beyond routine care in the children with special needs and how these three types of consequences contribute to parental strain and distress. Counselors also need to consider how the different types of disabilities and consequences can contribute to varied health and medical problems for the child (Beresford, 1995; Newacheck et al., 1998), behavioral problems in the child (Gray, 2002; Hassall, Rose, & McDonald, 2005; Saloviita, Italinna, & Leinonen, 2003), and parental burden and emotional distress for the parents (Gray, 2003). Newacheck et al. (1998) found that children with special needs had three times as many days, twice as many school absences, almost three times as many physician visits, and three times as many hospitalizations when compared to children without special needs.

Additionally, these increased visits contributed to increased healthcare costs and financial stressors (Beresford, 1995; Dobson & Middleton, 1998). Behaviors problems also presented problems for the child and contributed to distress in the parents. Gray (2002) found a greater level of distress in parents of adolescents with autism when aggressive and/or severely obsessive behaviors were present. Saloviita et al. (2003) found that the existence of behavior problems in the child was the greatest predictor of stress. Similar findings were also reported by Hassall et al. (2005) that supported the association between child behavior difficulties and parenting stress.

Parents of children with special needs experienced varied emotions including disappointment, sadness or depression, loneliness, fear, anger, frustration, shock, devastation ad numbness (Gray, 2003; Pelchat & Lefebre, 2003). Increased parental and caregiver demands also contributed to greater levels of overall distress (Ehrenkrantz, Miller, Vernberg, & Fox, 2001; Keller & Honig, 2004). For fathers, one specific predictor of stress was their perception of social acceptance (Saloviita et al., 2003). Another was irritability and demanding behavior of the child (Dyson & Fewell, 1986). Fathers also experience more difficulty than mother in accepting the disability diagnosis of their child (Lamb & Billings, 1997).

In response to this distress, fathers were more likely to suppress their feelings than mothers, who were able to engage in more productive coping behaviors (Gray, 2003). Men also tended to distance themselves, exhibit less confidence, greater difficulty in deriving meaning form the situation, and less mastery in coping strategies than women (Grant & Whittell, 2000). However, more research is needed to better understand the experiences of fathers for a child with a special need (Carpenter, 2002; Navalkar, 2004; Turbiville & Marquis, 2001).

When investigating fathers of a child who has special needs, adaptation and adjustment were important areas of inquiry (Lamb & Billings, 1997). Understanding fathers' reactions to the diagnosis and prognosis of the child are relevant elements to evaluate (Simmerman et al., 2001). According to Lamb and Billing (1997), fathers experience more difficulties than mothers in accepting their children's diagnosis as well as the long-term implications of the disability. For parents of a child with a disability, self-esteem, emotional stability, expectations along with hopes and dreams suffer (Pelchat et al., 2003; Wang et al., 2004). Caring for a child with special needs presents additional stresses for both parents. However, fathers and mothers may have different needs and cope differently with this stress. A need does exist to examine psychological and emotional impact caring for a child with a special need has on fathers.

During the last decade, coping has received quite a bit of attention in research (Blalock & Joiner, 2000; Houser & Seligman, 1991; Moos, 1993; Sears, Stanton, & Danoff-Burg, 2003). Indeed, focus has been given to understand the effects of stressful life events on psychological and emotional well-being (Sears et al., 2003). How does coping counteract the effects of stressful life events (Corbeil, Quayhagen, & Quayhagen, 1999)? And can coping mechanisms lower the impact of stressful life events (Miller, Cate, & Johann-Murphy, 2001)? If so, is there a relationship between coping and emotional levels of distress? Ways of coping have been explained as problem-focused or emotion-focused and approach-based or avoidance-based (Moos, 1993; Moos, Brennan, Fondacaro, & Moos, 1990; Sharkansky et al., 2000). Problem-focused coping addresses dealing with the precipitating stressor and emotion-focused addresses managing emotional responses. Approach-based coping involves direct attempts to resolve the problem and avoidance-based coping involves not thinking about the stressor. Some studies suggest that the avoidant coping strategies lead to increases in depressed moods more than approach and problem-emotion focused coping strategies (Billings & Moos, 1985; Blalock & Joiner, 2000; Moos et al., 1990).

CREATIVE INTERVENTIONS TO HELP PARENTS COPE

When working with fathers of children with special needs, creative approaches can be used to help them utilize positive strategies as they cope with multiple challenges. For example, one of the major and ongoing stressors, particularly at different developmental milestones, is realizing that one's child is not going to be able to do all the various things parents usually dream of during pregnancy. This realization contributes to the emotional distress already experienced by parents (Lamb & Billings, 1997; Wang et al., 2004). "Redreaming" is one coping response with potential for helping parents of children with special needs. As an intervention, "redreaming" is a cognitive reappraisal process that allows parents to establish news hopes, goals, accomplishments and dreams for their child. Clinically, one can think of "redreaming" as a way to enhance reframing. Three creative interventions to facilitate this "redreaming" process are creating a dream collage for their child, the use of drawings, and the use of journaling.

In creating a dream collage for their child, the parent creates a visual collection of what they dream for their child that helps them see and evaluate expectations, hopes, and desires for the child, considering their potentials and limitations. These "redreams" would include things they wish for their child and look forward to help their child attain. A dream collage brings a concrete and hopeful picture for the parents. The dream collage also allows parents to focus on positives they wish for the child's future.

When creating a dream collage, the parents are asked to bring copies of pictures that are representative of the child and are given a poster board, copies of magazines, glue and a pair of scissors. Clients look through the magazines and cut out phrases, words or pictures that are representative of what they dream for their child. Then, they can begin creating a dream collage. Like any creative activity, it is important to process the activity with the parents. This process involves examination and self-evaluation of their hopes, expectations, and desires for their child as well as the related emotional responses.

John, a 38-year-old father whose 4-year-old son was born with cerebral palsy, said the following in response to the counselor's question about the collage: "Well, here is Jonathan in the middle of the picture. On the outside, the symbol of medical pills represents doctors and medical facilities because that is so much a part of his life and will probably always be part of his life. I put a ball here on the outside because he and I

[handwritten marginalia: Collage of hope - magazines]

enjoy playing ball together and I hope he can enjoy sports despite his limitations. I also put a picture of my wife and me because this has been a stressful journey for all of us. But, we are both committed to take care of our son, even if we do so in our different ways." The collage helped John verbalize current challenges as well as new dreams he had for his child.

Another creative intervention involves the use of drawings. The counselor can ask the parents to draw a picture of the child's future; what they envision the child to be able to do. The parents are given drawing paper, crayons and markers and asked to draw a picture of their child engaging in a particular activity. The parents are instructed that they can draw more than one picture as they arrive at various activities for which their child could engage. After the parents complete their various drawings, the counselor would process the drawings with them. Again, the processing would involve examination and self-evaluation of their hopes, expectations, and desires for their child as well as the related emotional responses.

For example, Reggie was a 37-year-old man with a 5-year-old son, Lester, who was diagnosed with autism. Reggie was asked to draw a picture of Lester engaging in a particular activity. Reggie drew a picture of Lester swimming that included him helping his son in the pool. Afterwards, Reggie drew a picture of Lester playing basketball, and on the side of the picture there was a syringe that symbolized the different medications needed for the Lester to more effectively carry out normal activities. Reggie also drew a picture of Lester in a classroom studying and talking to the teacher about his homework. Reggie commented on the important role teachers would play in his child's life as they would monitor Lester throughout the day. When processing with the counselor, Reggie stated that Lester could engage in many activities throughout the day but that he needed constant monitoring and the use of medication on a daily basis. The use of drawings helped Reggie verbalize some of the activities that Lester could engage in despite the need for close monitoring that the illness required.

Another creative intervention that counselors can use with fathers is the use of journals. Parents can journal about the child's life and of the ways they want their child to know how special they are in the family. If the journal is guided, the counselor can give parents specific topics they may want to write about and the parents can also add their own entries. For instance, "The day you were born . . . ," "When we celebrated your first birthday . . . , " "You are special in so many ways . . . , " "What we hope for you . . . . " Parents also can include photos in their journal to make it a more visual and personal expression. Parents would then bring their journals to counseling and reflect some of their writings. As with the other two creative approaches to "redreaming," the counselor would process the activity with the parent. Additionally, the parent could read what they wrote to their child. After all, this is the child's personal story through the parents' eyes.

Bruce brought a sample of his journal entries to counseling. Bruce was a 41-year-old man whose five year-old daughter, Becky, was diagnosed with Down's syndrome. In discussing his journal, Bruce said: "The day you were born I felt a sense of happiness that is hard to describe, to think that somebody so beautiful would be part of our lives. When we found out about your disease we were scared but happy you were our daughter. What I hope for you is that we can find ways to make your world a beautiful place, the gift you have given us." The counselor processed the meaning of this journal entry with Bruce, helping him grieve the child's disability and "redream" the child's story. The use of journaling helped Bruce get in touch with new dreams he had for Becky and served as an empowering testimony that he could share with her in the future.

The integration of creative interventions when working with parents with children with disabilities can be empowering when focusing on "redreaming." Stories, images, metaphors, and symbols are tools that help parents represent their inner and outer worlds as they relate to their child. Creative and expressive interventions can facilitate change in how parents perceive the challenges of coping with a child with special needs.

Considering the emotional impact of caring for a child with special needs and the potential benefits of "redreaming" as a creative intervention, the authors sought to investigate the relationship between the emotional distress experienced by fathers of a child with a disability and the coping responses utilized in dealing with such stressors. The null hypothesis was that no relationship existed among participants with higher and lower levels of emotional distress and coping responses they used. Results from this study support the development of an intervention program for families of children with special needs and in particular, for the fathers.

METHODS

Instrumentation

Coping Resources Inventory. The Coping Responses Inventory (CRI-Adult Form) is a 58-item inventory that assesses approach coping responses and avoidance coping responses for individual coping with a variety of stressors (Moos, 1993). It consists of 10 items that evaluate the stressful event being rated and its outcome and the remaining 48 items compose the following eight coping responses:

1. Logical Analysis: cognitive attempts to understand the stressor and consequences;
2. Positive Reappraisal: cognitive attempts to construe a problem in a positive way;
3. Guidance and Support: behavioral attempts to seek information, guidance, and support;
4. Problem Solving: behavioral attempts to take action to directly deal with the problem;
5. Cognitive Avoidance: cognitive attempts to avoid realistically thinking about the problem;
6. Resigned Acceptance: cognitive attempts to accept the problem;
7. Alternative Rewards: behavioral attempts to create new sources of satisfaction through alternative activities.

Emotional Discharge: reducing tension by expressing negative feelings.The first 10 items that measure the focal stressor are on a 4-point Likert scale with 1 representing "Definitely No" and 4 representing "Definitely Yes." There are 6 questions for each of the 8 scales and items are rated on a 4-point Likert scale based on frequency from "not at all" to "frequently." Additionally, the first four subscales measure approach coping responses and the last four measure avoidant coping responses. An additional variable used in this study was a summary index of reliance on approach coping. Derived from summing the participants' scores on the approach coping subscales and dividing by the sum of all eight subscales, this index has been used in other studies utilizing the CRI (Holahan & Moos, 1991; Moos et al., 1990; Sharkansky et al., 2000).

Internal consistency scores range from .61 to .74 and were moderately intercorrelated ($r = .29$). Also, the reliability Coefficients of the CRI-Adult Form range from .58 to .74 (Plake, Imapra, & Murphey,

2001). Alpha coefficients for the four approach coping indices were .64 (logical analysis), .74 (positive reappraisal), .62 (guidance and support), and .66 (problem solving). For the avoidance coping indices, the alpha coefficients were .72 (cognitive avoidance), .62 (resigned acceptance), .71 (alternative rewards), and .61 (emotional discharge).

Brief Symptom Inventory. The Brief Symptom Inventory (BSI) is a 53-item inventory that measures psychological distress. Items are answered on a 5-point scale (0 = not at all, 1 = a little, 2 = moderately, 3 = quite a bit, 4 = extremely). In addition to the 9 subscales (Somatization, Obsessive-Compulsive, Interpersonal Sensitivity, Depression, Anxiety, Hostility, Phobic Anxiety, Paranoid Ideation, and Psychotism) the BSI has 3 global indices of distress: The Positive Symptom Total (PST), the Positive Symptom Distress Index (PSDI), and the Global Severity Index (GSI).

The GSI, which reflected the mean intensity ratings for all items on the BSI and indicated current level of distress, was the index of interest to measure emotional distress. Significant GSI scores were gauged by a t-score > 63 on the GSI or a t-score > 63 on 2 or more of the 9 subscales (Derogatis & Spencer, 1982). The test-retest reliability for the Global Severity Index (GSI) is .90 (Derogatis, 1993). In order to estimate the internal consistency of the GSI with these participants, an alpha coefficient was derived. The participant alpha coefficient was calculated at .96. The GSI was the first dependent variable in this study and provided a measure of each participant's distress.

Caregiver Survey Questionnaire. The Caregiver Survey Questionnaire was a researcher-designed questionnaire that consisted of 19 questions. It contained eight demographic questions about the participant and five demographic questions about their child with a disability. There also were six questions related to professional assistance received by participant and child, the amount of direct care provided by participant, and subjective response items on how the participant has been affected by the caregiving role.

Participants and Procedures

Participants in this study were fathers of a child with a physical or developmental disability living in the Southeastern United States. They were identified based on the following criteria of inclusion: (1) the father of a child with a physical or development disability and (2) the child resides in the father's household at least 50% of the time. Potential participants were limited to fathers of a child with special needs.

To solicit potential participants, invitation letters, copies of the Informed Consent, were mailed to a variety of community agencies that provide support to individuals with special needs and their families. The agencies forwarded invitation letters to families. Those who expressed interest and met the criteria of inclusion and consented to participate, via signing the Informed Consent Form, received a packet containing the Caregiver Survey Questionnaire, Coping Resources Inventory, Brief Symptoms Inventory, and a copy of the Informed Consent Form for their records. They were asked to complete the three instruments and return to the primary investigator in a stamped envelope included in the packet. Twenty-three (N = 23) individuals indicated they were interested in participating and all completed the study-related paperwork.

Participants' responses were coded in the Statistical Package for the Social Sciences (SPSS). Two groups were created using the cut point of the Global Severity Index's median score. Independent-Samples T Test analyses were then used to compare the means of individuals who fell above and below the median GSI cut point for the different Coping Responses Inventory scales.

RESULTS

Twenty-three participants contributed data to this study. Their ages ranged from 25 to 58 years old, with a mean of 38.5 years. Seventy-eight percent (n = 18) of the participants identified themselves as White, 13% (n = 3) identified themselves as Hispanic, 4.3% (n = 1) identified themselves as Black/Non-Hispanic, and 4.3% (n = 1) identified themselves as other. A variety of educational attainments were represented in this participant pool with 34.8% (n = 8) completing high school, 34.8% completing their Bachelor's degree, and 30.4% (n = 7) completing some level of graduate education. Additional demographic information has been provided in Table 1.

The age of the participants' children ranged from one year old to 20 years old with a mean age of 5.9 years. All participants except one shared the same residence as their child with a special need. The one that did not had their child in their residence at least 50% of the time. Table 2 presents demographic information on the participants' children.

T-tests analyses were used to examine the relationship among individuals with higher and lower levels of emotional distress and coping responses used. A comparison of mean scores for the eight coping responses yielded significant differences on two scales. Significant differences in positive re-

TABLE 1. Participants' Demographic Information

Variable		
Age	Mean: 38.5	
	Percentage	*Number*
Race		
White	78%	(n = 18)
Hispanic	13%	(n = 3)
Black/Non-Hispanic	4.3%	(n = 1)
Other	4.3%	(n = 1)
Marital Status		
Married	86.9%	(n = 20)
Single	4.3%	(n = 1)
Separated	4.3%	(n = 1)
Divorced/Widowed	4.3%	(n = 1)
Education		
High School	34.7%	(n = 8)
Bachelors	34.7%	(n = 8)
Graduate	30.4%	(n = 7)
Monthly Income		
< $2,000	8.7%	(n = 2)
$2,000-$4,000	52.2%	(n = 12)
$4,100-$6,000	17.4%	(n = 4)
$6,100+	17.4%	(n = 4)

appraisal ($t = -2.19, p = .02$) were found between individuals with higher and lower levels of emotional distress. This result suggested that participants with lower levels of emotional distress (scoring below the GSI median cut-point) relied more on the positive reappraisal coping response than those with higher emotional distress scores (scored above the cut-point). Also, significant differences in emotional discharge ($t = 2.40, p = .03$) were found between the groups. These results suggested that participants with higher levels of emotional distress relied more on the emotional discharge coping response than those with lower levels of emotional distress. Although differences existed between the two groups (higher and lower levels of emotional distress) on the other six coping responses, none of the other differences were significant at the .05 level.

TABLE 2. Demographics of Participants' Children

Variable		
Age	Mean: 5.9	
	Percentage	*Number*
Gender		
Female	34.8%	(n = 8)
Male	65.2%	(n = 15)
Race		
White	78%	(n = 18)
Hispanic	13%	(n = 3)
Black/Non-Hispanic	4.3%	(n = 1)
Other	4.3%	(n = 1)
Disability		
Cerebral Palsy	26.1%	(n = 6)
Developmental Delay	13%	(n = 3)
Down's Syndrome	21.7%	(n = 5)
Hydrocephalus	8.7%	(n = 2)
Visual Impairment	8.7%	(n = 2)
Other	21.7%	(n = 5)

Additionally, the t-test examining the index of reliance on approach coping and emotional distress was significant ($t = -2.33$, p = .03). This suggested that participants with lower scores on the GSI were more likely to rely on approach coping responses and those that rely less on approach coping responses had higher scores on the GSI. Table 3 presents a comparison of the mean scores for the CRI subscale scores and summary index for reliance on approach coping for the two groups of participants (those that fell above the Brief Symptoms Inventory's Global Severity Index median cut-point and those that fell below).

IMPLICATIONS FOR FUTURE RESEARCH AND CONCLUSION

One area of future research would involve replicating this study with a larger and more diverse participant sample. This would allow for more robust analyses of the data potentially controlling for demographic factors. Research also is needed examining gender differences in coping

TABLE 3. Means, Standard Deviations, and T-Test Analyses Results

Coping Response	n	Mean	SD	t	p
Approach Coping Responses					
Logical Analysis					
Higher Distress Group:	12	9.67	4.48		
Lower Distress Group:	11	11.18	2.71		
T-Test Results:				−.97	.34
*Positive Reappraisal					
Higher Distress Group:	12	9.17	5.22		
Lower Distress Group:	11	13.91	3.24		
T-Test Results:				−2.59	.02
Guidance and Support					
Higher Distress Group:	12	9.75	4.27		
Lower Distress Group:	11	9.82	4.62		
T-Test Results:				−.04	.97
Problem Solving					
Higher Distress Group:	12	9.92	4.72		
Lower Distress Group:	11	12.00	3.95		
T-Test Results:				−1.14	.27
Avoidance Coping Responses					
Cognitive Avoidance					
Higher Distress Group:	12	7.92	2.94		
Lower Distress Group:	11	7.45	4.68		
T-Test Results:				.27	.78
Resigned Acceptance					
Higher Distress Group:	12	7.50	3.48		
Lower Distress Group:	11	7.45	3.45		
T-Test Results:				.03	.98
Alternative Rewards					
Higher Distress Group:	12	6.00	3.44		
Lower Distress Group:	11	5.82	3.43		
T-Test Results:				.13	.90
*Emotional Discharge					
Higher Distress Group:	12	7.08	3.48		
Lower Distress Group:	11	4.36	1.75		
T-Test Results:				2.34	.03

* $p < .05$

responses between caregiving fathers and mothers. Additionally, these parents would also benefit from a demonstration research project examining short-term and long-term effects of redreaming and other creative interventions. Future research could also involve the evaluation of "redreaming" as an intervention with parents of children with special needs.

A significant contribution could be made through a study, with a control group that examines the three different approaches to facilitate the "redreaming" presented. Although many research opportunities exist in this area, it is most important that researchers continue to investigate and further understand caregiver distress and coping response along with the development of effective strategies to help parents cope more effectively so they can better attend to their children.

Conclusions and interpretations drawn from this study must be considered in the parameters of the study's representative sample. Thus, generalizability is not claimed considering the small size of the sample. However, caregiving fathers for children with special needs are a challenging population to engage in research endeavors (Carpenter, 2002; McConkey, 1994; Ricci & Hodapp, 2003). Subsequently, that challenge in obtaining a large sample size may well contributed to gaps in this research area. Further studies are needed to support these findings and expand understanding of the stress involved in fathering a child with special needs, its emotional impact on parents and the coping responses used to deal with such challenges. For mental health professionals, additional research may reveal understanding of how to provide adequate support to families of children with special needs.

In conclusion, the present study has shown that fathers of children with special needs with lower levels of emotional distress rely more on approach coping responses and positive reappraisal, and less on emotional discharge coping responses. On the other hand, fathers of children with special needs with higher levels of emotional distress relied less on approach coping responses and more on emotional discharge coping responses. Thus, teaching fathers strategies for responding to stressors by using positive coping responses could alleviate distress, help them cope more effectively, and be more helpful to their children. Additionally, redreaming and other creative interventions may prove beneficial in helping fathers utilize more effective coping responses. However, additional research is required to further understand the role of the use of coping responses in relationship to emotional distress for fathers of children with special needs and the use of creative interventions such as "redreaming."

DISCUSSION

A need existed for additional research exploring how fathers of children with special needs cope (Carpenter, 2002; Navalkar, 2004; Simmerman et al., 2001; Turbiville & Marquis, 2001). In this study, the Coping Responses Inventory and the Brief Symptoms Inventory's Global Severity Index were used to examine the relationship among coping responses and emotional distress in caregiving fathers for children with special needs. The findings suggest that individuals with lower levels of emotional distress in their caregiving role rely more on approach coping responses. As Moos (1993) stated, "In general, approach coping is problem-focused; it reflects cognitive and behavioral efforts to master or resolve life stressors" (p. 1). Similarly, this 'approach' to coping has been supported in other studies using the CRI (Holahan & Moos, 1991; Moos et al., 1990; Sharkansky et al., 2000). The results of this study, as well as previous work in the area, suggested that individuals with lower levels of emotional distress rely on positive reappraisal, an approach coping index that involves cognitive attempts to construe a problem in a positive way. Additionally, those with lower levels of emotional distress rely less on emotional discharge, an avoidance coping index that involves expressing negative emotions to reduce tension.

The results of this study do have positive implications for mental health professionals and others that work with caregiving fathers. A significant challenge exists in getting men to counseling and other interventions. Men also are more likely to participate in outcome-oriented interventions (Turbiville & Marquis, 2001). The development of problem-solving and cognitive-behavioral skills lends itself to psychoeducational approaches. Whether in a small group, large group, or in psychoeducational literature, individuals could be taught key problem-solving and cognitive-behavioral strategies. Additionally, these approaches could also address the potential shortfalls in reducing tension through the expression of negative emotions. This is not to suggest that individual and group therapeutic approaches would not be effective. However, more creative approaches that assist fathers of children with special needs to utilize positive reappraisal and directly address their emotional responses are needed.

REFERENCES

Administration for Children and Families (ACF). *ADD Fact Sheet*. Retrieved on April 9, 2006 from the World Wide Web: http://www.acf.hhs.gov/programs/add/Factsheet.html
American Psychiatric Association. (1994). *Diagnostic and statistical manual of mental disorders* (4th ed.). Washington, DC: Author.

Americans With Disabilities Act (ADA) of 1990, Pub. L. No. 101-336, 2, 104 Stat. 328 (1991).

Ballantine, J. H. (2000). Figuring in the father factor. *Childhood Education, 76,* 104-105.

Beresford, B. (1995). *Expert opinions: A national survey of parents caring for a severely disabled child.* Bristol: Policy Press.

Billings, A. G., & Moos, R. H. (1985). Psychosocial process of remission in unipolar depression: Comparing depressed patients with matched community controls. *Journal of Consulting and Clinical Psychology, 53,* 314-325.

Blalock, J. A., & Joiner, T. E. (2000). Interaction of cognitive avoidance coping and stress in predicting depression/anxiety. *Cognitive Therapy and Research, 24,* 47-65.

Carpenter, B. (2002). Inside the portrait of a family: The importance of fatherhood. *Early Child Development and Care, 172*(2), 195-202.

Corbeil, R., Quayhagen, M. P., & Quayhagen, M. (1999). Intervention effects on dementia caregiving interactions: A stress-adaptation modeling approach. *Journal of Aging and Health, 11*(1), 79-95.

Cummings, E., & O'Reilly, A. (1997). Fathers in family context: Effects of marital quality on child adjustment. In M. E. Lamb (Ed.), *The role of the father in child development, 3rd ed.* (pp. 179-190). Hoboken, NJ: John Wiley & Sons.

Derogatis, L. R. (1993). *Brief Symptom Inventory: Administration, scoring, and procedures manual–II.* Minneapolis, MN: National Computer Systems.

Derogatis, L. R., & Spencer, P. M. (1982). *Brief Symptom Inventory: Administration, scoring, and procedures manual–I.* Baltimore: Clinical Psychometric Research.

Dobson, B., & Middleton, S. (1998). *Paying to care: The cost of childhood disability.* London: YPS Joseph Rowntree Foundation.

Dyson, L., & Fewell, R. R. (1986). Stress and adaptation in parents of young handicapped and nonhandicapped children: A comparative study. *Journal of the Division of Early Childhood, 10*(1), 25-35.

Ehrenkrantz, D., Miller, C., & Vemberg, D. K., & Fox, H. (2001). Measuring prevalence of childhood disability: Addressing family needs while augmenting prevention. *Journal of Rehabilitation, 67*(2), 48-54.

Grant, G., & Whittell, B. (2000). Differentiated coping strategies in families with children or adults with intellectual disabilities: The relevance of gender, family composition and the life span. *Journal of Applied Research in Intellectual Disabilities, 13*(4), 256-275.

Gray, D. E. (2002). Ten years on: A longitudinal study of families of children with autism. *Journal of Intellectual Disability Research, 27*(3), 215-222.

Gray, D. E. (2003). Gender and coping: The parents of children with high functioning autism. *Social Science & Medicine, 56*(3), 178-192.

Hassall, R., Rose, J., & McDonald, J. (2005). Parenting stress in mothers of children with an intellectual disability: The effects of parental cognitions in relation to child characteristics and family support. *Journal of Intellectual Disability Research, 49*(6), 405-418.

Holahan, C. J., & Moos, R. H. (1991). Life stressors, personal and social resources, and depression: A 4-year structural model. *Journal of Abnormal Psychology, 100,* 31-38.

Houser, R., & Seligman, M. (1991). A comparison of stress and coping by fathers of adolescents with mental retardation and fathers of adolescents without mental retardation. *Research on Developmental Disabilities, 12*(3), 251-260.

Keller, D., & Honig, A. S. (2004). Maternal and paternal stress in families with school-aged children with disabilities. *American Journal of Orthopsychiatry, 74*(3), 337-348.

Lamb, M. E., & Billings, L. A. (1997). Fathers of children with special needs. In M. E. Lamb (Ed.), *The role of the father in child development, 3rd ed.* (pp. 179-190). Hoboken, NJ: John Wiley & Sons.

McConkey, R. (1994). Early intervention: Planning futures, shaping years. *Mental Handicap Research, 7*(1), 4-15.

Merchant, N. (1995). Wonder. On *Tigerlily* (CD). Seattle: Elektra/WEA.

Miller, A., Cate, I., & Johann-Murphy, M. (2001). When chronic disability meets acute stress: Psychological and functional changes. *Developmental Medicine & Child Neurology, 43*(3), 214-216.

Moos, R. H. (1993). *Coping Responses Inventory Adult Form: Professional Manual.* Odessa, FL: Psychological Assessment Resources, Inc.

Moos, R. H., Brennan, P. L., Fondacaro, M. R., & Moos, B. S. (1990). Approach and avoidance coping responses among older problem and nonproblem drinkers. *Psychology and aging, 5*(1), 31-40.

Navalkar, P. (2004). Fathers' perception of their role in parenting a child with Cerebral Palsy: Implications for counseling. *Internal Journal for the Advancement of Counseling, 26*(4), 375-382.

Newacheck, P. W., Strickland, B., Shonkoff, J. P., Perrin, J. M., McPherson, M., & McManus, M. et al. (1998). An epidemiologic profile of children with special health care needs. *Pediatrics, 102*(1), 117-123.

Pelchat, D., & Lefebvre, H. (2003). A holistic intervention programme for families with a child with a disability. *Journal of Advanced Nursing, 48*(2), 124-131.

Pelchat, D., Lefebvre, H., & Perreault, M. (2003). Differences and similarities between mothers' and fathers' experiences of parenting a child with a disability. *Journal of Child Health Care, 7*(4), 231-247.

Plake, B. S., Imapra, J. C., & Murphy, L. L. (2001). *The Fourth Mental Measurements Yearbook.* Lincoln, NE: University of Nebraska Press.

Ricci, L. A., & Hodapp, R. M. (2003). Fathers of children with Down's syndrome verses other types of intellectual disability: Perceptions, stress, and involvement. *Journal of Intellectual Disability Research, 47*(4), 273-284.

Saloviita, T., Italinna, M., & Leinonen, E. (2003). Explaining the parental stress of fathers and mothers caring for a child with intellectual disability: A double ABCX model. *Journal of Intellectual Disability Research, 47*(4), 300-312.

Sears, S. R., Stanton, A. L., & Danoff-Burg, S. (2003). The yellow brick road and the emerald city: Benefit finding, positive reappraisal coping, and posttraumatic growth in women with early-stage breast cancer. *Health Psychology, 22*(5), 487-497.

Sharkansky, E. J., King, D. W., King, L. A., & Wolfe, J., Erickson, J., & Stokes, L. (2000). Coping with Gulf War combat stress: Mediating and moderating effect. *Journal of Abnormal Psychology, 109*(9), 188-197.

Simmerman, S., Blacher, J., & Baker, B. L. (2001). Fathers' and mothers' perceptions of father involvement in families with young children with a disability. *Journal of Intellectual & Developmental Disability*, 26(4), 325-338.

Turbiville, V. P., & Marquis, J. G. (2001). Father participation in early educational programs. *Topics in Early Childhood Special Education*, 21(4), 223-231.

U.S. Department of Health and Human Services (USDHHS). (2004). *The National Survey of Children with Special Health Care Needs Chartbook 2001.* Rockville, Maryland: U.S. Department of Health and Human Services.

Wang, M, Turnbull, A. P., Summers, J. A., Little, T. D., Poston, D. J., Mannan, H. et al. (2004). Severity of disability and income as predictors of parents' satisfaction with their family quality of life during early childhood years. *Research & Practice for Persons with Severe Disabilities*, 29(2), 82-94.

Westbrook, L. E., Silver, E. J., & Stein, R. (1998). Implications for estimates of disability in children: A comparison of definitional components. *Pediatrics*, 101(6), 1025-1030.

doi:10.1300/J456v01n03_16

Chapter 17

Fictive Bibliotherapy
and Therapeutic Storytelling
with Children Who Hurt

Dale-Elizabeth Pehrsson

SUMMARY. This manuscript addresses the impact of traumatic events on children and the relevancy of treatment using books and stories with children in grief. It also addresses research, efficacy, and some limitations of these interventions. Finally, it recommends therapeutic strategies and suggests guidance for material selection, offering a listing of current Web related resources. doi:10.1300/J456v01n03_17 *[Article copies available for a fee from The Haworth Document Delivery Service: 1-800-HAWORTH. E-mail address: <docdelivery@haworthpress.com> Website: <http://www.HaworthPress.com> © 2005 by The Haworth Press, Inc. All rights reserved.]*

KEYWORDS. Bibliotherapy, therapeutic storytelling, creativity, counseling grief, trauma, children

---

Dale-Elizabeth Pehrsson is affiliated with the Oregon State University.
Address correspondence to: Dale-Elizabeth Pehrsson, 4802 NW Viola Place, Corvallis, OR 97331 (E-mail: dale.pehrsson@oregonstate.edu).

[Haworth co-indexing entry note]: "Fictive Bibliotherapy and Therapeutic Storytelling with Children Who Hurt." Pehrsson, Dale-Elizabeth. Co-published simultaneously in *Journal of Creativity in Mental Health* (The Haworth Press, Inc.) Vol. 1, No. 3/4, 2005, pp. 273-286; and: *Creative Interventions in Grief and Loss Therapy: When the Music Stops, a Dream Dies* (ed: Thelma Duffey) The Haworth Press, Inc., 2005, pp. 273-286. Single or multiple copies of this article are available for a fee from The Haworth Document Delivery Service [1-800-HAWORTH, 9:00 a.m. - 5:00 p.m. (EST). E-mail address: docdelivery@haworthpress.com].

Available online at http://jcmh.haworthpress.com
© 2005 by The Haworth Press, Inc. All rights reserved.
doi:10.1300/J456v01n03_17

When the children cry
Let them know we tried
'Cause when the children sing
Then the new world begins

(White Lion, 1987)

As a child, I loved when my teacher would read to us in class and typically requested a story at bedtime. I also remember how comforting stories were to children when I worked as a pediatric nurse. Later, as a school counselor, I would delight as children explored their minds and feelings in our readings of places and times far from our rural community. Since then, much of my research and therapeutic work has involved the use of bibliotherapy and storytelling in clinical practice. Although these approaches provide benefits for people of all ages, the focus of this manuscript addresses their use with children.

This manuscript will address childhood grief issues and clinical interventions that can be used to work through these issues. In particular, it will discuss the multidimensional clinical uses of bibliotherapy and storytelling. The reader will find historical perspectives on bibliotherapy and storytelling, including definitions, applications, treatment uses, benefits, theoretical frames, and therapeutic mechanisms. The manuscript will also address current research and efficacy findings on these interventions. The article provides an Appendix with a generous list of Web resources for counselors interested in using stories and books in their practices.

CHILDREN IN GRIEF

Children experience untold tragedies and grief experiences. There are times when they may not understand the pain they feel. Death of family members, friends, siblings, pets and neighbors are often shocking and agonizing events for children. Problems are exacerbated when families try to shield them from the experience by avoiding discussion on the event, loss or person (Pehrsson & Boylan, 2004). In the case of suicide, shame and social rules make support especially difficult (Ayyash-Abo, 2001, Pardeck & Pardeck, 1993).

Jeff was eight years old when his teenage brother, Jimmy, committed suicide. Jimmy's death brought with it shock, pain, fear, and a deadening disconnection among family members. Jeff recalls, with a sobering whisper, the day his parents returned from work to find Jim dead in the back yard. His older brother, the person who would make his eyes light up when he would enter a room; the person who let him play with his Nintendo; the person who taught him to tie his shoes had died of a self-inflicted gunshot wound.

After the panic, chaos, and debilitating pain the family experienced had become almost familiar, there came a time of acute loneliness. Jeff's father and mother became so quiet he hardly recognized them. Jeff, now an only child, would sit at the dinner table where the three would eat without a word. The sound of the silence and disconnection was excruciatingly profound. Memories of laughter, arguments, and his former life seemed eerily distant. Jeff had no words to speak, and for several months, he had no one who could listen if he had found the words to do so. Jeff and his family were living in a state of shame, silence, loneliness, and condemned isolation (Miller, 1988).

Children, like Jeff, experience trauma every day. Sometimes the trauma is a result of the death of a loved one. Other times it is a result of family dissolution, divorce, relocation and deportations. Any of these experiences and others impacts a child's feeling of connection, self-esteem, safety and trust. Whether reacting to a loved one's slow lingering illness, a tornado, or a community assault, traumatic events hurt children, impacting them cognitively, affectively, behaviorally and physiologically (Gil, 1991). Counselors working with children must consider the developmental needs of children and the relational and cognitive effects that trauma can bring to them.

For example, some children believe that an event can return and hurt them (Ayyash-Abo, 2001). Other times, children feel guilty or responsible when pain and tragedy hurts them or their families (Duffey, 2005). Disconnected from what they know, they experience confusion, become defocused, and may regress in learning. Developmental delays and communication deficits periodically emerge (Todahl, Smith, Barnes, & Pereira, 1998). After experiencing a form of trauma, children may feel upset, angry, fearful and anxious all at once. In addition, culture, religious and family norms all impact a child's response to loss (Pardeck & Pardeck, 1998a).

Though not an exclusive list, other affective responses to loss include nightmares, night fears and night sweats (Ayyash-Abo, 2001). Grieving children may be less able to manage stress and develop symptoms of depression. They may experience shock, withdrawal, anger, and refuse to leave home. Sometimes, children regress behaviorally and have problems with bedwetting, incontinence, fearful outbursts, anxiety sweats, and thumb sucking. They may begin to baby talk. In severe cases, they may harm themselves or others (Aiken, 1994; Ayyash-Abo, 2001).

Children, like adults, also experience physiological reactions to trauma, including headaches, stomachaches and gastrointestinal symptoms. Physiological or somatic symptoms may persist, creating conditions of nausea and vomiting, chronic fatigue, insomnia or hypersomnia, eating disorders, and chronic anxiety (Worden, 1991). When these are experienced, medical intervention becomes critical (Elliott & Place, 1998).

BIBLIOTHERAPY

When children experience periods of trauma and stress, a supportive therapeutic relationship where books and stories are collaboratively selected and shared can buttress their self-concept, cultivate their self worth and calm the storm. Shared stories can help children connect with the storyteller, identify how they feel about difficult life situations, and illuminate how their reactions differ from those of the protagonist. As a result, children feel less isolation in the identification and connection with the story characters (Adler & Foster, 1997; Butterworth & Fulmer, 1991).

Some children identify with a character in a story when they determine the character feels the same as they feel (Pardeck & Pardeck, 1997). For example, Sharon, 12, brought a book to therapy so the counselor could read with her. Sharon identified with the protagonist, Jay Berry Lee, in *Summer of the Monkeys* (Rawls, 1992). The main character in this book dealt bravely with severe family disability issues. Since Sharon's sister had recently experienced a severe automobile accident and was paralyzed, the story was particularly comforting to her.

Bibliotherapy also assists youngsters to release emotional pressures, provides multiple solutions, and promotes smoother dialogue about concerns. It models capable decision-making strategies and exposes children to divergent cultural views. Bibliotherapy generates opportunities for children to investigate other interests and produces fertile ground for self-reflection. Finally, reading books and listening to stories can be less threatening than holding direct conversations (Pardeck & Pardeck, 1998a; Pehrsson & McMillen, 2005).

In one example, Bill, 10, witnessed the accidental drowning death of his brother, Tommy. As part of the bibliotherapy process, Billy was asked whether he would like to read a book or whether he would like the counselor to read to him. He chose to listen while the counselor read a book he selected, *The Fall of Freddie the Leaf* (Buscaglia, 1985). During one session, Billy looked at the pages in the book and would occasionally stop and ask questions, such as, "Are people like leaves or are they more like the trees?"

In the next session, Billy selected another book, *Goodbye Rune* (Kaldhol & Oyen, 1987). This time, as he listened to the story, Billy walked to the table, sat, and started to draw. He drew pictures of a lake and trees, with leaves falling to the ground. Some leaves sank into the water. Quietly, he whispered, "This leaf is like Tommy." Billy experienced an empathic connection with his therapist and guided the therapy and the bibliotherapy process to match the fictive metaphor to his own relational and emotional needs.

Bibliotherapy, when matched to the needs of children, provides a developmentally specific counseling tool and strategy. Stories help children relate to situations that match their emotional, social, cultural and cognitive frame of reference. Books provide safety in a number of ways. Some children feel as if books are their "friends." They can read them at their own pace and at a distance that can feel safe. Through books, children often find a place of fantasy and freedom from the constant worries and hurts of everyday life (Bernstein & Rudman, 1989; Early, 1993).

Books can be therapeutically healing for children on a number of fronts. For one, children have a finely tuned capacity for imagination and identification. Their identification with stories gives children access to other worlds. Children easily connect with solutions and characters (Crenshaw, 2004; Gil, 1991). For example, Johnnie, 7, was initially drawn to the book, *Dinosaurs Divorce* (Brown, 1988) when he began therapy. However, he quickly identified with another book, *It's Not Your Fault, Koko Bear* (Lansky, 1998), which seemed to meet needs he could not articulate.

Johnnie needed to understand that his parents divorce was not his fault, and spontaneously repeated "it's not your fault" during session. In time, Johnnie was able to relate his feelings regarding the divorce to those of the protagonist, using the story as an anchor. The phrase "it's not your fault" and the story characters created a useful metaphor and served as a catalyst for helping Johnnie productively re-visit and re-story his experience.

The flexibility and autonomy involved in bibliotherapy creates wonderful opportunities for children. Children are able to associate story plots and characters with their own experiences and yield rich insights into the character and their own lives (Crenshaw, 2004; Pardeck &

Pardeck, 1993). When their counselors have the understanding, context, and resources to provide them with these opportunities, children gain experience with a coping strategy that can be used far after the immediate crisis is over.

However, several factors must be in place for this intervention to be successful. The topic, format, language, plot, cultural context, complexity of the text, and the children's needs and developmental level must be considered. Appealing illustrations, congruent with the storyline and emotional intent, also draw children into the tale. Ultimately, their needs should influence the literary genre selected.

Counselors must also consider practical considerations in the bibliotherapy process. Some of these considerations include how long it will take to read a story and if there are costs involved in obtaining books. When people are in grief, it may be helpful to have vivid metaphors and simple texts available. Another consideration relates to the appropriate length of book. It is also important to select books that are representative and respective of cultures. Racist and sexist attitudes can be insidious and counselors need be on alert in choosing materials that do not promote stereotypes and misconceptions.

STORYTELLING

Another intervention used with children is the process of storytelling. While bibliotherapy always involves books, storytelling also involves speaking, listening, writing, or pictures. Hug-Hellmuth (1921) first documented her approach and therapeutic constructs of storytelling with children. She postulated that children's stories were easier to analyze than dreams, free-associations and other verbal exchanges traditionally used with adult clients (Gardner, 1992). Storytelling transports events, feelings and beliefs to an accessible realm. Storytelling educates and entertains us; it calms us, comforts us, and connects us to one another.

Esperanza was six years old when her father was diagnosed with cancer. Esperanza loved her father and worried about him. Her mother, who was usually doting and quite affectionate, was gone much of the time accompanying her husband to the hospital. Esperanza's family immigrated from Mexico and few of her relatives lived close by. She did have one aunt who lived in town, however, her Tia Rosita. Her tia moved in with the family to help with their needs. At the recommendation of Esperanza's first grade teacher, her Tia Rosita made an appointment for Esperanza to attend a counseling session. Esperanza always enjoyed hearing the stories that her mother would tell her and her younger brothers, and welcomed the stories that her counselor would share with her. Esperanza felt a strong connection with the counselor and the stories they would share proved to be a source of healing for her.

Although the counselor did not share Esperanza's familial or cultural context, she was able to enter her world through the connection they shared. This helped the counselor learn more about Esperanza's unique experience relative to being a child in her family; and it helped Esperanza feel like she held a place of "mattering" to her counselor. It also gave Esperanza an opportunity to express her voice (see Gilligan, 1982) and to share it with a receptive and supportive adult (see Spencer, 2000).

Children display an intuitive ability to unravel the mysteries and understand the nuances of fictive stories and their characters. From this, they mine rich insights (Crenshaw, 2004). Indeed, stories guide children towards understanding the world and their place within it. Additionally, reading to or telling a story to children creates a bond between the storyteller and the child. Further, the telling of tales lets the child come to know the counselor in deeper ways. Children's books carry complex and beautiful illustrations and provide a visual opportunity for children to open a window to their imaginations (Adler & Foster, 1997; Bernstein, 1989). In addition, children have an uncanny way of leading counselors toward the right therapeutic path and to the right books. Very often we must simply observe, listen and follow their lead (Hynes & Hynes-Berry, 1994). For example, children who are in the midst of their own painful experience may write or illustrate their own story, tell their favorite tale, or create with the counselor a new fable. Below we see the resourceful coping strategies of a child whose family is experiencing divorce.

Ten-year-old Joanna gathered pictures of her family from around the house and glued them in a loose-leaf notebook. Below each picture, Joanna wrote a story that she narrated to describe her experience. Joanna's creative expression of loss was completely unsolicited. This was clearly one way for Joanna to invite communication with her mother and served to help her work through her experience of grief surrounding her lost dream. Counselors may offer tools such as dolls, puppets and other props thorough which a child may speak in telling their stories (Gil, 1991; Hynes & Hynes-Berry, 1994), or they may invite children to create stories much like Joanna's.

Another storytelling approach involves reading about a relevant topic and incorporating the new information into a fictive story (Crenshaw, 2004). Children can create poems, art or a song in response to the story. This concept builds upon a Mutual Storytelling technique (Gardner, 1993) which prompts children to create their own stories. The counselor and child take turns in the telling of the story. For example, after children complete their stories, the counselor uses the story created by the child and formulates another ending (Gardner, 1993). This gives children an opportunity to tell their story; it also gives the counselor an opportunity to hear the story and to offer an ending that would be supportive and facilitative.

Storytelling can also be conducted in group format. The collaborative nature of this group offers children opportunities to react and process grief and loss issues with others. It creates a context where children can be heard, validated, and supported. It also creates a context where their creativity can be used as resource and shared with others. In this setting, children listen to a story and respond either individually or with others. Some children choose to write another story in response to the story they just heard. Such story starters can work as icebreakers and build group trust.

THE PROCESS

The fictive bibliotherapy and storytelling process is collaborative and includes five steps or stages: preparation, selection, application, facilitation and follow-up (Hynes & Hynes-Berry, 1994). In the first stage, the counselor and client prepare for the process. During this stage, the counselor and client create a therapeutic connection and through the connection, the counselor assesses the viability of using bibliotherapy and storytelling in therapy. The therapeutic goals are specific: (a) to discover if the child has an interest in books and a desire to read; (b) to discover if the child has an interest in being read to; and (c) to discover whether the child has the ability to apply fiction to the client's life. Some children are uncomfortable or have limited interest in books or storytelling, making this intervention inappropriate. If bibliotherapy appears to be an appropriate therapeutic approach, the counselor and the child can begin to select relevant materials. Counselors must also determine how bibliotherapy and storytelling can be applied. With the children, they create an innovative follow-up activity and evaluate the effectiveness and impact of the intervention on the child's experience.

Although there are countless ways that these interventions can be used, most strategies fall into threes spheres: counselor-initiated, client-initiated, or interactive. Strategies also range from structured to unstructured, directive to non-directive and facilitative to non-facilitative (Bernstein, 1989; Hynes & Hynes-Berry, 1994; Pardeck & Pardeck, 1993). Regardless of how the intervention is employed, developmental (use in educational settings) and clinical (use in mental health settings) bibliotherapy practitioners seem to agree that shared processing of the material is an essential component of bibliotherapy (Hynes & Hynes-Berry, 1994).

Children may identify with or project their impression on the story, characters or plot. They may also experience abreaction or catharsis. Counselors then facilitate the process and assist clients to become more aware, gain insight, generalize, problem solve, and apply the material to personal issues. Pardeck and Pardeck (1998a) discuss how it may take time to apply this intervention, and insight and problem solving may come days and perhaps weeks after the end of treatment. For example, it was an important moment when Susan identified her feelings of hurt, fear, and uncertainty following the car accident she survived. She had initially remained indifferent to her experience and minimized its impact on her. Later, by connecting with her experience through story, she was able to deal productively with it. Stories can be like seeds that, in time, bear fruit in the form of insight and understanding.

RESEARCH AND DISCUSSION

Shrodes (1950) first conceptualized the framework used in bibliotherapy. Although her work is continually updated in the literature (Afolayan, 1992; Bernstein, 1989; Farkas & Yorker, 1993; Kramer & Smith, 1998; Morawski, 1997; Pardeck, 1998; Zaccaria & Moses, 1968), the research remains mixed. The majority of empirically based bibliotherapy studies focus on non-fiction practices that are disorder specific, often dealing with cognitive behavioral and self-help guides (Pehrsson & McMillen, 2005). Limited quality assessment tools exist, clearly demanding further development. Current research indicates that bibliotherapy and storytelling are often used as part of the therapeutic process, although some researchers question if these practices are effective (Riordan, 1991). Although a small amount of empirical research is available in this area, case studies, application techniques and anecdotal reports abound (Marrs, 1995). Given that, a need exists to further gather empirical data on the value of bibliotherapy and storytelling.

CONCLUSION

Children undergoing difficult times need a safe place to process their experiences. Spencer (2000) reports how children can overcome experiences of adversity if they have at least one adult who can support them in their experience. Children need a language they can relate to and they need a counselor who can be moved by their experience (Hartling, 2005); a counselor who can take their needs, interests, and development into account. Building on these relational connections, bibliotherapy and storytelling are two mediums that counselors can use in their work with children facing life crises and periods of grief and loss. Counselors must consider how they can best use reading materials and stories in their work with children (Hynes & Hynes-Berry, 1994; Pehrsson & McMillen, 2005). They must also consider other factors, such as theory base, clinical environment, presenting problem, therapeutic goal, diagnosis, treatment plan, budget, developmental, reading and emotional levels, and stages of therapy.

Zaccaria and Moses (1968) argued that bibliotherapy was not a panacea and cannot be utilized with all clients. Pioneer bibliotherapy researcher, Carolyn Shrodes (1950) emphasized that no two individuals related to the same material with the same interpretation and meaning. Titles can be deceiving and the content can be contraindicated in some situations. Further, counselors must be familiar enough with their clients to anticipate the state of their readiness for reading or listening. They should determine if the facts found in books are accurate and up to date. They also need to employ stories with characters and situations similar enough to the circumstances of their clients to facilitate some level of identification (Pehrsson & McMillen, 2005).

Still, bibliotherapy and storytelling can assist children to increase self-awareness, clarify emerging values and gain a greater empathic understanding of others (Morawski, 1997). These mediums help develop the ethnic/cultural identity of children and teach them to value cultures different from their own (Tway, 1989). Wisely chosen literature assists children to expand their viewpoints. Additionally, children learn coping skills and alternative responses to problems through books and stories. Children may also gain respite from feelings of isolation simply by learning that others share their experience. Some children find new hope in learning how other people have dealt with similar situations. In these cases, characters from a story become a welcomed friend; a trusting ally and companion. When children feel isolated and confused, and when they have a counselor who can be with them in the midst of their storm, this can be a particularly comforting experience and a catalyst for healing.

REFERENCES

Adler, E. S., & Foster, P. (1997). A literature-based approach to teaching values to adolescents: Does it work? *Adolescence, 32*(126), 275-287.

Afolayan, J. A. (1992). Documentary perspective of bibliotherapy in education. *Reading-Horizons, 33*(2), 137-148.

Aiken, L. R. (1994). *Dying, death and bereavement* (3rd ed.). Boston, MA: Allyn & Bacon.

Ayyash-Abo, H. (2001). Childhood bereavement: What school psychologists need to know. *School Psychology International, 22*(4), 417-433.

Bernstein, J. E. (1989). Bibliotherapy: How books can help young children cope. In M. K. Rudman (Ed.), *Children's literature: Resource for the classroom* (pp. 159-173). Norwood, MA: Christopher-Gordon Publishers, Inc.

Bernstein, J. E., & Rudman, M. K. (1989). *Books to help children cope with separation and loss: An annotated bibliography,* Volume 3. New York, NY: R. R. Bowker.

Brown, L. K., & Brown, M. (1988). *Dinosaurs divorce: A guide for changing families.* New York, NY: Little, Brown & Company.

Buscaglia, L. (1982). *The fall of Freddie the leaf.* Thorofare, NJ: Slack Inc.

Butterworth, M. D., & Fulmer, K. A. (1991). The effect of family violence on children: Intervention strategies including bibliotherapy. *Australian Journal of Marriage and Family, 12*(3), 170-182.

Crenshaw, D. A. (2004). *Engaging resistant children in therapy: Projective drawing and storytelling techniques.* Rhinebeck, NY: RCFC Publications.

Duffey, T. (2005). Grief, loss and death. In D. Comstock (Ed.), *Diversity and development–Critical contexts that shape our lives and relationships* (pp. 216-245). Belmont, CA: Wadsworth Publishing.

Early, B. P. (1993). The healing magic of myth: Allegorical tales and the treatment of children of divorce. *Child and Adolescent Social Work Journal, 10*(2), 97-106.

Elliott, J., & Place, M. (1998). *Children in difficulty: A guide to understanding and helping.* New York, NY: Routledge.

Farkas, G. S., & Yorker, B. (1993). Case studies of bibliotherapy with homeless children. *Issues in Mental Health Nursing, 14*(4), 337-347.

Gardner, R. A. (1992). *The psychotherapeutic techniques of Richard A. Gardner.* Cresskill, New Jersey: Creative Therapeutics.

Gil, E. (1991). *The healing power of play: Working with abused children.* New York, NY: Guilford Press.

Gilligan, C. (1982). *In a different voice.* Cambridge MA: Harvard University Press.

Gray, L. M. (1995). *My mama had a dancing heart.* New York, NY: Orchard Books.

Hartling, L. (2005). Fostering resilience throughout our lives: New relational possibilities. In D. Comstock (Ed.), *Diversity and development –Critical contexts that shape our lives and relationships* (pp. 337-354). Belmont, CA: Wadsworth Publishing.

Hug-Hellmuth, H. V. (1921). On the technique of child analysis. *International Journal of Psycho-Analysis, 2,* 287-305.

Hynes, A. M., & Hynes-Berry, M. (1994). *Biblio-poetry therapy, the interactive process: A handbook.* St. Cloud, MN: North Star Press of St. Cloud Inc.

Joosse, B. M. (1991). *Mama, do you love me?* San Francisco, CA: Chronicle Books.

Kaldhol, M. (1987). *Goodbye Rune.* La Jolla, CA: Kane/Miller Publishers.

Kramer, P. A., & Smith, G. G. (1998). Easing the pain of divorce through children's literature. *Early Childhood Education Journal, 26*(2), 89-94.

Lansky, V. (1998). *It's not your fault, Koko bear: A read together book for parents and young children during divorce.* Minnetonka, MN: Book Peddlers.

Marrs, R. W. (1995). A meta-analysis of bibliotherapy studies. *American Journal of Community Psychology*, 23(6), 843-870.

Miller, J. B. (1988). *Connections, disconnections, and violations*. Works in Progress, No. 33. Wellesley, MA: Stone Center Working Papers Series.

Morawski, C. M. (1997). A role for bibliotherapy in teacher education. *Reading Horizons, 37*(3), 243-259.

Pardeck, J. T. (1998). *Using books in clinical social work practice: A guide to bibliotherapy*. Binghamton, NY: The Haworth Press, Inc.

Pardeck, J. T., & Pardeck, J. A. (1993). *Bibliotherapy: A clinical approach for helping children*, Vol. 16. Langhorne, PA: Gordon and Breach Science Publishers.

Pardeck, J. T., & Pardeck, J. A. (1997). Recommended books for helping young children deal with social and development problems. *Early Child Development and Care, 136*, 57-63.

Pardeck, J. T., & Pardeck, J. A. (1998a). An exploration of the uses of children's books as an approach for enhancing cultural diversity. *Early Child Development and Care, 147*, 25-31.

Pehrsson, D. E., & Boylan, M. (2004). Counseling suicide survivors. In D. Capuzzi (Ed.), *Suicide across the lifespan* (chap. 11). Alexandria, VA: American Counseling Association.

Pehrsson, D. E., & McMillen, P. (2005). Bibliotherapy evaluation tool: Grounding counseling students in the therapeutic use of literature. *The Arts in Psychotherapy, 32*, 1.

Rawls, W. (1992). *Summer of the Monkeys*. London, UK: Random House Children's Books.

Riordan, R. J. (1991). Bibliotherapy revisited. *Psychological Reports, 68*(1), 306.

Shrodes, C. (1950). *Bibliotherapy: A theoretical and clinical-experimental study* (Doctoral dissertation, University of California, Berkeley, 1950). Dissertation Abstracts Online.

Spencer, R. (2000). *A comparison of relational psychologies*. Project Report, No. 6, Wellesley, MA: Stone Center Working Papers Series.

Todahl, J., Smith, T.E., Barnes, M., & Pereira, M. G. A. (1998). Bibliotherapy and perceptions of death by young children. *Journal of Poetry Therapy, 12*(2), 95-107.

Tway, E. (1989). Dimensions of multicultural literature for children. In M. K. Rudman (Ed.), *Children's literature: Resource for the classroom* (pp. 109-132). Norwood, MA: Christopher-Gordon Publishers, Inc.

White Lion. (1987). When the children cry. On *Pride* [Record]. Springfield: Atlantic/WEA.

Worden, W. J. (1991). *Grief counseling and grief therapy*. NY: Springer.

Wyeth, S. D. (1995). *Always my dad*. New York, NY: Random House.

Zaccaria, J. S., & Moses, H. A. (1968). *Facilitating human development through reading: The use of bibliotherapy in teaching and counseling*. Champaign, IL: Stipes.

doi:10.1300/J456v01n03_17

APPENDIX

Web Resources for Bibliotherapy

- A Guide to Children's Grief; PBS Home Program Series
  http://www.pbs.org/wnet/onourownterms/chapters/children.html

- About Children's Literature
  http://www.childrenslit.com/th_af.html

- African-American Voices in Children's Fiction: Arrowhead Library System
  http://als.lib.wi.us/AACList.html

- Carnegie Library of Pittsburgh
  http://www.clpgh.org/kids/booknook/bibliotherapy

- Celebrating Cultural Diversity through Children's Literature
  http://www.multiculturalchildrenslit.com

- Children and Grief: American Academy of Child & Adolescent Psychiatry
  http://www.aacap.org/publications/factsfam/grief.htm

- Children's Literature; Education Psychology Library
  http://www.lib.berkeley.edu/EDP/children.htmly Library UC Berkeley

- Disaster: Helping Children Cope: National Center for Mental Health and Education Center
  http://www.naspcenter.org/safe_schools/coping.html

- Eric Digest on Bibliotherapy
  http://www.ericdigests.org/2003-4/bibliotherapy.html

- Helping Children After a Disaster: American Academy of Children and Adolescent Psychiatry
  http://www.aacap.oorg/publications/factsfam/disater.htm

- Helping Children Cope with Disaster; Disaster Relief Organization
  http://www.Disasterrelief.org/Library/prepare/chilcope.html

- International Reading Association; Bibliotherapy Special Interest Group
  http://www.reading.org/dir/sig/sigbibl.html

- Multicultural Resources for Children
  http://falcon.jmu.edu/~ramseyil/multipub.htm

- National Center for Post Traumatic Stress Disorder
  http://www.ncptsd.org

- Resource Bibliography for the Study of African-American Children's Literature
  http://www.lib.usm.edu/~degrum/html/collectionhl/ch-afroamericanbib. shtml

- Ten Quick Ways to Analyze Children's Books for Racism and Sexism: The Council on Interracial Books for Children
  *http://www.birchlane.davis.ca.us/library/10quick.h*tm

- The Bibliotherapy Education Project; Oregon State University
  http://bibliotherapy.library.oregonstate.edu

Saying Goodbye:
Pet Loss and Its Implications

Thelma Duffey

SUMMARY. Pets can be loyal, loving, and entertaining members of a family. Their deaths are generally experienced as painful losses by the people who love them, even though the grief experience is often culturally disenfranchised. In this manuscript, we discuss the role that pets can play in a person's life, the effects that pet loss can have on the people who love them, and some creative rituals for memorializing a beloved pet. doi:10.1300/J456v01n03_18 *[Article copies available for a fee from The Haworth Document Delivery Service: 1-800-HAWORTH. E-mail address: <docdelivery@haworthpress.com> Website: <http://www.HaworthPress.com> © 2005 by The Haworth Press, Inc. All rights reserved.]*

KEYWORDS. Creativity, pet loss, counseling, grief

Mr. Bojangles, Dance

(Walker, 1968)

Family pets have been an important part of my life for as far back as I can remember. As a little girl, I had a dog I named Terry Calhoun, Jr. I

Thelma Duffey is the Counseling Program Director at the University of Texas at San Antonio.

Address correspondence to: Thelma Duffey, CEPAHE/DB, UTSA Downtown Campus, 501 West Durango Boulevard, San Antonio, TX 78207 (E-mail: tduffey@satx.rr.com).

[Haworth co-indexing entry note]: "Saying Goodbye: Pet Loss and Its Implications." Duffey, Thelma. Co-published simultaneously in *Journal of Creativity in Mental Health* (The Haworth Press, Inc.) Vol. 1, No. 3/4, 2005, pp. 287-295; and: *Creative Interventions in Grief and Loss Therapy: When the Music Stops, a Dream Dies* (ed: Thelma Duffey) The Haworth Press, Inc., 2005, pp. 287-295. Single or multiple copies of this article are available for a fee from The Haworth Document Delivery Service [1-800-HAWORTH, 9:00 a.m. - 5:00 p.m. (EST). E-mail address: docdelivery@haworthpress.com].

used to call him "Terry" for short. Terry was a mutt, although he looked very much like a Fox Terrier. The people who gave Terry to my family were the Calhoun's–thus the name. As a young girl I would walk home from school and as I was approaching my house, I would begin to call his name. I remember singing a song for Terry to the tune of "Daniel Boone was a Man." In my version, it was, of course, "Terry Calhoun was a Dog." We had a great time together.

A long time passed before I had another pet. When my children were small, someone gave us a cat my son named "Tiger." Tiger and I became fast friends for the almost 18 years of his life. So many of my memories involving children and family and major moves include adventures with Tiger. We had a number of other pets when my children were younger. There was Ruffles, our Cocker Spaniel; Madison, our Afghan Hound; Muffy, my friend, Dana's, cat that we adopted; Hot Dog, our dachshund; and now we have Bailey, our Collie dog.

Indeed, like the days of Terry Calhoun, we are again fortunate to come home to another warm welcome from Bailey, our 10-year-old Lassie look-alike. Bailey has initiated his own endearing rituals around our end of the day reconciliation. For example, when we return home, Bailey is waiting at the front window. His eyes perk up; he cocks his head to the left; and he stares intently. When we walk in the door, he runs up the stairs to beat us to the landing and holds out his paw to shake. Then, he excitedly begins to bark, as if in protest for our absence, and leans up next to us, as if to give us a hug.

It is no doubt that these pets have enriched our lives. And, when we lose them, we feel the loss of a loyal, faithful friend. With this writing, memories of our little Hot Dog come to mind. From the time he came home to live with us, we used to laugh at what a little personality he had. On occasion, Hot Dog would prance proudly toward the window with a poor squirrel in his mouth and never did quite understand why that did not please us. He had a best friend, a neighborhood cat named Steven, and the two would rest together side by side. Hot Dog was a character. Sadly, ever since he was a small pup, Hot Dog could not stay in the back yard. From time to time, he would dig holes and make his way out. We had a wooden fence across a yard too large to make foolproof. Within moments of getting out, Hot Dog would walk triumphantly to the front door where we would greet him and carry him back to safety. One day we were not as fortunate. He got out the back yard and a neighbor came by to tell us that he had been hit by a car. Hot Dog did not survive.

PETS AND THEIR PEOPLE

The research literature addresses the relationship between pets and the people who love them. Indeed, pets are known to provide unconditional love delivered with anticipation, innocence, and childlike delight. Pet lovers describe with much affection the bonds that can be formed between pets and their people. Comforting relationships with pets bring us companionship and fun, humor, playfulness, and an element of surprise. Pets can also positively affect our health and mental well being. For example, Siegel (1993) discusses human-animal relationships and reports that widowed elderly non-pet owners suffered more headaches, constipation, difficulty swallowing, cold sores, persistent fears, and feelings of panic than did widowed pet owners (Akiyama, Holtzman & Britz, 1986-87; Siegel, 1993). Additionally, the non-pet owner participants reported greater use of drugs, especially psychotropic drugs during bereavement (Akiyama et al., 1986-87; Siegel, 1993).

Further reports indicate that strong pet attachment is related to better physical health (Garrity, Stallones, Marx, & Johnson, 1989; Siegel, 1993). In addition, people with pets require fewer doctor visits than do people without pets (Siegel, 1990, 1993). Pets can also serve as supports during illness (Toray, 2004). Not surprisingly, pets help us stay healthy, and relax (Soares, 1985; Siegel, 1993). It is no wonder that pets are often considered best friend material.

SAYING GOODBYE TO A FRIEND

Given the benefits enjoyed by many pet owners and the shorter life cycle of pets, what, then, do people who love their pets do when they die? Donohue (2005) discussed pet loss and its implications. He reports that pet owners who are grieving the loss of their pet may be more susceptible to illness (Donohue, 2005). When people lose a beloved pet, they may suffer from a decrease in appetite, change in sleeping patterns, difficulties with social activities, and job performance (Quackenbush, 1984; Donohue, 2005). People who have bonded closely to their pets (Beck & Katcher, 1996; Gosse & Barnes, 1994; Donohue, 2005) and older pet owners who live alone may experience greater grief reactions to the loss of their pets (Donohue, 2005; Quackenbush, 1984). Additionally, Donohue (2005) reports how grieving the loss of a pet intensifies the grief feelings following the loss of connection from a significant other. This experience of loss is exacerbated when we do not have available to us adequate connection and support during our bereavement experience.

In another study, Archer and Winchester (1994) investigated the grief experience following the death of a pet. Approximately half of the participants in the study reported numbness or disbelief in learning of their loss. Over half of the participants were reportedly preoccupied with thoughts of their pets or the circumstances surrounding the loss. A quarter of the participants experienced anxiety and depression. Further, many participants reported an absence of social support (Archer & Winchester, 1994) because of the disenfranchised nature of the loss (Doka, 1989; Archer & Winchester, 1994).

Wrobel and Dye (2003) investigated the course of symptoms that pet owners suffer over the loss of a pet. Over half of the participants in the study experienced depression, feelings of loneliness, and guilt. Clements, Benasutti, and Carmone (2003) performed a review of the literature on the clinical implications of pet loss. The loss of a pet can create a grief response comparable to the grief experienced by the loss of a family member; a grief that is frequently misunderstood.

No doubt, pets can become important members of a family and hold a special place in our hearts. In fact, many of the losses that children first experience come in the form of a family pet. And as we grow older, these losses grow with us. The literature shows that people invest in their pets, and as people age, they become companions in unique ways. This issue is particularly salient as people age because of the loneliness that aging can bring. According to Peretti (1990), loneliness is often reported as the most difficult aspect of aging. Although a significant number of our elderly population is hospitalized or live in nursing homes, one third of the country's elderly live alone (Siegel, 1993).

Forming meaningful interaction and intimate relationships remains increasingly important (Peretti, 1990). However, as we age, we increase our chances of losing people we love. In some cases, pets become our willing and eager companions. Indeed, approximately one third of senior citizens live with pets (Garrity et al., 1989; Ory & Goldberg, 1983; Siegel, 1990, 1993). Given that, the loss of a pet in later life becomes increasingly significant.

Jake the Pup

Jake was a pup when Paul and Sheryl found him by the side of the road. He appeared to be homeless and seemed tired, thirsty, and hungry. After unsuccessfully trying to find his owner, they took him in and together they enjoyed a happy home for fifteen years. Paul and Sheryl would take Jake to the lake where he would mount the boat with them. With the wind blowing, they would laugh as he would bark and his ears would fly high. They had many such adventures, and, in time, Jake grew to be an old dog.

Paul and Sheryl were blessed with many happy years together. However, as Sheryl turned 70, she began to complain of headaches. Paul and Jake worried about her, and Jake would sit by her side. It was not long before Sheryl was diagnosed with a brain tumor. Paul, also 70, did everything he knew to make her comfortable. He gave her the best medical care available, and nursed her until the day came that Sheryl died. With Jake by Paul's side, together they grieved.

It was no surprise, then, that when Jake became ill and died, Paul grieved deeply. He knew Jake was an old dog and that they had enjoyed a good life. And, as he recalled their adventures, he missed Sheryl even more. Complicating matters, Paul and Sheryl had no children and his siblings lived in another state. Jake had been their only dog. Several of their friends had died or moved away through the years, and they had not invested time in making new ones. Paul, who remained in excellent health, felt eerily alone.

Paul needed to feel connected to others in his life and to find a place of belonging. After a period of withdrawal, he visited the local animal shelter. Paul had worked retail until retirement, and enjoyed being with people. He decided that volunteering at the shelter would help him connect with other people while also honoring Jake. The volunteer move was a good one for Paul. He made a few friends through his work and began to socialize again. In time, he brought home a pup that had been abandoned and clearly abused. Paul found a sense of belonging by forming connections with other people who shared his protective feelings toward animals. And as he connected with others, he rediscovered aspects of his own personality.

In time, Paul met and married a woman who also shares his love of pets. They delight in each other's company and appreciate the time they have with one another. Paul notes, "I am a lucky man to have met Ana at this point in my life. She is delightful, funny, and very loving. We have both suffered losses, so neither of us wants to take any day for granted. We have adopted Bud and Allie, two new additions to the family that we brought home from the shelter. They help keep us young. I thought my life was over. Happily, Ana, Bud, and Allie make it worth living again. I miss Sheryl and Jake every day. They are a part of me. But I've made room in my heart for Ana and our pups. Because of that, I'm a lucky man."

Not everyone is as fortunate–or resilient–in the face of loss. There are many factors that influence our ability to open our hearts and move beyond grief. Life circumstances, chance, luck, and opportunity certainly play a role in how our lives develop. Additionally, the way we have negotiated pain in our pasts is one predictor of resiliency after loss. Questions for us to consider include: Are we able to access and enjoy social supports? Do we form meaningful connections? Can we transcend our fears of future loss? Will we risk allowing ourselves to love again? These are simply some of the issues that people must reconcile in living life and coming to terms with loss.

COUNSELING CONSIDERATIONS AND CREATIVE INTERVENTIONS

Coming to terms with any loss is challenging. When people suffer losses of a disenfranchised nature (Doka, 1989), the losses can be even more challenging. Losing a pet is among these losses. Pets become ill, are hit by cars, and become wounded or hurt by other animals. Some are even terribly mistreated by people. Pet owners become witness to these experiences and are impacted by them. They can feel the same sense of helplessness, anger, disbelief, sadness, and loneliness that come with other forms of loss. Counselors who are not sensitive to the role that pets can play in a person's life may inadvertently minimize the experience or attempt to redirect sessions when their clients encounter these experiences. This can leave clients feeling even more isolated and alone.

In addition to having a therapist who can understand and be present in the face of pet loss, there are a number of interventions that be used to ritualize the experience. Clements et al. (2003) suggest the following: (1) creating a "wish list" based upon the needs a local animal shelter, (2) planting a tree or flower garden in memorial of the lost pet, (3) writing a letter expressing one's feelings for the pet (4) volunteering at the local animal shelter, (5) adopting another pet when one is ready, (6) holding a memorial for the pet, (7) and creating a scrapbook of the pet.

I have worked with a number of clients who have used these and other rituals to support them through their difficult time. In one example, I worked with a family that had long enjoyed the love and companionship of their pup, Missy. They bought Missy when she was a tiny puppy, before their first child was born. Four children and twelve years later, Missy was diagnosed with cancer. It was not long before it became obvious that she would have to be put to sleep.

Missy was cremated and the family held a service in her honor. Each child wrote a letter or poem to Missy during the service and erected a small marker under a Magnolia tree in their back yard. They also inscribed a nameplate with Missy's name, and years of birth and death, and attached it to a garden bench in their yard. Later, they organized a family scrapbook, which naturally included photographs of Missy. The children learned about grief through this experience, and more importantly, they learned about how comforting support can be during difficult times.

Comfort comes serendipitously. Soon after taking on a job at my former university, I, too, discovered that our 12-year-old dog, Madison, was very ill and would have to be put to sleep. I was in Florida at a convention when I heard the news, and the pain of hearing that Madison was sick, coupled with other unexpected losses that I encountered while at the convention, made the trip home a long one. Upon my return, I met with the veterinarian who explained my choices to me. Making and coming to terms with that decision was difficult.

One of my colleagues who taught a grief and loss course heard about Madison and organized a ritual for her. The students decided that everyone in the class would bring bags of dog food and related items to class. The plan was that, as a group, they would donate the food to a local animal shelter. The class formed a line, as if they were marching in a parade in honor of the pup. Together they made the trip to the shelter and distributed gifts in Madison's name. The generosity of my colleague and the goodwill of the students were moving. Seeing what they did for Madison touched my heart and helped bring comfort to what was a sad situation.

CONCLUSION

Human beings have a yearning to form connections with others. We are social, relational, and emotional creatures. Many of us feel energized, happy, and fulfilled when our relationships develop in growth-fostering ways. Indeed, few experiences can compete with the warmth and joy that caring, reciprocal, and supportive relationships can bring. In addition to these experiences, family pets also add to the quality of our lives, and our relationships with them can be endearing, playful, and important. As a result, losing a pet is a painful experience; and when un-acknowledged or disenfranchised, it can be an especially lonely one. By understanding the needs of clients who speak of their pet-related losses, counselors are able to help them give dignity to their pet's life and ritualize their loss. In so doing, their memories are given a mean-ingful place in their histories, to be affectionately recalled and en-joyed.

REFERENCES

Akiyama, H., Holtzman, J. M., & Britz, W. E. (1986-87). Pet ownership and health sta-tus during bereavement. *Omega, 17,* 187-193.

Archer, J., & Winchester, G. (1994). Bereavement following death of a pet. *British Journal of Psychology, 85,* 259-271.

Beck, A., & Katcher, A. (1996). *Between Pets and People.* West Lafayette, IN: Purdue University Press.

Clements, P. T., Benasutti, K. M., & Carmone, A. (2003). Support for bereaved owners of pets. *Perspectives in Psychiatric Care, 39*(2), 49-54.

Doka, K. J. (1989). Disenfranchised grief. In K. Doka (Ed.), *Disenfranchised Grief: Recognizing Hidden Sorrow,* (pp. 3-11). Lexington, MA: Lexington Books.

Donohue, K. M. (2005). Pet loss: Implications for social work practice. *Social Work, 50*(2), 187-190.

Garrity, T. F., Stallones, L., Marx, M. B., & Johnson, T. P. (1989). Pet ownership and attachment as supportive factors in health of the elderly. *Anthrozoos, 3,* 35-44.

Gosse, G. H. & Barnes, M. J. (1994). Human grief resulting from the death of a pet. *Anthrozoos, 7*(2), 103-112.

Ory, M., & Goldberg, E. (1983). Pet ownership and life satisfaction in elderly women. In A. H. Katcher & A. M. Beck (Eds.) *New Perspectives in Our Life with Companion Animals,* (pp. 803-817). Philadelphia: University of Pennsylvania Press.

Peretti, P. O. (1990). Elderly-animal friendship bonds. *Social Behavior and Personal-ity, 18*(1), 151-156.

Quackenbush, J. E. (1984). Pet bereavement in older owners. In R. K. Anderson, B. L. Hart, & L. A. Hart (Eds.), *The Pet Connection,* (pp. 292-299). Minneapolis: Univer-sity of Minnesota Press.

Siegel, J. M. (1990). Stressful life events and use of physician services among the el-derly: The moderating role of pet ownership. *Journal of Personality and Social Psy-chology, 58,* 1081-1086.

Siegel, J. M. (1993). Companion animals: In sickness and in health. *Journal of Social Issues, 49*(1), 157-167.

Soares, C. J. (1985). The companion animal in the context of the family system. *Marriage and Family Review, 8,* 49-62.

Toray, T. (2004). The human-animal bond and loss: Providing support for grieving clients. *Journal of Mental Health Counseling, 26*(3), 244-259.

Walker, J. J. (1968). Mr. Bojangles. [CD]. New York, NY: Atlantic.

Wrobel, T. A., & Dye, A. L. (2003). Grieving pet death: normative, gender, and attachment issues. *Omega, 47*(4), 385-393.

doi:10.1300/J456v01n03_18

Index

Bermudez & Bermudez 8-Step
    Therapy Model, 175
Bermudez, J. M., & Bermudez, S.,
    174,175,176,181
Bernstein J. E., 279,281,283
Bernstein, J. E., & Rudman, M. K.,
    277,283
Betrayal, feelings of, 43,109,142,214
Bettleheim, B., 243,251
Bibliotherapy, 273-284, *see also*
    Storytelling
  benefits of, 276-278,282
  case examples, 276-278
  considerations for counselors, 282
  cultural representation, 278
  developmental needs of children,
    277,282
  empirical research, 281
  factors to consider, 278
  practical considerations, 278
  racist and sexist attitudes, 278
  stereotypes, 278
  Web resources, 285-286
Billings, A. G., & Moos, R. H., 257,269
Biological parents, 238
Birren, J. E., 6,21
Bissler, Jane, 123-134
Bitar, George, Springer, Paul, 185-204
Black, C., 17,21
Blalock, J. A., & Joiner, T. E., 257,269
Blatner, A., 49,51,53
Blinde, E. M., & Stratta, T. M., 92,100
Bloom, B., Asher, S. J., & White, S. W.,
    136,151
Blume, S., 46,54
Borg, S., & Lasker, J., 157,169
Bosco, A. F., 221
Boss, P., 63,64,65,69
Boundaries, 141-143
Bowlby, J., 157-160,169
Bowman, T., 174,177,179,181
Brende, J. O., & Goldsmith, R., 207,221
Brent, D. A., Johnson, B. A., Perper, J.,
    Connolly, J., Bridge, J., &
    Bartle, S. et al., 211,221

Brent, D. A., Perper, J. A., Moritz, G.,
    Allman, C., & Liotus, L.,
    207,221
Brief Symptom Inventory (BSI),
    262-265,268
Brigham Young University, 253
Bright, R., 132,133,174,178,181
Brin, D. J., 166,169
Brock, G. W., & Barnard, C. P., 221
Brodzinsky, D., Schecter, M., &
    Henig, R., 240,241,243,251
Brodzinsky, D., Smith, D., &
    Brodzinsky, A., 239,241,251
Broken dreams, recovery from,
    146-150
Broken hearts, recovery from, 146-150
Bronstein, P., 74,86
Brook, D. W., Brook, J. S., Richter, L.,
    Whiteman, M.,
    Arencibia-Mireles, O., &
    Masci, J. R., 44,54
Brooks, J. L., Mark, L., & Sakai, R.,
    151
Brouwers, M., 110
Brown, D. R., & Blanton, C. J., 209,
    221
Brown, G. K., Beck, A. T., Steer, R. A.,
    & Grisham, J. R., 209,221
Brown, L. K. & Brown, M., 277,283
Brown, R. S., 78,86
Bruce, E. J., & Shultz, C. L., 93,100
Brumels, C., 226,234
Brunner, J., 243,251
Budman, S. H., & Gunman, A. S.,
    125,133
Buhrmeter, D. N., & Furman,
    P.,139,151
Bunim, M., & Murray, J., 228,234
Bureau of Justice Statistics, 188,201
Burning out, 61
Buscaglia, L., 277,282
Buser, Juleen K., 173-183
Buser, Trevor J., 173-183
Busseri, M. A., Tyler, J. D., & King,
    A. R., 75,86

Nelson, D., & Weathers, R., 130,133
Nelson, M. L., Englar-Carlson, M.,
    Tierney, S. G., & Hau, J. M.,
    74,87
Nerenberg, A., 46,55
Neugarten. B., 125,133
Neugebauer, R., Kline, J., O'Connor,
    P., Shrout, P., Johnson, J., &
    Skodol, A., 160,170
New Freedom Commission on Mental
    Health (NFCMH), 188,203
New life story, 179-181
New Orleans, 58,59,60,61,62,64
Newacheck, P. W., Strickland, B.,
    Shonkoff, J. P., Perrin, J. M.,
    McPherson, M., & McManus,
    M. et al., 256,270
Nickerson. R. S., 190,203
Nightmares, 275
Nock, A. J., 227,228,234
Non-diagnostic, 3
Non-professional significant others,
    220
Normal response, 68
Normalcy, sense of, 62,63
Norms, 104,275
Notification to supervisor of clients
    suicidal intent, 219
Novel Approach, 103,110-120
Nybo, A., Wohlfahn, J., Christens, P.,
    Olsen, J., & Melbye, M.,
    157,170

O'Harra, D. M., Taylor, R., &
    Simpson, K., 222
Obiwan-Kenobi, 247
Object Relations Theory, 176
    and artwork, 176
Odle, T. G., 226,234
Ogilvie, & Howe, 91,92
Ohio State University (The), 205
Oliver, M., Berstein, J., & Anderson,
    K., 76,87
Olkin, R., & Gaughen, S., 75,77,87

Olson, M. J., & McEwen, M. A.,
    190,203
Optimism, loss of, 126
Orbinson, R., 13,23
Oregon State University, 263-284
Orford, J., 43,45,55
Ory, M., & Goldberg, E., 290,294
Osterweis. M., Solomon, F., & Green,
    M., 207,222
Overdose, suicide, 215
Oxygen, 215

Pain, 106,112,207,210-214,274-275,
    287,292
    externalized, 192
Paralysis, sense of, 68
Paralyzed, 276
Parasuicide plan, 212
Pardeck, & Pardeck, 274,275,276,
    277-278,281,284
Parent/child relationship, 123-132,230
Parent's perspectives, 28
Parental
    bereavement, 124-127
    grief patterns, 164
    closure, 166
    re-telling, 166
    story, 166
    substance use, 44
    telling, 166
    grief, 123-127
    models of grief, 127
    projection, 126
Parental-child bonding issues, 44
Parents, 27,28,35,36
    drug use, 44
    of children with disabilities,
    253-271
Parham, W. D., 91,101
Parker, Peter, 245-246
Parkes, C. M., 90,101
Parkes, C., Launagni, P., & Young, B.,
    4,23
Partner, 32
    their challenge, 32
Partnership, loss of, 105

power, 26
practice, 76
process, 67
rituals, 65,67
Therapist, 19,26,27,66,77,82
created symbols, 67
developed symbols, 67
Therbert-Wright, C., 170
Thibault, J. M., Ellor, J. W., & Netting,
F. E., 6,23
Third Eye Blind, 14,15,23
Thompson, R. A., 223
Thompson. C. L., & Rudolph, L. B.,
106,107
Thought Field Therapy (TFT), 96
Thoughts of death, 213
Thumb sucking, 276
Timmerman. G. P. M., 139,153
Todahl, J., Smith, T. E., Barnes, M., &
Pereira, M. G. A., 275,284
Toedter. L, Lasker. N., & Alhadeff, J.,
164,171
Toray, T., 289,295
Trained, athletes, 89,94
Trainee, 78,79
Trauma, 44,57,61
and children, 273-284
chronic, 65
histories, 45
immediate, 58
large scale,180
physiological reactions in children, 276
relational and cognitive effects on
children, 275
wake, 63
Traumatic event, 57,63
Treatment approach, 65
Treatment, 32,33,43,47
goals, 65
status, 52
team, 33
Trepal, Heather,155-171
Turbiville, V. P., & Marquis, J. G.,
257,268,271
Turetsky, C. J., & Hays, R. E., 174,
180,183
Tway, E., 282,284

Twelve step programs, 46,49,140

U. S. Department of Education,
206,223
U. S. Department of Health and
Human Services (USDHHS),
188,203,206,223,255,271
U2, 16,23,104,119
Unacknowledged grief, 160
Unconditional love, 289
University, 60,72,73,78
administrators, 81
community, 60
Louisiana State, 57
of Akron, 155
of Central Florida, 135,253
of Colorado at Boulder, 225
of North New Orleans, 59
of Texas at San Antonio (UTSA),
1,41,103,155,205,287
of Wisconsin-Oshkosh, 25
president of the, 72
Southeastern Louisiana, 57
St. Mary's, 89
Unrealistic professional goals, 219
Unrealized promise, relationship is,
137
Unrequited
dreams, 11,13,19
experiences, 20
hope, 3
Vacha-Haase, T., Davenport, D. S., &
Kerewsky, S. D., 73,76,77,88
Valadez, Albert A., 103-121
Values clarification, 225
process, 231
group process, 231-233
guiding questions, 232
Values, 146,167,175,225,226
Van Dongen, C. J., 207,223
Van, P., 164,171
Verrier, N. N., 241,252
Videka-Sherman, L., 134
Videography, 173,176
Viorst, J., 3,23,37,39
Visual arts, 173